Antibody Therapy

Paul Imbach
Editor

Antibody Therapy

Substitution – Immunomodulation – Monoclonal Immunotherapy

Springer

Editor
Paul Imbach
Department of Pediatrics
Medical Faculty of the University of Basel
Basel
Switzerland

ISBN 978-3-030-09819-3 ISBN 978-3-319-68038-5 (eBook)
https://doi.org/10.1007/978-3-319-68038-5

Softcover re-print of the Hardcover 1st edition 2018

Printed on acid-free paper

This Springer imprint is published by the registered company Springer International Publishing AG part of Springer Nature
The registered company address is: Gewerbestrasse 11, 6330 Cham, Switzerland

The path of antibodies therapy from substitution to immunomodulation to the development/use of monoclonal antibodies for patients with immune deficiencies, inflammatory, autoimmune and oncological diseases – based on the similarities of the immune pathogenesis, namely the loss of immune tolerance – is presented

Foreword

In 1735, Werlhof described a clinical syndrome of bleeding and purpura long before platelets were identified as the cellular component of blood that play an essential role in primary hemostasis. Werlhof's disease, as it became known, was later renamed idiopathic thrombocytopenic purpura, from which the acronym ITP originally derives. Little followed from these observations until the early 1900s, and we have just passed the centenary of the first successful treatment for the condition. In 1916, a medical student in Prague, Paul Kaznelson, proposed that, in an analogy with hemolytic anemia, essential thrombocytopenia, as it was also known, resulted from increased platelet destruction in the spleen. Kaznelson convinced his tutor to perform a splenectomy in a 36-year-old woman with a history consistent with our current definition of chronic ITP. The platelet count was 2×10^9/l prior to splenectomy and rose to 500×10^9/l within four weeks from surgery with complete resolution of the purpura. This confirmed the role of the spleen in the pathophysiology of ITP, and splenectomy has remained a mainstay of treatment ever since. The pathophysiology of ITP remained elusive for many decades. Although some intriguing observations by Dameshek and Miller in 1946 suggested reduced megakaryocyte function, the "increased platelet destruction, reduced production" debate appeared to have been settled by the classic Harrington-Hollingsworth experiments in 1951 that unequivocally demonstrated that ITP was characterized by reduced platelet survival due to a humoral factor that was soon identified as an antiplatelet antibody. In his historical review of ITP in 2002, Paul Imbach reported that Harrington et al. had also observed a child with purpura born to a mother with chronic ITP that resolved in the child 3 weeks after birth, although the mother still had ITP, indicating that a humoral antiplatelet factor had been passed from mother to child.

At the same time, the successful use of corticosteroids and adrenocorticotropic hormone (ACTH) in elevating the platelet count was described by Wintrobe (1951), and standard-dose prednisolone has been considered the initial treatment for newly diagnosed ITP since then. Immunosuppressive agents were introduced in the 1960s, when the autoimmune nature of ITP was clarified.

A milestone in the treatment of symptomatic ITP in children, however, was the introduction of intravenous immunoglobulin by Paul Imbach in 1981. The efficacy of this treatment was subsequently validated both in adults and in pregnancy by Adrian Newland in 1983. Abdulgabar Salama introduced anti-D treatment and the concept of macrophage blockade in 1984. James Bussel and his group later expanded the knowledge about the modalities of treatment with anti-D in various settings.

With an increasing understanding of the underlying molecular biology and with advances in pharmacological technologies, targeted therapy became more attractive and has been investigated since the 1980s in many conditions. In ITP, the most consistent results with monoclonal antibody therapy have been obtained with rituximab, an anti-CD20 chimeric antibody inducing B-cell depletion. Roberto Stasi first reported the successful use of rituximab in adults with chronic ITP in 2001. This agent has become the standard (albeit unlicensed) treatment for patients with this condition in many countries, and its use has been extended to a variety of autoimmune conditions.

There is no doubt that in recent years, we have seen a major breakthrough in the treatment of chronic ITP, with the introduction of the thrombopoietin receptor agonists. The pioneering work of David Kuter with these agents has shown response rates unequalled by previous medical therapies. These agents are almost as efficacious in splenectomized patients as in the non-splenectomized ones, and recent studies have confirmed the efficacy and safety following long-term usage.

The second half of the twentieth century brought recognition on the autoimmune components of ITP, hence the need for a new standard nomenclature, which has been widely accepted. ITP currently stands for immune thrombocytopenia, a name that more appropriately reflects the low platelet count rather than purpura as the main feature of the disease and defines its underlying nature.

Advances in our knowledge of the disease have paralleled the burgeoning availability of new therapeutic agents, and we are now entering an era of treatment options based on pathophysiological principles. There is no doubt that the enormous expansion in our understanding of the condition and its treatment was stimulated by the observations of Paul Imbach in children with thrombocytopenia. A relatively rare disease with few treatment options, the disease suddenly became totem for clinical study and laboratory investigation and a marker for the possibilities in other autoimmune diseases. It was Imbach's realization that intravenous immunoglobulin was more than a replacement treatment but that it had a major impact on both immunological and phagocytic functions that had implications in a wide variety of conditions. This book systematically charts the history and the development of immunoglobulin and its association with ITP while highlighting how treatment and understanding of the latter has changed and how the former has developed into an important therapeutic option. Our forebears would be astounded at the progress over the last 50 years which is admirably described in these chapters.

Adrian Newland, CBE, MA, FRCP, FRCPath
Academic Haematology Unit
Barts and The London School
of Medicine and Dentistry
Queen Mary University of London
Turner Street, London, E1 2AD, UK

Contents

About the Editor

Paul Imbach is a highly respected pediatric oncologist-hematologist who has developed worldwide clinical research on the indications for intravenous immunoglobulin. Dr. Imbach graduated in Medicine in 1972. He went on to structure the Swiss Pediatric Oncology Group (SPOG) and in 1978 performed the first autologous stem cell transplantation in Switzerland. He discovered the immunomodulatory effects of human immunoglobulin G concentrate (IVIG) in childhood immune thrombocytopenia (as reported in *Lancet* in 1981). In 1990, Dr. Imbach began working at the University Children's Hospital Basel, where he started stem cell transplantation in children and was appointed Head of Pediatric Oncology-Hematology. He was subsequently elected as full professor and also as Dean of Education introducing a thorough curriculum reform at the medical faculty of the University of Basel. In parallel to his other activities, he co-founded the International Cooperative ITP Study (ICIS) group (www.itpbasel.ch), which now has more than 90 centers worldwide. He has served as president of medical societies and foundations, is a member of medical editorial boards, and has published over 350 peer-reviewed articles, textbook chapters as well as the textbook *Pediatric Oncology – A Comprehensive Guide* (3rd edition 2014) in German and English. In 2015 he was awarded the Guido Fanconi Prize, the highest award of the Swiss Society of Pediatrics.

Introduction

The book starts with a narrative description including citations of the first clinical observation of immunoglobulin (IgG) administration in children with "idiopathic" thrombocytopenia. This highlights the importance of clinical observation, inquisitiveness and translational clinical research. This leads into a discussion of the fundamental discovery (Chap. 2).

Written in a practical fashion as manual, Chap. 3 describes some main indications of substitution by IgG in primary and secondary immune deficiencies and Chap. 4 summarizes many of the new immunomodulatory indications, some of which remain quite controversial.

Autoimmune disorders are characterized by complex heterogeneity of clinical presentation and pathophysiological abnormalities of the innate and adaptive immune system. Immunomodulatory IgG indications are rarely evidence based and in general are disorder oriented with specific individual indications. Based on the very large number of clinical and laboratory studies in the literature—over 40,000 peer-reviewed articles in Pubmed—a categorization of the indications is proposed in the manual of autoimmune disorders.

One specific IgG preparation is Anti-D, which is a targeted product specifically binding to the Fc receptors as its mechanism of action; in contrast the polyclonal IgG concentrate induces a broad spectrum of synergistic immune challenges to the imbalanced immune system in patients with autoimmune disorders.

Chapter 6 is dedicated to the general immunomodulatory effects of IgG followed by a chapter that covers classical drugs, IgG and monoclonal antibodies with exploration of their mechanisms of action. The combination of the different immunomodulators often results in a more effective clinical outcome in the individual patient. The first part concludes with two expert reviews of the current use of IgG in conjunction with other therapeutic options in both neurology and dermatology.

The second part of the book updates the basic knowledge of the IgG molecule starting with historical aspects of polyclonal IgG. Currently production and the regulations for a safe and effective IgG product are complex. Many such preparations are now available internationally, and these are listed highlighting their specific characteristics with a consideration of the future perspectives of IgG preparations.

Since 'idiopathic', now immune thrombocytopenia ITP was the key disorder of the first observation of immunomodulatory effects of IgG, the third part summarizes ITP as the model syndrome of autoimmune disorders. In the majority of children with ITP the condition will resolve within weeks, months or very occasionally years. In adults the position is more complex with few spontaneously remitting and many developing chronicity. There has therefore been much interest in identifying prognostic factors, studying clinical outcomes and reviewing health-related quality of life issues in mild, moderate or severe disease. In order to standardize treatment approaches guidelines have been developed and regularly updated. There is increasing interest in secondary ITP and how it relates to the primary condition.

Newer aspects of platelet function are being recognized. Before 1980 the platelet was mainly thought to be responsible for coagulation, but now it is increasingly recognized as having an active role within the immune system (Chap. 17).

For many years the role of megakaryocytes has been suspected in the pathology of ITP, and the recognition of reduced platelet production led to the development of platelet stimulation by recombinant thrombopoietin and thrombopoietin receptor agonists, which is the focus of Chap. 18. For patients with severe, chronic ITP, e.g. with recurrent or at risk of life-threatening bleeding, thrombopoietin receptor agonists have become a major option with a low adverse event profile and increasingly have a place early in the treatment of refractory or relapsed disease. Chapter 18 summarizes the development and the characteristic of this long-term approach.

Nevertheless, in patients with acute, life-threatening bleeding immediate high dose IgG and/or corticosteroid administration and occasionally platelet transfusion remain the first choice.

The heterogeneity and immunological complexity of autoimmune diseases was the reason to start worldwide online registries of patients with ITP. The first endpoint of these registries is to distinguish subgroup of patients concerning demographics and follow up of this rare disease (for details see Chap. 19 and www.itpbasel.ch). There is also a large adult registry in the UK (www.ukitpregistry.com). Through recognition of subgroups of an autoimmune disease, evidence-based trials might become feasible.

We are now entering an exciting new phase of a "bridge" from antibody therapy of human origin progressing to monoclonal, engineered (or human adapted, e.g. CAR cell) treatment as an immunomodulatory approach to both autoimmune disorders and cancer. In a critical overview Chap. 20 explains the definitions, methods and adverse effects of monoclonal antibodies and presents an extensive list of those currently available monoclonal antibodies and their possible indications. One of the first antibodies introduced into clinical use, anti-CD-20, is described in Chap. 21. The anti-CD 20 antibody was initially developed as an adjunct in the treatment of Non-Hodgkin Lymphoma NHL, but its activity against immune competent B lymphocytes led to its exploration in many immunological and oncological disorders—based on the similarities of the immune pathogenesis, namely the loss of immune tolerance.

In summary the use of IgG, monoclonal antibodies and a variety of combinations with other immunomodulatory approaches has opened up the path from translation to more targeted biological, therapeutic approaches for patients with unresolved immune and malignant disease.

We thank all our contributing authors and the staff of Springer, especially Mrs. Meike Stoeck and Mrs. Dr. Isabelle Arnold, for their commitment to this extraordinary book.

Basel, Switzerland Paul Imbach

The Clinical Translation of Intravenous Immunoglobulin from Substitution to Immunomodulation

1

Paul Imbach

The subject of the book highlights 37 years of experiences following the first observation emphasizing the importance of the skill of critical medical observation, the development and production of a safe human blood extracts with minimal adverse effects, and research on how the administration of IgG intravenously or subcutaneously benefits patients with other autoimmune disorders and the potential mechanisms of action.

1.1 History of New Observations

1980 Pediatric Hematology-Oncology, University Children's Hospital Berne, Switzerland: On January, during a ward visit PI (the abbreviation of names relates to the full names in the reference list) and his colleagues observed a minimal increase in platelet count after each intravenous immunoglobulin G (IVIG) substitution in a child with typical Wiskott-Aldrich syndrome who also had thrombocytopenia in addition to hypogammaglobulinemia. On the same ward, there was a 12-year-old boy (M) with severe, refractory immune thrombocytopenia ITP of 9 years' disease duration with many complications despite splenectomy and cytotoxic treatment. The latter treatments resulted in secondary hypogammaglobulinemia and recurrent infections. Discussion with visiting colleagues led to the decision to ask for permission from the medical director ER to administer IVIG, and for consent from the patient with ITP and his parents. The first dose of 0.4 g IVIG/kg body weight was administered on the next Monday. During the evening visit, the boy said: "I am feeling much better, and I am sure that my platelet count will be much better tomorrow." This was the reality: his platelet count increased remarkably from 2 to 21 × 10^9/L. Now, PI discussed the observation with the chief immunologist SB treating adults with primary immunode-

P. Imbach
Medical Faculty of the University of Basel, Basel, Switzerland
e-mail: paul.imbach@unibas.ch

P. Imbach (ed.), *Antibody Therapy*, https://doi.org/10.1007/978-3-319-68038-5_1

ficiency with IVIG at the cancer research institute, who recommended to empirically continue the daily administration of the same dose of IVIG. On Friday of that week and after 5 × 0.4 g IVIG/kg body weight, the boy's platelet count was higher than 150×10^9/L.

In the following PI asked for permission to administer the same IVIG treatment regimen to other patients with severe, chronic ITP with platelet counts of less than 30×10^9/L and without hypogammaglobulinemia and as a control for two children with aplastic anemia. The IVIG was provided by the Swiss Red Cross, who were the local producers of the product. At this time, gamma globulin was the former name of IVIG.

In this pilotstudy children with ITP consecutively responded to IVIG, but children with aplastic anemia did not. Following these observations, the first manuscript was produced with input of his consultant HpW (Imbach et al.; see some citations (in cursive letters) and the Fig. 1.1 from the very first article below):

Summary

A new immunoglobulin (IgG) for intravenous use was given in high doses to 4 children with refractory idiopathic thrombocytopenic purpura (ITP) and 2 children with idiopathic aplastic anemia (IAA). Within 5-10 days after initiation of IgG therapy the platelets of the children with ITP rose to 300,000-650,000/mm3 and could be maintained at normal levels with one IgG infusion every 1-3 weeks. No response of platelet counts, was observed in the 2 patients with IAA… The IgG treatment was tolerated without complication by all patients.

The effect of intravenous IgG on the number of platelets is shown in Fig. 1. (see below). The platelets of all patients with ITP rose to a maximum between 300,000 and 650,000 within 5 to 10 days and returned to values between 100.000 and 300,000/mm 3 within the next 10 days.

The platelet count of patients with aplastic anemia was not influenced by the IgG therapy during the period of observation.

Discussion

We do not know how i.v. IgG administration influences the elimination of platelets. One could postulate that IgG acts primarily on the reticuloendothelial system and diminishes its platelet-eliminating effect. This hypothesis would also explain why the non-splenectomized child with chronic ITP (patient 3) required more frequent IgG infusions than the two splenectomized patients with chronic ITP in order to maintain adequate platelet levels. We also do not know whether infused lgG has a different effect on platelets of children with chronic versus acute ITP. It should be noted that the child with acute ITP resistant to prednisone, after a single 5-day course of IgG, remained in unmaintained remission for at least 6 weeks.

Despite the fact that IgG had no effect on the platelet counts of our 2 patients with aplastic anemia, further trials, particularly in patients with immune aplastic anemia may be rewarding.

Finally, since the intravenous IgG therapy described was well tolerated and had a striking effect on the platelet count of 4 children with chronic or acute ITP, the question arises whether the use of intravenous IgG should be considered for other autoimmune diseases as well. Obviously, the mechanism by which intravenous IgG exerts its effects should be known more precisely (end of citation).

In parallel with the first publication, the investigators continued to treat a total of 13 children with acute (7 patients) and chronic (6 patients) ITP using the same treatment regimen. Because all children in this pilot study showed responses to IVIG, the statistician determined the consecutive response rate to be a new phenomenon.

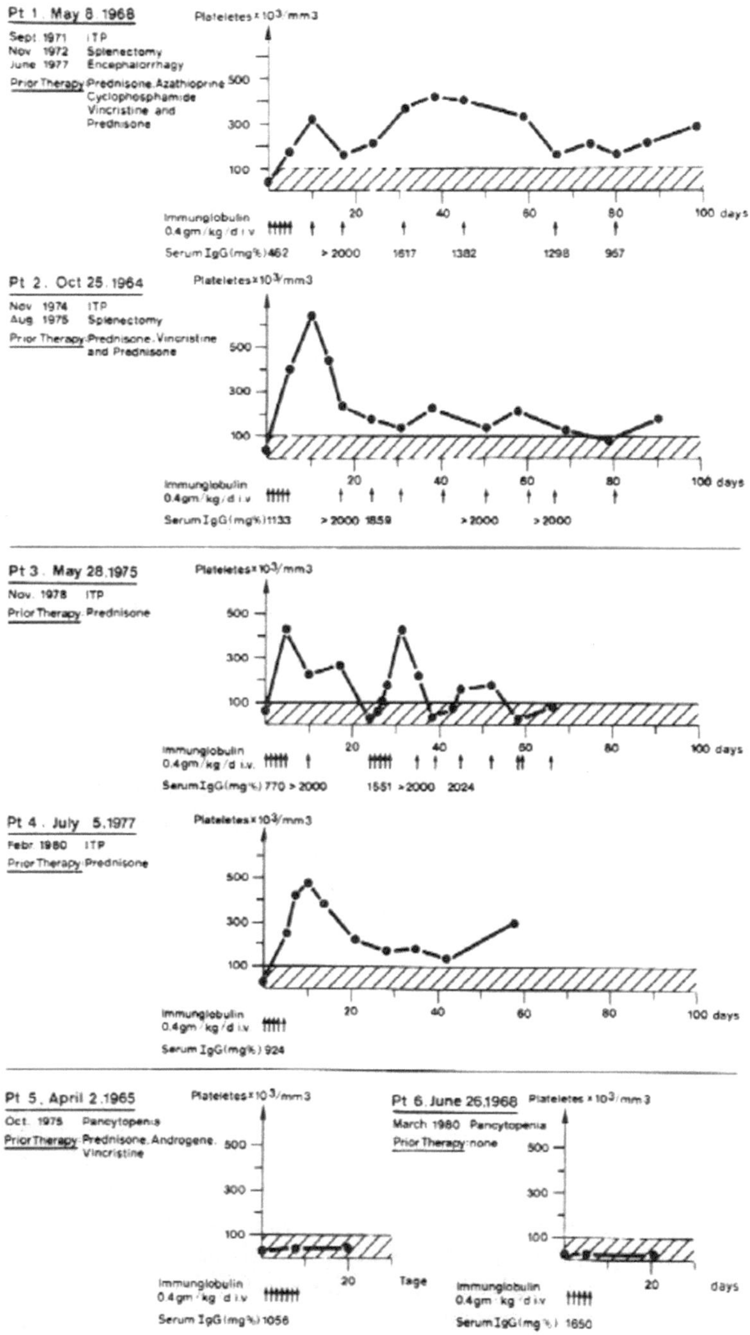

Fig. 1.1 Effect of i.v. IgG: Patients 1–4 with refractory ITP: 0, 4 g i.v. IgG/kg body weight/day x 5 rose to 300–650 x 103/mm3 platelet counts within 5–10 days and could be maintained at normal levels with one dose of i.v. IgG every1–3 weeks. Patients 5 and 6 with idiopathic aplastic anemia: no reaction of platelet counts to the same doses of i.v. IgG

The group sent their manuscript to The Lancet. The editor in chief of The Lancet, made confirmation of the originality of the new observation, published it as a rapid communication. In the article and Fig. 1.2a and b (Imbach et al. 1981), it was stated (citations slightly modified):

> ***'Patients and Methods'***
>
> *All patients first received, on 5 consecutive days, 0.4g IVIG/kg body-weight/day. IVIG is a polyvalent Ig concentrate obtained by modified alcohol cryoprecipitation, including mild acidification at pH4. The similarity of its in vivo biological half-life with that of normal serum IgG, and its intact Fc-receptor mechanisms reflect the structural and functional integrity of the 7S-IgG.*
>
> ***'Results'***
>
> *No patient had adverse effects during and/or after immunotherapy.*
>
> *IVIG induced a dramatic initial response in all patients (Figs. 1 and 2). In twelve of the thirteen children, the platelet count rose from pretreatment counts of <30x109/l platelets to a maximum of 150–600 x 109/l within 5-10 days of onset of treatment and returned to 80-400/ during the next ten days. In the thirteenth patient (patient 7), maximum counts were achieved after 10 days. Serum IgG levels rose to >2000mg/dl 10-20 days after onset of IVIG treatment (Figs. 1 and 2).*
>
> ***'Discussion'***
>
> *The dramatic response to IVIG in patient 1 prompted us to give IVIG to other patients with chronic ITP and, later, to patients with acute ITP.*
>
> *Although all of our patients showed a dramatic initial response to IVIG, the rates of increase and decrease and the maximum platelet counts differed between patients.*
>
> *In view of the large IgG doses given, the mode of action of IVIG could be the overloading and blocking of the reticuloendothelial system by IgG catabolism. This explanation might account for the differences in the response patterns between splenectomized and non-splenectomized children with chronic ITP. Reaction with and inactivation of circulating antiplatelet factor or interference with platelet-bound IgG and/or C-3, could be responsible for immediate effects, and activation of T and suppression of B cells for late effects of IVIG. In one patient with acute ITP (not included in this study) 0.5 g of a pepsin-treated gammaglobulin (Fab')2/kg body-weight/day on 3 consecutive days did not influence the platelet count, whereas a single dose of 0,4 g of IVIG/kg body-weight raised counts from 1.7 to 6x109/l within 6 h and to 12.6x109/l within 18 h.*
>
> *How IVIG works still needs to be investigated. The most effective and economic dose will also have to be determined.*

This article has been followed up by one for adults with ITP at the neighboring university (Fehr et al. 1982), by two other hemato-immunologists (Newland et al. 1983; Abe et al. 1983), and another colleague (Bussel and Hilgartner 1984). All confirmed the effects reported in the first publications. The observations led to much speculation on the many potential mechanisms of action and stimulated worldwide interest and study from clinical and laboratory investigators (see part III).

The nonprofit producer of IVIG was met with a high demand for the product and proposals for IVIG studies. Sandoz (later named Novartis), as a professional, worldwide distributor and coordinator of IVIG, took over that demand, while the local Red Cross expanded human-derived IVIG production, development, and research. The name changed from intravenous IgG to Sandoglobulin.

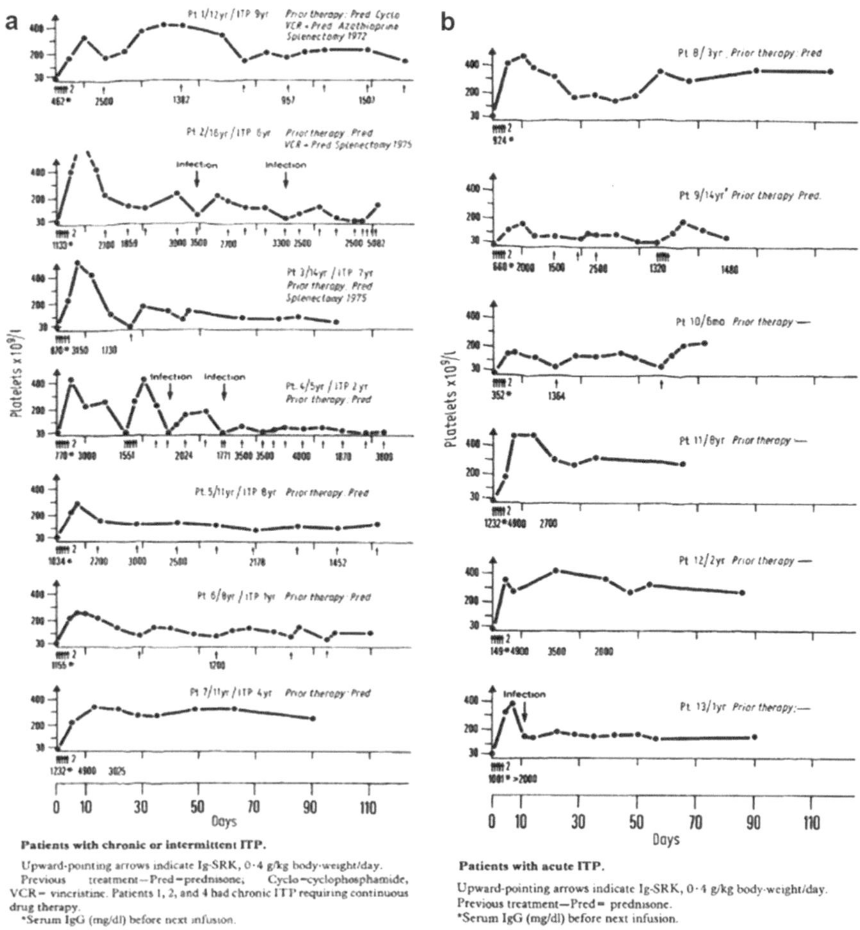

Fig. 1.2 (**a**) Patients with chronic or intermittent ITP (**b**) Patient with acute ITP

1981–1985 During a consultation at the University Children's Hospital Basel, the author met a well-known European expert of pediatric hematology EK, in Ulm, Germany, to whom he presented his data described above. This hematologist showed a great interest in the new, therapeutic possibility of IVIG. At that meeting, a proposal of an international cooperative study for administering IVIG to children with acute, newly diagnosed ITP was agreed (see below). This study was analyzed by BM and later published in "The Lancet" (Imbach et al. 1985). The article is entitled "An international cooperative, randomized study comparing IVIG with the classic corticosteroid treatment." Here are some citations:

Summary

In a randomized, multicentre study treatment with intravenous IgG was compared to oral corticosteroids in 108 children with untreated acute immune thrombocytopenic purpura. IVIG was an efficient treatment with no severe adverse reactions reported. The effects of corticosteroids and IgG were identical for rapid responders, who accounted for 62% of all patients. In contrast, patients requiring more than initial treatment responded better if randomized to IgG. The serum levels increased two-fold after IgG. A significant rise in IgM levels was observed after both IgG and corticosteroids.

Introduction

In a pilot study, the same preparation at a comparable dose was found to have a similar effect in children with acute or chronic ITP and normal serum immunoglobulin levels. A randomized trial was set up to compare the efficacy in raising platelet count, potential side-effects, and the relapse rate and number of patients progressing to chronic ITP in previously untreated children with ITP given intravenous IgG or oral corticosteroids.

Patients and Methods

After informed consent had been obtained from the parents, the patients were randomized according to a computer-generated code to receive either IgG 0.4 g/kg body weight intravenously on 5 consecutive days or oral prednisone 60 mg/m2 daily for 21 days (initial treatment). If the platelet count did not rise within the first 7 days (non-responder) or fell below 30x109/l during the following 14 days (relapse), the patient was switched to the other treatment regimen.

Results

47 children randomized to IgG and 47 to corticosteroids could be evaluated. The two groups were well matched (see table below and Fig. 1.3)

CHARACTERISTICS OF TWO STUDY GROUPS

—	Corticosteroids	IgG
n	47	47
M/F	22/25	23/24
Mean age	6 yr 3 mo	6 yr 10 mo
Mean initial platelat count ($\times 10^9$/1) (range)	9.8 (0.1–28)	9.3 (0.2–28)
Mean time from first symptom to therapy (days)	16.8	13.0
*History**		
Postinfectious	33	38
Insidious	14	9

*No significant difference (p=0.337)

36 of 47 (77%) patients randomized to corticosteroids and 39 of 47 (83%) randomized to IgG responded to the initial treatment (i.e., the platelet count rose to >100x109/l). The mean time to the peak count was 12 days with corticosteroids and 9 days with IgG.

Of the 47 patients randomized to corticosteroids, 27 needed initial treatment only. 12 of the 20 who required more than initial treatment crossed over to IgG, and in 5 patients the platelet count rose to >100x109/l. Of the 47 patients randomized to IgG, 31 received initial treatment only. 16 of 16 patients who required more than initial treatment were crossed over to corticosteroids and 6 responded.

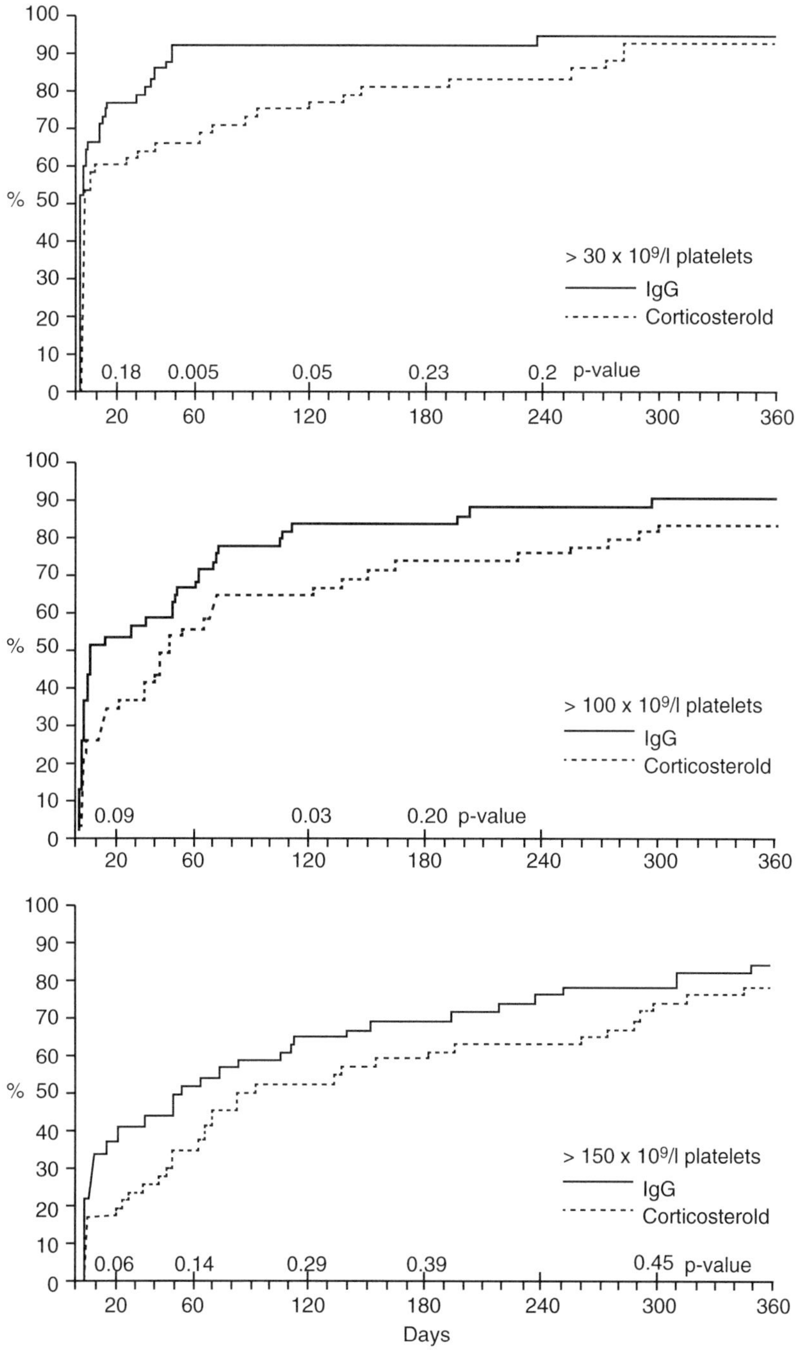

Fig. 1.3 Percentage of patients with platelet count >30, >100, and >150 × 10^9/l

The percentage of patients with a platelet count of >30x109/l, >100x109/l, or >150x109/l at various times after starting therapy is shown for both treatment arms in Fig. 1. Significant differences were found at days 60 and 120.

The serum IgG concentration increased by a factor of two from an average pretreatment level of 12.5+/- 0.6 g/l to an average peak level of 25.9+/-0.9 g/l after five doses of IgG (fig. 3). Peak values were observed between days 4 and 7. During the next 4 weeks the serum IgG gradually returned to pretreatment levels.

In patients randomized to corticosteroids, the serum IgG concentration fell significantly over 5 weeks from average levels of 12.0+/-3.7 g/l to 7.8+/-2.8 g/l- After initiation of therapy, the difference in serum IgG concentration between the IgG and corticosteroid groups was significant.

The serum IgM level increased significantly in both groups, but the rise was greater (33%) in patients randomized to IgG (Fig. 1.4). 35 days after initiation of therapy the IgM concentration had returned to pretreatment values.

Adverse reactions were observed during or shortly after 14 of 474 (2.9%) IgG infusions; they consisted of headache (8 infusions) and/or fever (6), vomiting (3), and vertigo (3). These reactions were observed in 14 of 63 (22%) of the children treated with IgG. In 47 of 61 (77%) children who received corticosteroids a Cushing's syndrome developed initially or later with an increase in body weight of more than 10% (28 patients), acne (3), and other side effects (3).

Discussion

The best treatment for acute childhood ITP remains to be defined. The main aim is to prevent potentially fatal central nervous system haemorrhage, which occurs in less than 1% of all children with ITP admitted to hospital. 1 of the 108 children entered into our study died from CNS haemorrhage, despite receiving three doses of IgG. Thus, if there is no rise in platelets after one or two doses of IgG, the treatment does not prevent intracranial hemorrhage. At necropsy, this child had evidence of active disease.

In the prospective, randomized, double-blind, multicenter study Sartorius found that corticosteroids, compared with placebo, accelerated the initial rise of platelet count but did not significantly influence the further evolution of the disease.

Our results show that the intravenous administration of large quantities of structurally and functionally intact IgG is an efficient treatment for acute ITP, including a rapid rise in the platelet count in the majority of patients. Chronic ITP, defined as thrombocytopenia (platelet count < 150x109/l) for more than 6 months, developed in 43% of patients randomized to corticosteroids and 32% of those randomized to IgG. If the platelet count defining chronic ITP is reduced to <30x109/l, only 9 (19%) versus 4 (9%) patients met the criteria. Indeed, this latter group of patients with platelet counts below 30x109/l required treatment for longer.

The mechanisms by which corticosteroids and IgG act are unclear. Blockade of the reticuloendothelial system (e.g., by modulation of Fc receptor expression or by Fc receptor blockade), protection of platelet surface structure by monomeric IgG, or interference with free or platelet bound antigen and/or immune complexes have been postulated.

There was no correlation between platelet-associated IgG index and the platelet count of the serum IgG or IgM concentrations.

Despite IVIG treatment leading to significantly fewer side-effects and inducing a faster response in slow responders than corticosteroids for ITP patients, IgG has not yet become a generally accepted treatment for ITP, mainly because of the high costs.

In a preliminary study, we found that two infusions of 0.4 g IgG/kg body weight for rapid responders achieved a satisfactory response and Bussel et al have shown that hospital admission could be prevented by a single infusion of 1g IgG/kg body weight in about half of children with acute ITP.

In the above-cited randomized study, it was not clear why IgM increased after both IVIG and corticosteroid treatment. Additionally, the results on

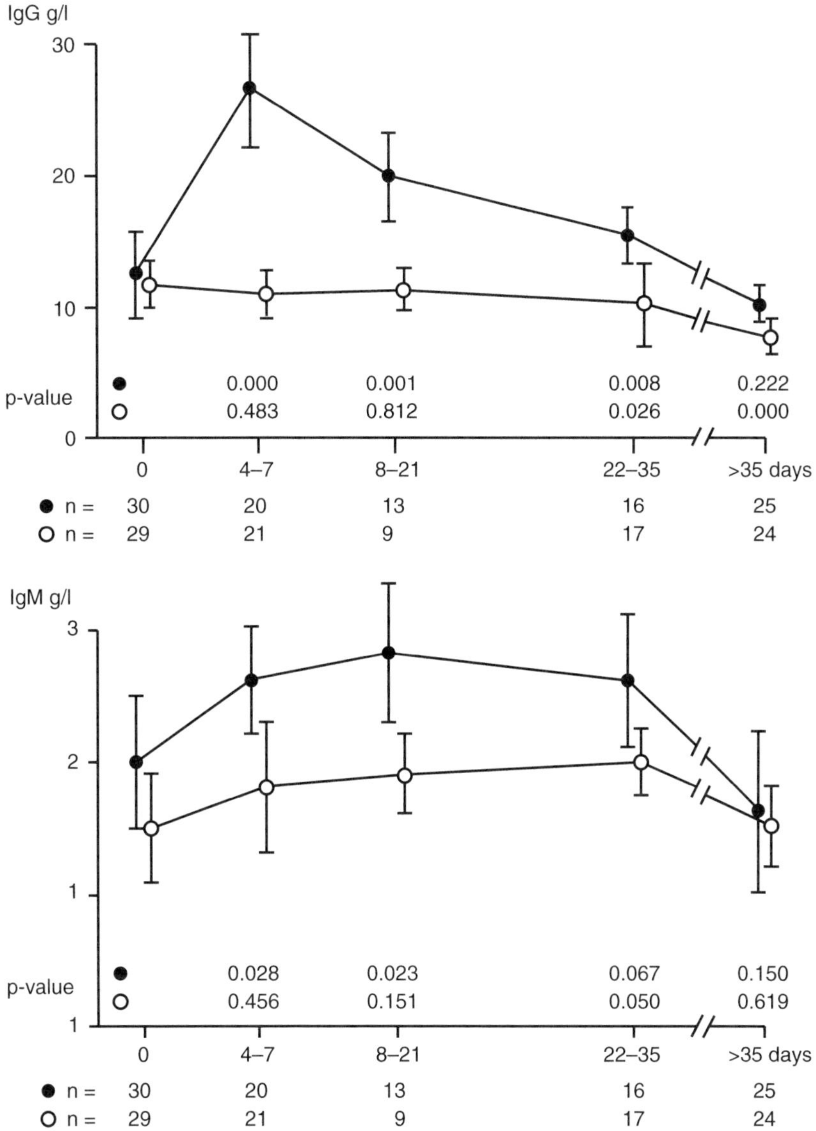

Fig. 1.4 Serum IgG and IgM before, during, and after IgG (●) and corticosteroid (○) therapy. p-values indicate significance of differences between initial values and values at various times after initiation treatment

platelet-associated IgG (PAIgG, not cited above: see original article) are questionable; the sensitivity of the PAIgG test is high, but the specificity is low. Therefore, the author began to collect serum samples from children with ITP, and supplemented these with samples from adults provided by a colleague AN in the UK. With these samples, the author traveled to the Scripps Institute in La

Jolla, CA, where he could analyze PAIgG under supervision of RMcM (Imbach et al. 1991).

As mentioned above, after the pilot study was published in The Lancet in 1981, and after the start of the randomized study (Imbach et al. 1985), it was evident that "the high-dose IVIG treatment" had similar effects as 2 × 0.4 or 1 × 0.8 g IVIG/kg body weight in patients with ITP, doubling their serum IgG levels. A large, 4-arm, randomized, cooperative study was organized by Canadian colleagues, comparing 0.8 g IVIG/kg and 2 × 1 g IVIG/kg body weight with a higher dose (4 mg/kg body weight/day of corticosteroids during a short duration (4 days, then tapering) and anti-D IgG treatment, which confirmed the lower dose of IVIG treatment in ITP (Blanchette et al. 1994).

1986 After completing the analysis of the randomized study in children cited above and the UK study in adults, the FDA in the USA and, later, the EMA in Europe accepted IVIG treatment as a new therapeutic for ITP. Thus, ITP became the first immunomodulary indication of IVIG as an autoimmune disorder.

1990 PI transferred to the University Children's Hospital, Basel, where he continued his innonative work as head of pediatric oncology, hematology, and stem cell transplantation, earned the title of full professor and as dean of education performed a throughout curriculum reform at the medical faculty of the University of Basel. 1997 PI together with his colleague TK (Chap. 19) started the ongoing Intercontinental Cooperative ITP Study (ICIS) group which now has over 90 cooperating centers worldwide (www.itpbasel.ch).

1.2 The Translation of IVIG From ITP to Other Autoimmune Disorders

Since the immunopathophysiology of ITP is similar in many other autoimmune and chronic inflammatory disorders, IVIG became the subject of worldwide clinical and laboratory studies and of its mechanisms of action. PI as an independent consultant started to supported the clinical research and development group of the central laboratory of the Swiss Red Cross and Novartis. Many peer reviewed articles, symposia and presentations at congresses reflect the pros and contras the efficacies of IVIG which the present book critically update.

1.3 The Bridge of Polyclonal and Monoclonal Antibodies

Furthermore the bridge to the engineered, monoclonal antibodies is in the focus of this book by a basic knowledge, a updated list of target antibodies, their indication and adverse effects. PI would like that the monoclonal antibodies would be combined with the polyclonal IVIG in clinical trials with the endpoints of lower the side effects and probably the increase of the efficacy. The high demand, the shortage of IVIG and the high costs of polyclonal and monoclonal antibodies might be the hindrance of such studies of antibodies combination.

Acknowledgment The author thanks Adrian C. Newland, London, UK, for his corrections and suggestions of the chapter text.

References

Abe T, Matsuda J, Kawasugi K, Yoshimura Y, Kinoshita T, Kazama M. Clinical effect of intravenous immunoglobulin on chronic idiopathic thrombocytopenic purpura. Blut. 1983;47(2):69–75.

Blanchette V, Imbach P, Andrew M, Adams M, McMillan J, Wang E, Milner R, Ali K, Barnard D, Bernstein M, Chan KW, Esseltine D, de Veber B, Israels S, Kobrinsky N, Luke B. Randomised trial of intravenous immunoglobulin G, intravenous anti-D, and oral prednisone in childhood acute immune thrombocytopenic purpura. Lancet. 1994;344:703–7.

Bussel JB, Hilgartner MW. The use and mechanism of action of intravenous immunoglobulin in the treatment of immune haematologic disease. Br J Haematol. 1984;56(1):1–7.

Fehr J, Hofmann V, Kappeler U. Transient reversal of thrombocytopenia in idiopathic thrombocytopenic purpura by high-dose intravenous gamma globulin. N Engl J Med. 1982;306:1254–8.

Imbach P, Barandun S, Baumgartner C, Hirt A, Hofer F, Wagner HP. High-dose intravenous gammaglobulin therapy of refractory, in particular idiopathic thrombocytopenia in childhood. Helv Paediatr Acta. 1981a;46:81–6.

Imbach P, Barandun S, d'Apuzzo V, Baumgartner C, Hirt A, Morell A, Rossi E, Schoeni M, Vest M, Wagner HP. High-dose intravenous gammaglobulin for idiopathic thrombocytopenic purpura in childhood. Lancet. 1981b;317:1228–31.

Imbach P, Wagner HP, Berchtold W, Gaedicke G, Hirt A, Joller P, Mueller-Eckhardt C, Müller B, Rossi E, Barandun S. Intravenous immunoglobulin versus oral corticosteroids in acute immune thrombocytopenic purpura in childhood. Lancet. 1985;2(8453):464–8.

Imbach P, Tani P, Berchtold W, Blanchette V, Burek-Kozlowska A, Gerber H, Jacobs P, Newland A, Turner C, McMillan R. Different forms of chronic childhood immune thrombocytopenic purpura defined by antiplatelet autoantibodies. J Pediatr. 1991;118:535–9.

Newland AC, Treleaven JG, Minchinton RM, Waters AH. High-dose intravenous IgG in adults with autoimmune thrombocytopenia. Lancet. 1983;1(8316):84–7.

Further Reading

Imbach P, Lazarus AH, Kühne T. Intravenous immunoglobulins induce potentially synergistic immunomodulations in autoimmune disorders. Vox Sang. 2010;98(3 Pt 2):385–94. Review.

Imbach P, Crowther M. Thrombopoietin-Receptor Agonists for Primary Immune Thrombocytopenia. N Engl J Med. 2011;365:734–41.

Imbach P, Kabus K, Toenz O. Successful treatment of a severe drowning accident after 20 minutes submersion. Schweiz Med Wochenschr. 1975;105(48):1605–11.

Imbach P, Odavic R, Bleher EA, Bucher U, Deubelbeiss KA, Wagner HP. Autologous bone marrow reimplantation in children with advanced tumor. First experiences of feasibility. Schweiz Med Wochenschr. 1979;109(8):283–7.

Imbach P, Kuehne T, Arceci RJ. Pediatric Oncology: A Comprehensive Guide, Third Edition, Springer 2014.

Part I

Update of Substitutive and Immunomodulatory Antibodies/ Drugs Indications

From Immune Substitution to Immuno-modulation

2

Volker Wahn

2.1 History

The description of agammaglobulinemia by Bruton (1952) was a milestone in the history of medicine. For the first time it was shown that the absence of immunoglobulins was associated with recurrent mainly bacterial and viral infections and that the administration of Cohn fraction II subcutaneously (!) had the potential to reduce the number and severity of such infections. Today, the treatment of severe humoral immunodeficiencies consists in lifelong immunoglobulin replacement. Intramuscular administration has become obsolete because of injection site-related side effects but especially because only insufficient amounts of immunoglobulin can be administered.

Intravenous administration of Cohn fraction II probably as a consequence of complement activation by IgG aggregates offered no perspective. Thus, methods had to be developed to make products well tolerated by patients. After appropriate achievements, intravenous IgG (IVIG) replacement became the most widely used route of administration since the 1980s and allowed the administration of adequate immunoglobulin doses. IVIG treatment may be limited due to risk of anaphylactoid reactions and poor vein access in small children and because health-care personnel must, at least in Germany, directly supervise the infusions. As an alternative for iv IgG replacement, rapid administration (up to 50 mL/h) pumps for subcutaneous infusion (SCIG) are now generally accepted. SCIG was successively used for clinical trials in the Scandinavian countries since the early 1990s. Both intravenous and the subcutaneous administration achieve therapeutic IgG levels, and the clinical efficacy is comparable. One SCIG uses local administration of human recombinant hyaluronidase prior to IgG in order to increase the amount of IgG infused

V. Wahn
Department of Pediatric Pneumology and Immunology, Charité University Hospital, Augustenburger Platz 1, 13353 Berlin, Germany
e-mail: Volker.Wahn@charite.de

P. Imbach (ed.), *Antibody Therapy*, https://doi.org/10.1007/978-3-319-68038-5_2

subcutaneously and to reduce infusion numbers. All preparations are now approved by many authorities, and the mode of treatment can be chosen on the basis of the patients preferences.

2.2 IgG for Replacement: How Much?

Maintenance doses for IgG of between 400–1000 mg/kg body weight per month are recommended. The major goal of treatment is the reduction of severe infections like chronic rhinosinusitis or pneumonia and the avoidance of irreversible organ damage like bronchiectases. The doses of IgG and the trough levels achieved vary among patients depending on the underlying disease, the response to treatment, and the presence or absence of chronic lung disease (Lucas et al. 2010). Probably, an individualized approach comes closest to the patient's needs.

Some general principles of treatment may reflect our current knowledge:

- There is a clear pharmacokinetic difference between iv and sc administration. The trough level in iv therapy persists only a few days before the next peak level is reached. In sc therapy peak and trough level hardly differ from each other. From a recent meta-analysis (Orange et al. 2010), it was shown that the incidence of pneumonia with IVIG declines up to a trough level of 1000 mg/dl. Similar results were obtained with SCIG. A recent analysis from Holland (Janssen et al. 2017) shows that, at least in patients with CVID, trough levels >1000 mg/dl may be required in order to prevent silent progression of airway disease. The authors, however, state that randomized prospective trials would be necessary to prove that trough levels >1000 mg/dl are, in fact, more effective. This illustrates that current recommendations may have to be updated in the future.
- For now, if a patient with an IgG of 500–800 mg/dl is free from infections, the maintenance of these trough levels is sufficient. If a patient with 1000 mg/dl still suffers from severe infections, this trough level is not sufficient, and a higher dose should be chosen. Thus, the optimum is reached with a biological and individual IgG level that provides effective infection control (Bonagura et al. 2008).
- Most IgG licensing studies were done with XLA (X-linked agammaglobulinemia) and CVID (common variable immunodeficiency) patients together. Lucas et al. (2010) have shown that an XLA patient needs significantly higher IgG levels to be free from infections compared to patients with CVID. Thus, the underlying disease must be taken into account.
- In patients with bronchiectases, all experts in the world agree that they require higher doses of IgG than patients without this complication. Retrospective data from Lucas et al. (2010) showed that patients with bronchiectasis require twice as much replacement doses to achieve the same IgG level compared with those free of bronchiectasis. Prospective trials, however, addressing this question, have never been performed.

For further details of replacement therapy, I would like to refer to existing national and international guidelines for the use of immunoglobulins in antibody-deficient patients.

2.3 Immunomodulation in Autoimmune Diseases

The second milestone in the history of the clinical use of immunoglobulins was the publication by Imbach et al. (1981). The authors described seven children with chronic and six with acute ITP in whom the platelet count was markedly increased through high-dose administration of immunoglobulins. The course was variable, with some patients needing IVIG infusions on a regular basis. Several publications by other authors confirmed these initial observations in controlled clinical trials.

As Imbach's paper had shown that certain immunopathological reactions may be modified by IVIG, it encouraged many authors worldwide to exploit the potential of IVIG treatment in other diseases too. The number of diseases where this mode of treatment was attempted may now exceed 100. Not all attempts were successful, and only a few turned out to be "indications" on the basis of randomized controlled trials (RCT). However, in some very rare diseases, the call for RCT may be inadequate because the number of patients is simply too small. Keeping this in mind even case reports may be meaningful. Many results and "indications" are summarized in a small booklet (Wahn and Orange 2013) and in a recent review (Perez et al. 2017).

Imbach et al. (1981) used a 7S preparation of IV gamma globulin (Sandoglobulin), which had an intact Fc fragment. Later publications showed the poorer effect of F(ab′)2 fragments (=5S IgG) (Burdach et al. 1986). In contrast, a good clinical effect could be achieved with purified Fc fragments devoid of F(ab′)2 (Debré et al. 1993). A substantial part of the biological effect of IgG is thus dependent on the presence of the Fc portion suggesting that the interaction of IVIG with the various types of Fc receptors is crucial for its efficacy (Fig. 2.1).

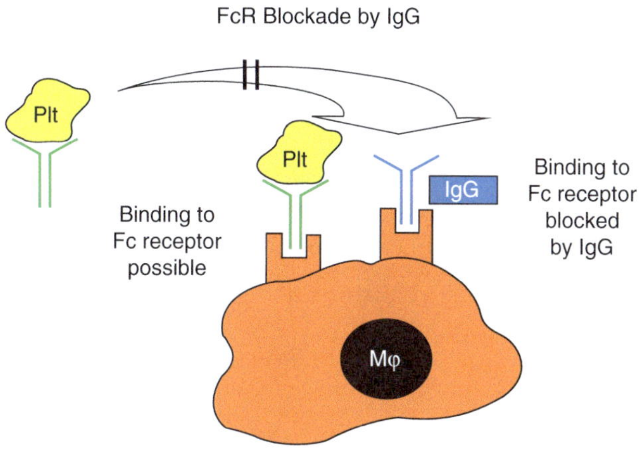

Fig. 2.1 In ITP, induced by known or unknown triggers autoantibodies bind to platelets which are taken up by cells of the reticuloendothelial system via Fc receptors expressed at the surface. If such receptors are blocked my therapeutic IgG, antibody-coated platelets remain in the circulation

Beyond these interactions many other mechanisms may be effective either alone or in concert which have been discussed in detail (Imbach et al. 2010; Matucci et al. 2015).

2.4 Immunomodulation in Alloimmune Diseases

After having studied Imbach's work, my colleagues and I were inspired to study the potential role of IVIG in another pediatric disease affecting newborn babies, rhesus hemolytic disease. The pathomechanism of disease can be illustrated as follows (Fig. 2.2):

If so we hypothesized that IVIG could decrease the degree of hemolysis and thus reduce the number of exchange transfusions required, the first three cases (Rübo and Wahn 1990) suggested that, in fact, IVIG modified the course of bilirubin incline and allowed us to avoid exchange transfusions. This observation motivated us to study the effects of IVIG in a larger group of babies in a randomized controlled trial (Rübo and Wahn 1991; Rübo et al. 1992). In this setting, we were able to show that the number of exchange transfusions could be significantly reduced if IVIG was given early enough in babies at risk for bilirubin encephalopathy.

As IVIG does not reduce the number of antibody-coated red blood cells but only slows down their uptake by the RES, we followed all children for the development of late anemia. In fact, a few IVIG-treated babies required blood transfusions for late anemia. Because, however, the risk of a blood transfusion is by far lower than the risk of an exchange transfusion, we considered this risk acceptable.

Our observation has been confirmed in later publications reporting results in babies with rhesus and ABO hemolytic disease. In 2004, the American Academy of Pediatrics recommended prophylactic IgG as an alternative for blood exchange transfusions.

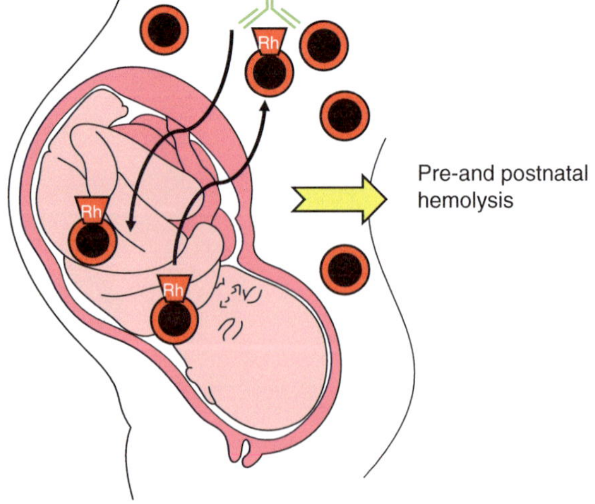

Fig. 2.2 During pregnancy, fetal rhesus D+ red blood cells stimulate the generation of maternal anti-Rh D alloantibodies. These can cross the placenta and may destroy Rh D+ red blood cells in the baby by Fc receptor mediated uptake by cells of the reticuloendothelial system. This is the major mechanism as anti-D antibodies do not bind complement

2.5 Immunomodulation in Inflammatory Diseases

While the two previous examples are associated with disease-causing specific antibodies, the experiences in Kawasaki disease (KD; for review see Agarwal and Agrawal 2017) expanded the spectrum of IVIG efficacy to a pediatric vasculitis with unknown etiopathogenesis but with massive proinflammatory cytokinemia. The disease may be based on a complex interplay of genetic factors, infections, and immunity. KD mainly affects infants and toddlers. The major problem is the development of coronary artery aneurysms which are responsible for fatal courses. Initially, the disease was treated with aspirin at high doses. However, despite such treatment, aneurysms still occurred, and new modes of treatment had to be developed.

Keeping this background in mind, the paper by Newburger et al. (1986) for the first time showed that IVIG had an anti-inflammatory potential. In randomized trial, aspirin alone was compared to the combination of aspirin + IVIG at a dose of 4 × 400 mg/kg bw given on four consecutive days. Combination therapy reduced the number of coronary artery aneurysms significantly after 2 (from 23 to 8%) and after 7 weeks (from 18 to 4%). In a subsequent trial (Newburger et al. 1991), the administration of 2 g/kg bw given on 1 day compared to 4 × 400 mg/kg bw on 4 days further reduced the risk for aneurysms by another approximately 50%. Since then 2 g/kg bw is an effective treatment for most of the kids. If symptoms persist based on data from appropriate trials, German guidelines recommend the addition of oral steroids. For resistant cases German Guidelines recommend infliximab.

The mode of action of IVIG is not quite clear. Maybe that like in ITP several mechanism may act in concert. The following figure illustrates only one of the mechanisms described in the literature (Fig. 2.3).

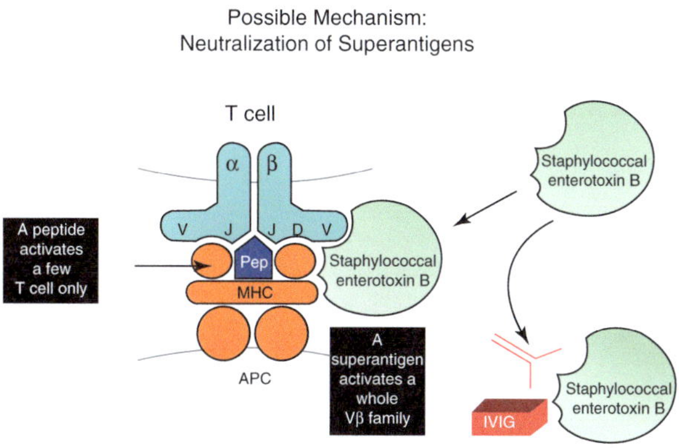

Fig. 2.3 In specific T-cell responses the antigen-presenting cell presents peptides which are recognized by a single clone of antigen-specific T cells using α- and β-chain of the T-cell receptor. In KD the so-called superantigens expressed by certain bacteria may activate a whole Vß family of T cells leading to a massive cytokine response. IVIG may neutralize these superantigens and, thus, reduce the inflammatory response

Whatever the mechanism of disease and the mode of action of IVIG may be, the fact remains that in addition to some autoimmune and alloimmune disorders also some disorders characterized by massive inflammation can be influenced by IVIG.

2.6 Expansion to New Indications

Inspired by the fascinating chance to modify immunopathology by IgG as a kind of treatment associated with a relatively low-risk clinicians worldwide looked for possible further indications. Figure 2.4 tries to illustrate that.

Not all attempts were successful. However, some clear indications have emerged making IgG treatment indispensable in clinical practice.

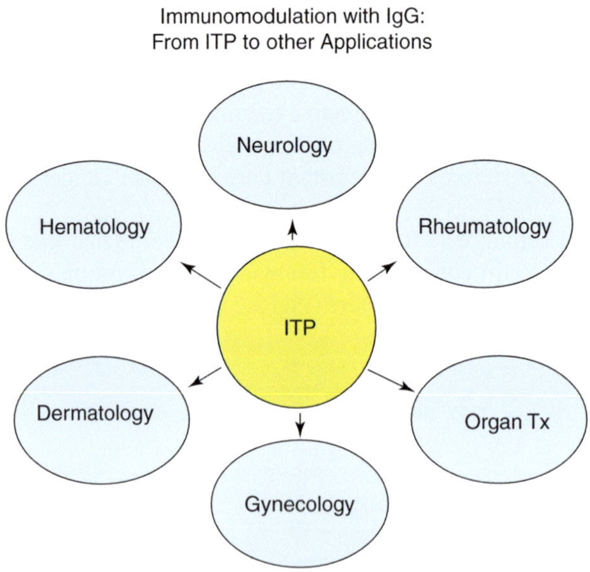

Fig. 2.4 The efficacy of IgG treatment as a mode to modify abnormal immune responses was first demonstrated in children with ITP. Since the several other potential applications have emerged (summarized in Wahn and Orange (2013) and Perez et al. (2017))

Disclosures In the last years, the author has received honoraria for scientific lectures from Octapharma, CSL Behring, Biotest, PPTA and the FIND-ID network. He was also paid for his work in an advisory board (Pharming) and data safety monitoring board (Octapharma, Pfizer).

References

Agarwal S, Agrawal DK. Kawasaki disease: etiopathogenesis and novel treatment strategies. Exp Rev Clin Immunol. 2017;13(3):247–58.

Bonagura VR, Marchlewski R, Cox A, Rosenthal DW. Biologic IgG level in primary immunodeficiency disease: the IgG level that protects against recurrent infection. J Allergy Clin Immunol. 2008;122(1):210–2.

Bruton OC. Agammaglobulinemia. Pediatrics. 1952;9(6):722–8.

Burdach SE, Evers KG, Geursen RG. Treatment of acute idiopathic thrombocytopenic purpura of childhood with intravenous immunoglobulin G: comparative efficacy of 7S and 5S preparations. J Pediatr. 1986;109(5):770–5.

Debré M, Bonnet MC, Fridman WH, Carosella E, Philippe N, Reinert P, Vilmer E, Kaplan C, Teillaud JL, Griscelli C. Infusion of Fc gamma fragments for treatment of children with acute immune thrombocytopenic purpura. Lancet. 1993;342(8877):945–9.

Imbach P, Barandun S, d'Apuzzo V, Baumgartner C, Hirt A, Morell A, Rossi E, Schöni M, Vest M, Wagner HP. High-dose intravenous gammaglobulin for idiopathic thrombocytopenic purpura in childhood. Lancet. 1981;1(8232):1228–31.

Imbach P, Lazarus AH, Kühne T. Intravenous immunoglobulins induce potentially synergistic immunomodulations in autoimmune disorders. Vox Sang. 2010;98(3 Pt 2):385–94.

Janssen WJ, Mohamed Hoesein F, Van de Ven AA, Maarschalk J, van Royen F, de Jong PA, Sanders EA, van Montfrans JM, Ellerbroek PM. IgG trough levels and progression of pulmonary disease in pediatric and adult CVID patients. J Allergy Clin Immunol. 2017;140(1):304–306.e4.

Lucas M, Lee M, Lortan J, Lopez-Granados E, Misbah S, Chapel H. Infection outcomes in patients with common variable immunodeficiency disorders: relationship to immunoglobulin therapy over 22 years. J Allergy Clin Immunol. 2010;125(6):1354–60.

Matucci A, Maggi E, Vultaggio A. Mechanisms of action of Ig preparations: immunomodulatory and anti-inflammatory effects. Front Immunol. 2015;5:690.

Newburger JW, Takahashi M, Burns JC, Beiser AS, Chung KJ, Duffy CE, Glode MP, Mason WH, Reddy V, Sanders SP, et al. The treatment of Kawasaki syndrome with intravenous gamma globulin. N Engl J Med. 1986;315(6):341–7.

Newburger JW, Takahashi M, Beiser AS, Burns JC, Bastian J, Chung KJ, Colan SD, Duffy CE, Fulton DR, Glode MP, et al. A single intravenous infusion of gamma globulin as compared with four infusions in the treatment of acute Kawasaki syndrome. N Engl J Med. 1991;324(23):1633–9.

Orange JS, Grossman WJ, Navickis RJ, Wilkes MM. Impact of trough IgG on pneumonia incidence in primary immunodeficiency: a meta-analysis of clinical studies. Clin Immunol. 2010;137(1):21–30.

Perez EE, Orange JS, Bonilla F, Chinen J, Chinn IK, Dorsey M, El-Gamal Y, Harville TO, Hossny E, Mazer B, Nelson R, Secord E, Jordan SC, Stiehm ER, Vo AA, Ballow M. Update on the use of immunoglobulin in human disease: a review of evidence. J Allergy Clin Immunol. 2017;139(3S):S1–S46.

Rübo J, Wahn V. A trial with high-dose gamma globulin therapy in 3 children with hyperbilirubinemia in rhesus incompatibility. Monatsschr Kinderheilkd. 1990;138(4):216–20.

Rübo J, Wahn V. High-dose intravenous gammaglobulin in rhesus-haemolytic disease. Lancet. 1991;337(8746):914.

Rübo J, Albrecht K, Lasch P, Laufkötter E, Leititis J, Marsan D, Niemeyer B, Roesler J, Roll C, Roth B, et al. High-dose intravenous immune globulin therapy for hyperbilirubinemia caused by Rh hemolytic disease. J Pediatr. 1992;121(1):93–7.

Wahn V, Orange JS. Clinical use of immunoglobulins UNI-MED science. 2nd ed. Bremen: UNI-MED Verlag AG; 2013.

3 Manual of Primary and Secondary Immunodeficiencies

Paul Imbach and Volker Wahn

3.1 Introduction

This chapter focuses on practical issues of management. A short summary presents the characteristics of the distinct disorders (for details see reviews).

Replacement with human polyclonal immunoglobulin concentrate is one of the main modes of treatment for the majority of patients with primary immunodeficiencies (PID). PID may present with life-threatening or severe infections, autoimmune diseases, lymphoproliferation, and malignancies. Many deficiencies are associated with impaired antibody production in addition to dysfunction of other components of the immune system.

To date, over 300 monogenetic PID have been described in the literature. Here, only a few classical examples are characterized.

3.2 X-Linked (Bruton's) Agammaglobulinemia

3.2.1 Definition and Prevalence

X-linked agammaglobulinemia is an autosomal recessive disorder characterized by severe reduction of plasma immunoglobulins and absence of B cells. The prevalence is estimated at 1:100,000.

P. Imbach
University of Basel, CH 4031, Basel, Switzerland
e-mail: paul.imbach@unibas.ch

V. Wahn (✉)
Department of Pediatric Pneumology and Immunology, Charité University Hospital, Augustenburger Platz 1, 13353 Berlin, Germany
e-mail: Volker.Wahn@charite.de

P. Imbach (ed.), *Antibody Therapy*, https://doi.org/10.1007/978-3-319-68038-5_3

3.2.2 Pathophysiology

The disease is caused by various mutations of BTK (Bruton's tyrosine kinase) which results in the absence of mature B lymphocytes, profound reduction of all classes of Immunoglobulins, and, lastly, the absence of antibody production. Precursor B cells (PreB) remain present in the bone marrow.

3.2.3 Clinical Manifestations

Recurrent infections: pneumonia, sinusitis, otitis, later on bronchiectases and gastrointestinal disorders, arthritis, viral meningoencephalitis, and autoimmune diseases.

After live vaccination with oral polio vaccine: vaccine-derived poliomyelitis.

Lymphatic tissue (tonsils, lymph nodes) small or absent.

3.2.4 Diagnostics

IgG, IgA, IgM, and IgE absent or very low. Absence of specific antibodies (tetanus, pneumococci) despite regular vaccinations. Absence of CD19/CD20 positive B cells. Typical mutations in the BTK gene.

3.2.5 Differential Diagnosis

Severe combined immunodeficiency (SCID, see 3.3), transient hypogammaglobulinemia of infancy.

Hypogammaglobulinemia due to loss of IgG (enteric, renal).

3.2.6 Therapy

IV- or SC-IgG substitution to obtain a plasma level >8 g/l IgG, usually achieved by doses of 0.3–0.6 g IgG/kg body weight every 3–4 weeks. Patients with bronchiectasis may require higher doses.

Aim of treatment: prevention of severe infections, survival, and improved quality of life.

3.2.7 Prognosis

With IgG substitution from early life onwards: normal to slightly reduced life expectancy

Without substitution: fatal infections in childhood

3.3 Severe Combined Immunodeficiency (SCID)

3.3.1 Definition and Prevalence

Combined cellular and humoral immunodeficiency with absent T cells and absent or dysfunctional B cells. Prevalence: 1:50,000 (USA). Without treatment, usually fatal within the first year of life.

3.3.2 Pathophysiology

3.3.2.1 Different Forms

T-B + Variants
Several mutations in genes for cytokine receptors, subunits of the T-cell receptor complex, other membrane proteins, signal transduction molecules and coronin 1A (necessary for thymic release of mature T cells).

T-B-Variants
Several mutations in genes responsible for stem cell maturation, B-/T-cell DNA recombination, and purine metabolism (ADA)

3.3.3 Clinical Manifestations

- Severe recurrent and opportunistic infections within the first months of life.
- Chronic graft-versus-host disease caused by maternal T cells, severe CMV, bacterial and fungal infections, *Pneumocystis jiroveci* pneumonia, chronic diarrhea and/or failure to thrive, and complicated infections by live vaccines (rotavirus, BCG)

3.3.4 Diagnostics

- Reduced lymphatic tissue, i.e., lateral thorax X-ray with small or absent thymus in some genetic variants
- FACS: Absence of T cells, some variants also lack B cells. Atypical findings with maternal engraftment, Omenn phenotype, or leaky SCID variants
- Serum IgG, IgM, IgA all markedly reduced
- Impaired T-cell proliferation with mitogens and antigens, absent antibody production after vaccinations

3.3.5 Treatment

Sterile environment, avoidance of live vaccines, avoidance of non-irradiated blood transfusions

- Antibacterial, antifungal, and antiviral treatment of infections
- IgG substitution as under A as long as B cells are not reconstituted by stem cell transplantation
- Parenteral nutrition if required
- Stem cell transplantation from matched family or unrelated donor. Haploidentical Tx less effective
- Somatic gene therapy only approved for ADA deficiency in cases where a matched family donor is not found

3.4 Hyper-IgM Syndromes

3.4.1 Pathogenesis

- Antibody class-switch defects: (a) X-chromosomal, recessive type with gene mutation of CD40 ligand (CD40L) and (b) autosomal recessive types (CD40 deficiency, uracil N-glycosylase deficiency (UNG), activation-induced cytidine deaminase (AID) deficiency, and several others)
- Presence of B cells, but low serum levels of IgG and IgA and normal or high levels of IgM

3.4.2 Clinical Presentation

CD40 and CD40L deficiencies are regarded as combined B-/T-cell deficiencies, while UNG and AID are predominantly B-cell deficiencies.

- Bacterial respiratory infections
- *Pneumocystis jiroveci* infection (CD40 and CD40L), especially in the first year of life
- Diarrhea, infections with cryptosporidium
- Lymphadenopathy, neutropenia, thrombocytopenia, anemia

3.4.3 Treatment

- Treatment of existing infections
- IgG substitution as under Sect. 3.2.6
- Stem cell transplantation in selected patients with CD40 or CD40L deficiencies

3.5 Common Variable Immunodeficiency (CVID)

3.5.1 Incidence and Diagnosis

Common variable immunodeficiency (CVID) is the most frequent symptomatic PID. 10–20% are monogenetic disorders, some with autosomal dominant and some with autosomal recessive inheritance. Estimated prevalence 1:10,000–1:50,000.

(a) Reduction of IgG and IgA
(b) IgM may be normal
(c) Impaired antibody response to vaccines
(d) Other causes excluded

The diagnosis can be made in the absence of recurrent infections if (a)–(d) are met (according to International Consensus 2016).

3.5.2 Clinical Manifestations

- Infections similar to agammaglobulinemia (A.1), development of bronchiectasis, and chronic lung disease
- Noninfectious manifestations: diarrhea, malabsorption, high rate of autoimmune disorders such as rheumatoid arthritis, autoimmune hemolytic anemia, thrombocytopenia, neutropenia granulomatous and lymphoproliferative complications, malignancies

3.5.3 Treatment

- IgG substitution as in Sect. 3.2.6

  Treatment of infections
  Immunosuppression for autoimmune and granulomatous complications
  Stem cell transplantation is not a standard treatment

3.6 Selective Antibody Deficiency

3.6.1 Definition and Diagnosis

- Immunoglobulins IgG, IgA and IgM normal, B cells normal
- Impaired vaccine antibody production to pneumococcal polysaccharide vaccine (Pneumovax®)
- Recurrent infections with encapsulated bacteria

3.6.2 Treatment

- Antibiotic prophylaxis and/or treatment
- IgG substitution as Sect. 3.2.6 in severe cases

3.7 Transient Hypogammaglobulinemia of Infancy

3.7.1 Definition and Diagnosis

- Delay of B-cell maturation
- Affects mainly infants and toddlers <6 years of age
- Usually no abnormal susceptibility to infections
- Hypogammaglobulinemia with normal antibody responses

3.7.2 Management

- Usually no IgG substitution required

3.8 Isolated IgG 1–3 Subclass Deficiency

- Some patients with recurrent infections
- Minority with deficient antibody response to polysaccharide vaccines, especially in the absence of IgG2

3.8.1 Management

- Antibiotic treatment of infections
- IgG-substitution when polysaccharide responses are absent

3.9 Selective IgA Deficiency with or without IgG2 Deficiency

- Selective IgA deficiency usually asymptomatic, slightly increased risk for celiac disease, rheumatic diseases and allergies
- Increased susceptibility to infections if associated with IgG2 deficiency
- In rare cases, risk of anaphylactic reaction to IgG substitution or blood transfusions due to the presence of autoantibodies to IgA
- If IgG substitution is indicated: use of IgG-preparation with low IgA content

3.10 Wiskott-Aldrich Syndrome (WAS)

3.10.1 Pathogenesis/Etiology

- X-chromosomal inheritance
- Combined immunodeficiency with high levels of serum IgE and IgA and low serum IgM, impaired polysaccharide responses
- Defective protein (WASP) leads to impaired signal transduction and actin poly-merization following lymphocyte activation

3.10.2 Clinical Manifestations

- Thrombocytopenic bleeding, eczema, recurrent infections, and increased risk for malignancies

3.10.3 Treatment

- Administration of IVIG, antibiotic, and antiviral treatment.
- Allogenic stem cell transplantation may be curative.
- Somatic gene therapy is still experimental.

3.11 Ataxia Telangiectasia

3.11.1 Pathophysiology/Etiology

- Autosomal recessive disorder with ATM-gene mutations. ATM is involved in repair of DNA strand breaks and control of cell cycle. Radiosensitive disorder with chromosomal instability.
- Some patients present with combined ID, variable expression of hypogamma-globulinemia, low IgG subclasses, low IgA and IgE, low antibody responses.
- Some patients have a hyper-IgM phenotype. Alpha-1 fetoprotein usually elevated.

3.11.2 Clinical Manifestation

- Susceptibility to all kinds of infections. Development of telangiectases and cerebellar ataxia in the first year of life, later on high risk for lymphatic and other malignancies

3.11.3 Treatment

- Treatment of infections
- IgG substitution may be useful if severe infections occur and specific antibody responses are markedly impaired
- Prognosis is still poor

3.12 Secondary Immunodeficiency

3.12.1 Chronic Lymphocytic Leukemia (CLL), Multiple Myeloma (MM) and Treatment of Related Secondary Immunodeficiency in Patients with Hematologic or with Solid Tumor Malignancy with or without Transplantation

General Aspects

- Due to novel treatment regimens with immunosuppressive, anticancer drugs, anti-inflammatory drugs, and monoclonal antibodies, which have significantly prolonged malignancy-related survival and also increased the risk of morbidity and mortality due to severe infection and the underlying diseases, the indication of IVIG has to be reconsidered.
- The cumulative treatments lead to immune defects such as severe neutropenia, mucosal lesions, T-cell dysregulations, natural killer cell dysfunction, cytokine alterations, phagocytic dysfunctions, complement activation, apoptotic changes, and many other immune response alterations. In addition, hypogammaglobulinemia due to defective B-cell production of polyvalent antibodies may be present.
- The combined treatment regimen with monoclonal antibodies such as alemtuzumab, anti-CD20, chimeric antigen receptor (CAR) T cells, Bcl-2 antagonist, tyrosine kinase inhibitor ibrutinib, Syk inhibitor fostamatinib, and others increase the risk of reactivation of herpes virus, hepatitis B infections, the risk of opportunistic infections, such as *Pneumocystis jiroveci*, listeria, mycobacteria, and candida, and the risk of encapsulated bacteria (*Staphylococcus pneumoniae*, *Staphylococcus aureus*, *Haemophilus influenzae*) infection/pneumonia and bronchiectasia.
- Since the majority of patients with these diagnoses have secondary immunodeficiency, analyses are recommended prior to, during, and after specific treatment, namely, history of infections and vaccinations, clinical examinations, differential blood analyses, FACS including CD4 and CD8 T cells and B cells, and quantitative analysis of serum IgG with subclasses, IgM, IgA, and IgE, antigen-specific antibody production (e.g., to polysaccharide antigens (T-cell-independent response) as by the 23-valent pneumococcal vaccines), and antibody responses to tetanus toxoid or influenza virus.

Supportive Management

- Vaccinations (all live vaccinations are contraindicated!) before specific treatment (if possible) and after completion of treatment, when indicated by the results of analyses (see above).
- IVIG replacement as prophylaxis and treatment in selected patients with defective immunity and those with recurrent infection refractory to or insufficiently responding to antibiotics/antiviral/antifungal treatment.
- IVIG may also influence the defense against the underlying disease.
- Dosage of IVIG: As in primary immune deficiencies with the aim to reach a serum IgG level of 6–8 g/l, as long as necessary/as recovery of the immunological functions.

3.12.2 Specific Aspects

3.12.2.1 CLL and MM

- In the past, patients with CLL, hypogammaglobulinemia, and recurrent infections have been significantly protected from infections by administration of IVIG in several controlled studies, it rarely is used, today with the conventional treatment.
- For new combined treatment see "Gemeral aspects" above.

3.12.2.2 Hematopoietic Stem Cell Transplantation HSCT

- Currently, IVIG prevention treatment of graft-versus-host disease (GVHD) and infection during the peritransplantation time is no longer recommended in patients with HLA-identical HSCT except in patients with severe secondary immunodeficiency/complications (see above).
- Patients with HSCT due to severe combined immunodeficiency and other primary or secondary immunodeficiencies with a- or hypogammaglobulinemia are candidates for IgG preventive treatment. Additionally, infants should be substituted by IVIG before and after HSCT as long as reconstitution of the immune functions is established. Thus, individual IgG administration is indicated in these groups of patients.

3.12.2.3 Solid Organ Transplantation

- IgG treatment is beneficial for sensitized patients exposed to ABO blood group antigens, including from platelet transfusions, during the wait time for organ transplantation, i.e. kidney transplantation, and for patients after non-identical HLA antigen exposure due to transplantation.
- High dose IVIG administration with or without monoclonal B-cell depletion (i.e. rituximab) and/or plasma exchange reduces the level of anti-HLA antibodies and improves the rate of transplantation.

- IVIG and monoclonal B-cell depletion (i.e. rituximab) can be useful for desensitization, especially before, during and after allogenic heart and/or lung transplantation due to donor-specific HLA antibodies. Donor-specific HLA antibodies are an important risk factor of bronchiolitis obliterans.
- In patients with antibody-related rejection of a transplantation, the combination of IVIG, monoclonal B-cell depletion (i.e., rituximab), and eventually plasma exchange is the recommended approach.
- Patients during and after non-HLA-identical or haploid HSCT may benefit from IgG preventive treatment for a limited time, i.e., until reconstitution of the immune functions.

3.12.3 HIV Infection in Children

- IgG substitution has shown positive effects for HIV infected children with CD4 T cells >200/µl in controlled clinical studies. However, these studies have been performed before highly active antiviral treatment (HAART) became available. Today, children with HIV infection treated with HAART show reconstitution of T cells and normalization of antibody responses. Thus, IgG administration in HIV infected children is an approved indication which is no longer practiced.

3.12.4 Preterm Infants

- IgG substitution in premature babies has been studied in many trials using a prophylactic or therapeutic design. Based on the latest large trials, it became clear that babies do not benefit from IgG treatment.

3.12.5 Geriatrics: Immunosenescence

- Elderly people may have deficient adaptive and innate immune responses.
- Evaluation of the immune state and function is indicated, if recurrent, severe, or difficult to treat infections are present, i.e., by anomalies of FACS, IgG, and subclasses, antibody responses to vaccines.
- IgG substitution may be considered in elderly patients with immune deficiencies. Dosage as in Sect. 3.11.3.
- Adverse effects to IgG treatment see Chap. 10 are higher in patients over 60 years of age.
- Serious adverse effects in older patients include higher risk of acute, transient renal failure and venous thrombosis depending on comorbidities.
- Recommendation of administration of IVIG in elderly patients: sufficient hydration prior to IVIG, slow infusion rate, IVIG preparation with low concentration of sucrose, and monitoring renal function.
- In the future: subcutaneous Ig SCIG administration may have less adverse effects.

3.13 Other Combined Immunodeficiency

- Among the over 300 monogenetic disorders leading to immunodeficiency, there are many with impaired antibody responses where affected patients benefit from IgG replacement. Several of these combined ID, however, can be corrected by stem cell transplantation. If thereafter the B-cell compartment is fully reconstituted, IgG administration may become dispensable.

Manual of Intravenous and Subcutaneous IgG Indications in Autoimmune Diseases

4

Paul Imbach

4.1 Introduction

This manual is a brief summary of extensive reviews of the literature extracted from PubMed and a recent review by Perez et al. (2017), which mainly categorizes the indications according to FDA/EMA approvals and evidence-based findings.

The manual is written by a physician involved in the clinical care of patients considering the different individual manifestations and the complex characteristics of the autoimmune and inflammatory diseases. It focuses on the clinical options of recommended therapeutic, immunomodulatory effects of administration of IVIG and categorizes them in respect to other treatment approaches.

4.2 General Characteristics of Autoimmune Disorders

Autoimmune disorders are characterized by:

- Clinical manifestations and follow-ups of inflammatory and autoimmune diseases are heterogenous and variable.
- The disorders are often associated with pathogenic antigen(s), antibodies, or immune complexes.
- The immune system is imbalanced, and the innate and/or adaptive immune responses differ from patient to patient.
- A minority of common autoimmune diseases, where controlled (randomized and/or blinded) clinical studies could be performed leading to evidence-based recommendation (category A, see below).

P. Imbach
University of Basel, CH 4031, Basel, Switzerland
e-mail: paul.imbach@unibas.ch

P. Imbach (ed.), *Antibody Therapy*, https://doi.org/10.1007/978-3-319-68038-5_4

- The majority of autoimmune disorders which are rare and controlled clinical studies often are not feasible; therefore, rare inflammatory or autoimmune diseases are off-label indications of IVIG (category B, see below).
- Continuous discussion and assessment of each indication of administration of intravenous or subcutaneous immunoglobulin (IVIG or SCIG) concentrate are necessary.

4.3 General Characteristics of IVIG as an Immunomodulatory Biological Agent

In contrast to substitutive administration of IVIG for primary and secondary immunodeficiencies, immunomodulatory administration of IVIG is characterized:

- By high dosage of IVIG usually 2 g/kg within 1–5 days per course (named HD IVIG in the following texts); for other dosage recommendations and for the new possibility of SCIG administration, see text of the respective disorder.
- By adverse effects of HD IVIG which are mild or moderate at a rate of 5%; however, some severe side effects are known.
- By the high demand of IVIG, and this limits the potential indications because of the shortages, of the costs, etc.
- By the immunomodulatory mechanisms of action of IVIG, which involves the whole innate and adaptive immune response in a synergistic and complex way (Imbach et al. 2010) and, therefore, remains unclear and often unexplained.
- By the health authorities, and the insurance providers who may disagree on covering the cost of this biological agent for certain indications.

4.4 Clinical Categorization of IVIG Indications of Autoimmune and Inflammatory Disorders

In the above respect, the following categorization of the various IVIG indications will be used:

- According to evidences, guidelines, and literature reviews/updates
- According to the need of individual indications due to efficacies; due to the failure of other treatments, which may induce secondary immunodeficiency or other unacceptable adverse effects or which may be contraindicated; due to comorbidities, or as an adjuvant to first-line treatment, etc.: For details: See Table 4.1
- Always keeping in mind that indications may change by development of new biological drugs (e.g., monoclonal antibodies) or by new recognition of the complex pathophysiology of the diverse diseases

The following categories are indicated prior to each below-mentioned indication (Suggestion to the reader; Copy table 4.1 for your convenience):

Table 4.1 Categories for the below mentioned indications

A a	Evidence due to controlled (randomized and/or blinded) trials and approved by authorities
A b	Guidelines/recommendations by experts/committees and reviews/updates (e.g. Cochrane, others)
A c	Association with primary/secondary immune deficiencies
B a	Efficacies in individual patients or cohorts with very rare diseases with any possibilities of reliable clinical studies
B b	Efficient alternative – to other treatments, – to few or no treatment alternatives, – to contraindications of drugs with adverse effects, – with drug sparing effects (e.g. corticosteroids, other immunosuppressives)
B c	Adjuvant treatment in combination with other drugs (e.g. corticosteroids, other immunosuppressive drugs, monoclonal antibodies)
B d	Failure of conventional/first line treatment (e.g. corticosteroid, other immunosuppressants, antiepileptics)
B e	High fatality of a disease
B f	Relevance of improvement of quality of life
C	Historical studies with some specific, efficient aspects, but insufficient evidence
D	Documentation of any efficacies

4.5 Hematology

4.5.1 *A, a** Immune Thrombocytopenia (ITP) (*See Table 4.1)

- IVIG prevents or fastly controls patients with bleedings.
- This disorder was the "door opener" for the immunomodulatory effects of IVIG (see Chap. 1 and Part III).

4.5.2 *A, a** Alloimmune Thrombocytopenia (*See Table 4.1)

1. **A, a** *Fetomaternal alloimmunization (*See Table 4.1)
   - Rare disease, high risk of intraventricular, fatal hemorrhages.
   - Maternal alloantibodies against platelet antigen HPA-1a (responsible for 80% of fetomaternal alloimmunization).
   - Recurrence rate during subsequent pregnancy is 79%.
   - Diagnosis: paternal genotype of HPA-1a involved in the preceding fetomaternal alloimmunization; when paternal heterogeneity is present, maternal incompatibility must be analyzed by cell-free fetal DNA.
   - Treatment: no longer invasive fetal analyses (fetal blood sample) or treatment (intrauterine fetal platelet tr\ansfusions); complication rate is 11%.
   - 2 × 1 g IVIG/week to the mother, repetitions weekly, starting at the 20th week of gestation.

- Prognosis: 3% intracranial hemorrhage (retrospective result of $n = 839$, and 4% mortality of $n = 821$).

(Winkelhorst et al. 2017; Rayment et al. 2005, 2011)

2. **A, a**[*] Postnatal alloimmune thrombocytopenia ([*]See Table 4.1)
   - IVIG administrations in neonates until platelet counts remain <30 × 109/l.
3. **A, a**[*] Rhesus hemolytic anemia ([*]See Table 4.1)
   - Fetal Rhesus D+ red blood cells stimulate maternal anti-Rh D alloantibodies, which cross the placenta and destroy Rh D+ blood cells in the baby.
   - IVIG modifies the course of bilirubin incline and significantly reduces the number of exchange transfusions and decreases the risk of bilirubin encephalopathy.

(Rübo et al. 1992, see also Chap. 3 in this book.)

4. **B, a, c**[*] Posttransfusion purpura ([*]See Table 4.1)
   - Thrombocytopenia occurs 7–10 days after transfusion of platelet-containing blood products with positive platelet antigen 1 or anti-HLA class 1 to a patient with negative antigen 1 or anti-HLA class 1 antigen, which may cause life-threatening bleeding.
   - Treatment: HD IVIG, individually or together with IV corticosteroids, plasmapheresis, and/or rituximab.

(Mueller-Eckhardt and Kiefel 1988)

4.5.3 *B, a*[*] Pure Red Cell Anemia Associated with Chronic Parvovirus B19 Infection ([*]See Table 4.1)

- Rare, severe anemia (<7 g/l hemoglobin).
- Occurs often, but not always in immunocompromised patients (HIV infection, posttransplantation, primary immunodeficiency, hematologic malignancy).
- Treatment: HD IVIG, corticosteroid, cyclosporine A, rituximab (in patients with associated disease).
- Prognosis: response rate to first course of IVIG is 93%; relapse rate is 33.9% within 4.3 months.

(Crabol et al. 2013)

4.5.4 *B, a, e*[*] Thrombotic Thrombocytopenic Purpura (TTP) (*See Table 4.1)

- Rare microangiopathic coagulopathy, observed in patients with mutations of ADAMTS13 or with para-/postinfectious and immune dysregulated conditions.
- Prognosis may be fatal.
- Treatment: daily plasma exchange, HD IVIG, corticosteroids, rituximab, and immunosuppressive drugs.

(Moore et al. 2007)

4.5.5 *B, a, c*[*] Autoimmune Neutropenia (*See Table 4.1)

- Severe form: ANC <0.5 × 109/l.
- Pathogenesis: autoantibodies against neutrophils, spontaneous recovery possible.
- First-line treatment: G-CSF, GM-CSF.
- In patients with infection or immunodeficiency including patients after stem cell transplantation, HD IVIG as adjuvant treatment is effective.

(Marriotti et al. 2014) See comment in PubMed Commons below (Marriotti et al. 2014).

4.5.6 *B, a, d*[*] Autoimmune Hemolytic Anemia (AIHA) and Evans Syndrome (affecting 2–3 Hematopoietic Lineages) (*See Table 4.1)

- AIHA is a rare disease (1–3:100,000 people per year).
- Autoantibodies against red blood cells.
- Classified as warm (wAIHA), cold (CAD), or mixed/paroxysmal form depending on the thermal range of autoantibodies. It may be as secondary AIHA associated with other concomitant disorders such as infection, immunodeficiencies, lympho- or myeloproliferative disorder or cancer, and drugs.
- Evans syndrome (±35%) is an autoimmune destructive disorder of 2–3 hematologic lines (mostly erythrocytes and thrombocytes).
- Diagnosis is based on hemolysis, detectable by the direct antiglobulin test (DAT):
  - Warm AIHA (wAIHA) by anti-IgG antisera (Cd3) (rate 65–70%/).
  - Cold AIHA (CAD) by IgM autoantibodies/Cd3 agglutinating at 37 °C (rate 20–25%).

  - The third form binds IgG autoantibodies to erythrocytes in the cold, but not at 37 °C, named paroxysmal cold hemolysis due to Donath-Landsteiner antibodies (rate 1–3%).
- First-line treatments are corticosteroids, rituximab or other immunosuppressive drugs, splenectomy (in adults with severe wAIHA only), or plasma exchange:
  - CAD: avoidance of cold; if symptomatic (hemolysis), rituximab as monotherapy or in combination with fludarabine
  - Evans syndrome: IVIG, corticosteroids; when refractory, rituximab
- HD IVIG is frequently administered in children with wAIHA due to less adverse effects and benefits with or without immunosuppressants.
- Prognosis: 40–64% complete recovery, 30–40% chronic/relapsing forms, and 4% mortality in case series.

(Liebman and Weitz 2017)

4.5.7 *B, a, c** Acquired Hemophilia (*See Table 4.1)

- Rare autoimmune disorder with severe, life-threatening bleeding.
- Inhibitory autoantibodies against coagulation factor, mainly directed against FVIII.
- Occurs in postpartum patients, with connective tissue disease, with paraneoplastic syndrome, and drug and herbal related.
- Spontaneous recovery within 14 months is possible.
- Treatment:
  - Emergency: FVIII replacement or recombinant FVII administration; new: emicizumab activating FIX and FX with longer half-life (administration weekly)
  - Long-term treatment: immunosuppressive drugs; in refractory patient, HD IVIG or a combination of immunosuppressants and HD IVIG

(Mo and Bao 2017)

4.5.8 *B, a, c** Acquired Autoimmune Coagulation Factor Inhibitors and Acquired von Willebrand Syndrome (*See Table 4.1)

- Common hereditary form and rare acquired form, mainly associated with lympho- or myeloproliferative disorders with prolonged bleeding time.
- Deficiency of FVIII associated with hemostatic disorder or of von Willebrand factor (VWF).
- Diagnosis: low levels of VWF and FVIII due to specific or non-specific autoantibody forming immune complexes.
- Treatment for acute bleeding: desmopressin (DDAVP) and VWF/FVIII concentrate; when refractory, recombinant FVII.
- IVIG together with corticosteroids is effective in 70% of patients.

(Yamamoto 2007)

4.5.9 B, b, d* Antiphospholipid Syndrome (APS) (*See Table 4.1)

Different forms of primary APS:

a. Venous and arterial thrombosis
b. Recurrent spontaneous abortion
c. APS associated with other autoimmune disorders (e.g., SLE)
d. Catastrophic APS with widespread thrombotic disease (CAPS)

Pathogenesis:
- Activation of endothelial cells, monocytes, and platelets leads to procoagulation serum.
- Presence of antiphospholipid (aPL) antibodies , also named lupus anticoagulant, anticardiolipin antibodies, or beta2-glycoprotein-1.

- Diagnosis: in a. often mild thrombocytopenia, hemolytic anemia or skin alterations, heart valve disease, and nephropathy.
- Treatment: the results are controversial.
  a. **B, d*** Venous and arterial thrombosis: low-dose aspirin and low-molecular heparin; when refractory, HD IVIG (*See Table 4.1)
  b. **B, c, d*** Recurrent spontaneous abortion: low-dose aspirin, rituximab, eculizumab; adjuvant or in patients with refractory to conventional treatment, 1 g IVIG/kg and repetition every 2 weeks, eventually after apheresis (*See Table 4.1)
  c. **B, d*** APS associated with other autoimmune disorders: treatment as under a (*See Table 4.1).
  d. **B, c, d*** CAPS: triple therapy with anticoagulants, corticosteroids, plasma exchange, and/or HD IVIG and/or rituximab (*See Table 4.1)
- Women with systemic lupus erythematosus (SLE) and recurrent abortion may have higher rate of regular birth after HD IVIG than with corticosteroid or NSAIDs.

(Ata et al. 2011; Tenti et al. 2016; Asherson et al. 2003)

4.5.10 *B, a, c, d** Antineutrophil Cytoplasmic Autoimmune (ANCA) Disorders (*See Table 4.1)

- Granulomatosis with polyangiitis (Wegener), eosinophilic granulomatosis with polyangiitis (Churg-Strauss) and microscopic polyangiitis.
- Treatment: first line with immunosuppressives (corticosteroid, cyclophosphamide, methotrexate, azathioprine, or monoclonals (rituximab, infliximab)).
- HD IVIG as an adjuvant treatment in patients with refractory or relapsing ANCA disorders demonstrated beneficial response.

(Jayne et al. 1993; Levy et al. 1999; Crickx et al. 2016)

4.6 Vascular Diseases/Rheumatology

4.6.1 *A, a** Kawasaki Syndrome (KS) (*See Table 4.1)

- Acute infectious or postinfectious, vascular/endothelial condition, high fever, and with high levels of proinflammatory serum cytokines, leading to coronary aneurysm in about 25% of children in the absence of treatment.
- Incidence is variable worldwide; in North America circa 25:100,000 children <5 years of age per year, highest in Asia.
- Conjunctivitis, skin rash, strawberry tongue, erythema of oral and pharyngeal mucosa, and palmar and plantar erythema.
- One dose of 2 g IVIG/kg within the first 10 days together with aspirin (<80 mg/kg b.w.) reduces the frequency of coronary artery anomalies significantly (to under 10%). The addition of 2 mg/kg b.w. per day corticosteroids further reduced the complication rate (under 5%).
- In patients with persistent or recurrent fever, the risk of developing coronary abnormalities remains. Repetitions of the combined treatment (see above or, instead of corticosteroids, use infliximab) or HD methylprednisolone may be indicated.

4.6.2 *B, a** Henoch-Schönlein Purpura (*See Table 4.1)

- Vasculitis with purpura of the skin, sometimes with gastrointestinal, renal, and rarely cerebral hemorrhage.
- HD IVIG is effective in patients with bleeding.

4.6.3 *B, b, d, C** Juvenile Idiopathic Arthritis (JIA) (*See Table 4.1)

- JIA is a clinically heterogeneous, common chronic rheumatic disease (see below).
- Children with no sufficient response to classic treatment (nonsteroidal anti-inflammatory drugs (NSAIDs), glucocorticosteroids, methotrexate) may be considered for treatment with HD IVIG.
- IVIG may serve as a corticosteroid-sparing option, when adverse effects are disturbing.
- Monoclonal antibody treatment is a new line: etanercept, infliximab, adalimumab, tocilizumab, rituximab.

4.6.4 *B, a, b, c, d** Systemic Juvenile Chronic Arthritis (Still's Syndrome) (*See Table 4.1)

- Vasculitis with fever, skin lesions, and arthritis.
- In severe disorders associated with HLA-DR4.
- Laboratory: CRP high, hemoglobin low, and ANA not increased.

- HD IVIG is effective in 50%, but often transient—spontaneous recovery possible/remission; in patients with severe, long-term disease, IVIG leads to more adequate results than immunosuppressive treatments.

4.6.5 B, a* Felty Syndrome (*See Table 4.1)

- Variant of rheumatoid arthritis.
- Systemic inflammatory process with splenomegaly, neutropenia, occasionally lymphadenopathy and hepatomegaly.
- HD IVIG is effective in individual patient.

(Breedveld et al. 1985)

4.6.6 B, a, e* Macrophage Activation Syndrome (*See Table 4.1)

- Severe, life-threatening variant of JLA, of SLE, of postviral infection, or after medication or toxin exposure.
- HD IVIG may be effective, especially in early disease states.

(Stephan et al. 2001; Boom et al. 2015)

4.6.7 B, a, d* Polyarteritis Nodosa (PAN) (*See Table 4.1)

- Vasculitis of the medium and large arterioles (not capillaries as in SLE).
- Treatment: first line with immunosuppressives (corticosteroid, cyclophosphamide, or monoclonals (rituximab, infliximab)).
- HD IVIG demonstrated responses in reports.

(Asano et al. 2006; Breda et al. 2016).

4.6.8 *B, a, b, c, d, f** Systemic Lupus Erythematosus (SLE) (*See Table 4.1)

- SLE is a systemic autoimmune connective tissue disease with various presentations and diverse clinical courses and prognosis.
- Standardization of treatment is difficult, and controlled studies with homogeneous cohort groups are not feasible.
- Different expert groups published recommendations (EULAR, ERA-EDTA, ACR).
- First-line therapeutics are hydroxychloroquine, corticosteroids, belimumab, and aspirin.
- In patients with severe disease: cyclophosphamide, mycophenolate mofetil, and azathioprine.

- HD IVIG or rituximab has been effective in individual, organ-specific disorders such as SLE-associated nephritis, myocarditis, polyradiculopathy, bone marrow suppression, and multi-organ disease.
- HD IVIG treatment of general SLE resulted in transient improvement of 65% of patients, in some responding patients after 6 monthly courses only.
- HD IVIG mainly remains an adjuvant treatment, a steroid sparing, and an option for patients who are refractory to conventional treatments or in patients with contraindication for conventional treatment.
- HD IVIG may cause prothrombotic effects in SLE, especially in SLE with neurologic involvement.

(Sakthiswary and D'Cruz 2014)

4.6.9 D* Carditis in Rheumatic Fever (*See Table 4.1)

- IVIG did not show effects in prevention of cardiac sequelae of acute rheumatic fever.

(Voss et al. 2001)

4.7 Infection-Related Diseases

4.7.1 *A, c, C** Secondary Infections in HIV Infection of Children with B- and/or T-Cell Deficiencies Despite Taking Highly Active Antiretroviral Treatment (HAART) or Not Taking HAART (*See Table 4.1)

- IVIG as adjuvant treatment was effective for reducing the rates of lethality, see also Chap. 3.12.3.

(Deener et al. 2008)

4.7.2 *B, c** Bacterial Sepsis, Septic Shock, and Streptococcal Toxic Shock (*See Table 4.1)

- IVIG as adjuvant treatment was effective for reducing the rates of lethality; however, the result is controversial, especially in:
  - Neonatal sepsis, suspected bacterial or fungal infection in neonates
  - Group B streptococcal disease in newborn
  - Invasive streptococcal syndrome
  - Postoperative sepsis
  - Trauma-associated sepsis

- Streptococcal toxic shock: evaluations from large controlled IVIG studies of streptococcal shock as an adjuvant treatment for children and adults (exception: newborns; see below) demonstrated divergent results with respect to lethality.
- IVIG preventive treatment of sepsis of neonates is no longer recommended.

(Alejandria et al. 2002; Crowley and Gropper 2016; Di Rosa et al. 2014; Sallam et al. 2016)

4.7.3 *B, a, b** Pediatric Autoimmune Neuropsychiatric Disorder Associated with Streptococcal Infection (PANDAS) (*See Table 4.1)

- Streptococcal infections may lead to behaviors of obsessive-compulsive tic disturbances.
- IVIG was successful in a case-controlled study; there is an ongoing study.

(Williams et al. 2016)

4.7.4 *B, c, f** Parvovirus B19-Associated Chronic Fatigue (*See Table 4.1)

- The prevalence of B19 infections is high in the general population and in patients with autoimmune disorders.
- IVIG or SCIG may decrease viremia and proinflammatory cytokine levels and improve chronic fatigue syndrome.

(Kerr et al. 2003; McGhee et al. 2005)

4.8 Neurology (See Also Chap. 8)

Overview: Ref. Lünemann et al. (2015)

4.8.1 A, a* Guillain-Barré Syndrome (GBS) (*See Table 4.1)

- Pathogenesis: mostly postinfectious (systemic CMV infection, gastroenteritis by *Campylobacter jejuni*) polyneuroradiculitis with antibodies cross-reacting with ganglioside antigen activating complement and causing demyelination of peripheral nerves.
- Clinical diagnosis: ascending acute progressive motor weakness, often starting in the lower extremities, autonomic nerve dysfunction (diaphragmatic muscles with lung dysfunction resulting in mechanical ventilation), and bulbar and facial muscle dysfunction, the latter with inability to walk.

- GBS variants are the acute axonal motor or motor sensory form (Miller Fisher syndrome) and the acute dysautonomia form.
- Treatment: IVIG (0.4 g/kg b.w./day × 3–5) and/or corticosteroids or plasma exchange depending on the grade of severity of the progression.

(Hughes et al. 2007, 2014; van Koningsveld et al. 2004; van Doorn et al. 2010)

4.8.2 *A, a** Chronic Inflammatory Demyelinating Polyneuropathy (CIDP) (*See Table 4.1)

- Most common autoimmune peripheral neuropathy.
- Pathogenesis: immunological progressive destruction of the myelin sheaths of peripheral nerves.
- Any target antigen is detectable, electrophysiological signs of demyelination with conduction block.
- Clinical diagnosis: slow onset of symmetrical weakness of muscles with areflexia and sensory loss, progressive over months.
- Treatment: IVIG or SCIG 16 (2 g/kg within 5 days) with repetitions (1 g/kg) every 3 weeks improves disabilities within 2–6 weeks and increases quality of life; response rate of 60% is not only transient but also long-term improvement with strong impacts of quality of life.
- Alternative treatments are plasma exchange and/or high-dose methylprednisolone.

(Dalakas et al. 2011; Dalakas et al. 2015; Berger et al. 2008; Eftimov et al. 2009; Hughes et al. 2008)

4.8.3 *A, a** Multifocal Motor Neuropathy (MMN) (*See Table 4.1)

- Pathogenesis: chronic progressive inflammatory disease asymmetrically affecting the motor nerves.
- The weaknesses mainly occur at radial, ulnar, and common peroneal muscle nerves.
- Treatment: IVIG or SCIG (0.4 g/kg/day × 5) with 60–80% improvements of muscle strength and scores.
- An alternative is subcutaneous IgG (SCIG) administration, which had the same efficacy as IVIG in a small treatment study.
- IV/SCIG repetitions with 1–2 g/kg, if unsatisfactory or unsustained response.
- In contrast to GBS and CIDP, corticosteroids and plasma exchange are not effective in MMN.

(Hahn et al. 2013; Leger et al. 2001; Harbo et al. 2010)

4.8.4 *B, a, b, d, f*[*] **Myasthenia Gravis** ([*]See Table 4.1)

- Pathogenesis: neuromuscular junction deficiency of stimulation of muscles resulting in muscle weakness including occasionally bulbar or respiratory failure.
- Associated with antibodies against the acetylcholine receptor or against muscle-specific kinase.
- Two patterns of clinical manifestation: early onset without thymoma, mostly in women, and late onset with thymoma.
- Clinical symptoms: asymmetric ptosis, diplopia; less common, oropharyngeal and limb weakness.
- Treatment: individual approach.
- First line: cholinesterase inhibitors.
- Among corticosteroids and plasma exchange, HD IVIG had equal or higher response rates of decrease in acetylcholine receptor antibodies and clinical efficacies 6 weeks after IVIG administration.
- The tolerance of IVIG is higher, adverse effects are lower, and IVIG has steroid-sparing effects.
- Efficacy of IVIG has been demonstrated in juvenile myasthenia and myasthenic exacerbations.
- IVIG is indicated in preparation of thymectomy.

(Alabdali et al. 2014; Wolfe et al. 2002; Gajdos et al. 2012)

4.8.5 *B, a*[*] **Lambert-Eaton Myasthenic Syndrome (LEMS)** ([*]See Table 4.1)

- Rare disease of neuromuscular, presynaptic signal transmission in patients with autoantibodies against the presynaptic calcium channel at the motor end plates.
- Also observed as paraneoplastic conditions, mainly in patients with small-cell lung cancer.
- Symptoms: proximal muscle weakness, with low tendon reflexes.
- HD IVIG showed transient efficacies (clinical, antibody level, and in nerve stimulation) within 2–4 weeks. It is an alternative therapy for immunosuppressive treatments with less adverse effects (see above).

(Skeie et al. 2010)

4.8.6 *B, a*[*] **Dermatomyositis** ([*]See Table 4.1)

Dermatomyositis is described in Sect. 4.9.1.

4.8.7 *B, a, d, f*[*] **Multiple Sclerosis (MS)** ([*]See Table 4.1)

- Clinical manifestation (wide variety): optic neuritis, dizziness, bladder dysfunction, sensory impairment.

- Treatment is complex with individualized approach; corticosteroids and/or beta-interferon still are the first-line treatment.
- In some early studies, long-term administration of 0.2–2 g IVIG/kg b.w. monthly reduced the relapse rate, the disability scores, the rate of progress/deterioration, and the number and volume of detected lesions by MRI; later on, controlled studies showed any significant improvement within IVIG in remitting-relapsing and progressive MS.
- IVIG is recommended as a second-line treatment along with beta-interferon and/or corticosteroids.
- IVIG treatment in patients with early stages of MS and pregnant women with MS showed less relapses.
- In patients with severe progressive or refractory MS, rituximab may be considered.
- New immunomodulators such as monoclonal antibodies (alemtuzumab, natalizumab) and drugs will define the role of IVIG

(Sorensen et al. 2002; Fazekas et al. 2008).

4.8.8 *B, a, d, f** Neuromyelitis Optica (*See Table 4.1)

- Central nervous inflammatory, demyelinating disease with autoantibodies against components of astrocytes (aquaporin-4).
- IVIG as first- or second-line long-term treatment (similar as in multiple sclerosis) decreases the rates of relapses and the progression of disabilities.

(Magraner et al. 2013)

4.8.9 *B, a, d, e, f** Intractable Epilepsy in Children and Refractory Pediatric Epilepsy (*See Table 4.1)

- Lennox-Gastaut syndrome, West syndrome, and myoclonic encephalopathy are the classic examples in children with imbalanced immune responses.
- HD IVIG reduced the frequency of seizures.
- Children with refractory epilepsy and low quality of life profit from a treatment with IVIG.

(Billiau et al. 2007)

4.8.10 *B, a, d, f** Rasmussen Syndrome (*See Table 4.1)

- Characterized by focal seizures, progressive neurological and intellectual deterioration, chronic encephalitis, and hemispheric atrophy.

- HD IVIG reduces seizures, but not the progression of the disease, compared with HD corticosteroids in children and adults.

(Hart et al. 1994)

4.8.11 *B, a, c, e, f** Neuroimmunological Conditions, Disorders with Autoantibodies Against Nervous Tissues/Receptors/Other Antigens (*See Table 4.1)

- Examples are acute disseminated encephalomyelitis, autoimmune encephalitis, demyelinating brain stem encephalitis, subacute rhombencephalitis optica, opsoclonus-myoclonus syndrome.
- Besides immunosuppressive treatment in patients with one of the treatment mentioned above, rare diseases associated with autoantibodies IVIG may justify a trial for severe or treatment refractory, for individual patients.
- Even small controlled studies are not feasible in those conditions.

(Nosadini et al. 2015)

4.8.12 *C* D* Polyneuropathy Associated with Monoclonal IgM Gammapathy (*See Table 4.1)

- Inclusion myopathy, idiopathic neuropathies, brachial plexopathy, diabetic amyotrophy, adrenoleukodystrophy, autism without primary immunodeficiency.
- These disorders didn't show evidence of improvement after IVIG administration.

4.8.13 *B, a, f** Stiff Person Syndrome (SPS) (*See Table 4.1)

- Stiff person syndrome is characterized by muscle rigidity and spasms and with high anti-glutamic acid decarboxylase antibodies.
- Patients may benefit from IVIG administration resulting in reduced stiffness and daily activities as well as improved quality of life.

(Dalakas et al. 2005)

4.8.14 *B a (A c)** Chronic Fatigue Syndrome Associated with Immune Dysfunctions (*See Table 4.1)

- Case and anecdotal reports of patients with disorders associated with immune dysfunctions (e.g., ITP) may profit from IVIG administration.

(Twisk et al. 2014)

4.8.15 *C D** Alzheimer's Disease (*See Table 4.1)

- The studies on IVIG in Alzheimer's disease are controversial.
- The clinical disease assessment Scale-Cognition demonstrated reversal of disease progression, decreased beta-amyloid peptide levels in the cerebrospinal fluid, and improved cognitive function.
- Another controlled study did not support the efficiency of IVIG.

(Dodel et al. 2013; Relkin et al. 2017)

4.9 Dermatology

Overview: Enk et al. 2017

4.9.1 *A, b, B, b** Dermatomyositis (*See Table 4.1)

- Rare, heterogenous conditions of mostly acquired inflammatory muscle diseases classified as:
  - Dermatomyositis (DM)
  - Polymyositis (PM)
  - Necrotizing myositis (NM)
  - Inclusion body myositis (IBM) (category **C**)
  - Overlapping disorder with SLE, Sjögren's syndrome, rheumatic arthritis (RA), systematic vasculitis
- Incidence: DM 2–9/1 Mio. population/year, IBM 4.5–9.5/1 Mio. population/year increasing to over 35/1 Mio. in over 50-year-old persons.
- Pathogenesis: T-cell-mediated autoimmunity and antibody-mediated effector mechanisms with endomysial capillary destruction.
- Symptoms:
  - Cutaneous: rash on the face and extremities (DM), periorbital edema, dystrophic nails, alterations of hairy scalp.
  - Cutaneous manifestations are variable, also present without muscle involvement = amyopathic DM (3–20%).
  - Muscles: symmetrical proximal muscle weakness; also pharyngeal, respiratory, cardiac, and neck muscles may be affected (pulmonary function test!).
  - Thirty percent of adults with DM are associated with malignancy.
- Laboratory/radiologic diagnosis: high creatine kinase (CK), CRP, and muscle aldolase and low serum complement (by consumption), EMG, muscle biopsy, and MRI.
- Different myositis-specific antibodies can be detected (not yet part of routine diagnosis).
- Treatment:
  - First line: Corticosteroids.
  - Adjuvant: azathioprine in adults, methotrexate in children.

  - In patients with fulminant progressive disease, with refractory/insufficient response, HD IVIG courses every 1–2 months.
  - In responders to IVIG, maintenance therapy for 1–3 years.
  - In some patients antimalaria agents (hydrochloroquine) in combination with the conventional regimen may be indicated.
  - HD IVIG led to significant improvement in muscle strength within 3 months, occasionally in combination with rituximab, and with corticosteroid-sparing effects, especially in children.
  - HD IVIG is used in patients who are unresponsive to conventional treatment or to avoid side effects.
  - In the future, subcutaneous IG (SCIG) with smaller doses/week is feasible, effective, and safe.
  - Cutaneous manifestation: in addition to systematic treatment, topical corticosteroids and ultraviolet light.
  - Long-term management with physical exercise.
- Prognosis: remission in 40%, partial remission in 43%, and exacerbation in 17%.
- In patient with IBM, IVIG and corticosteroids are ineffective.

(Dalakas 1995, 2015; Dalakas et al. 1993; Sunderkötter et al. 2016; Cherin et al. 2016)

4.9.2 *A, a, B, f (C)** Dermatologic Mucocutaneous Autoimmune Disorders (*See Table 4.1)

- Pemphigus vulgaris, pemphigus foliaceus, mucous membrane pemphigoid, and epidermolysis bullosa (blistering skin diseases).
- Mucocutaneous bullous conditions in which intraepidermal or subepidermal layers of the skin are separated due to antibodies against intracellular adhesion molecules, such as desmoglein.
- Chronic, relapsing-remitting autoantibody-mediated skin lesions with life-threatening complications.
- Treatment: IVIG as a parallel adjuvant treatment of immunosuppressive therapies (corticosteroid, azathioprine, mycophenolate mofetil, rituximab).
- Dosage and duration of IVIG administration: 2 g/kg b.w. in 2–5 doses initially and then monthly for a period of 6 months. If efficacious the interval of administration may be increased to 5–6 weeks. In parallel, the dosage of concomitant immunosuppressants (corticosteroid, cyclophosphamide, azathioprine, and others) can often be reduced.
- IVIG as a second line treatment in patients with relapsing disease or refractory to other first-line treatments.
- Regular intervals without IVIG should be attempted. And after 6 months washout period of responders should be considered.
- IVIG as first-line treatment with low or any immunosuppressants should be considered during pregnancy, in infants, and adolescents, if immunosuppressive treatment is contraindicated or in disorders with immunodeficiencies.

(Enk et al. 2017)

4.9.3 *B, a, c, d, e** Stevens-Johnson Syndrome and Toxic Epidermolysis (*See Table 4.1)

- Severe, occasionally fatal disorder associated with Fas (CD95) apoptosis.
- Early administration of HD IVIG (together with corticosteroids) is effective with no further progression and reduction of lethality.

(Viard et al. 1998; Huang et al. 2012)

4.9.4 *B, a, e, f** Photodermatosis/Solar Urticaria (*See Table 4.1)

- This rare skin disorder showed recovery with IVIG after 3–6 courses of 0.4 g/kg b.w.

(Adamski et al. 2011)

4.9.5 *B, a, d** Scleromyxedema and Variants: Systemic Sclerosis/Scleroderma with Skin Involvement, Linear Scleroderma, Morphea, Mixed Connective Tissue Disease, Sjögren's Syndrome (*See Table 4.1)

- Scleromyxedema is a severe condition characterized by fibroblast proliferation and mucin deposition in the skin and organs, often associated with monoclonal gammopathy.
- Symptoms: thickening of the skin with debilitating alterations.
- Treatment: often refractory to immunosuppressive treatment.
- HD IVIG is often the treatment of choice in severe, refractory situations, over a period of months in responding patients.

(Bidier et al. 2012; Jolles and Hughes 2006)

4.9.6 *B, a** Chronic Urticaria and Delayed Pressure Urticaria (*See Table 4.1)

- One third of patients with chronic urticaria have a related autoimmune process.
- HD IVIG may play a role in the aforementioned patients.

(Mitzel-Kaoukhov et al. 2010)

4.9.7 *B, b, c, d, f** Atopic Dermatitis (AD) (*See Table 4.1)

- In children and infants with severe, refractory to first-line treatment of AD, HD IVIG (2 g/kg b.w./4 weeks) for 3–6 months showed significant clinical improvement, decreases of eosinophils and serum IgE after 3 months, and remissions at 6 months.
- Children with severe, refractory AD and recurrent *Staphylococcus aureus* or herpes simplex superinfection had partial or complete remissions within 6–>12 months after HD IVIG treatment (dosage similar as mentioned above).
- Adults with severe atopic dermatitis show less dramatic results as reported in children (see above).

(Jee et al. 2011)

4.10 Organ-Specific Diseases

4.10.1 *A, c** Cystic Fibrosis (*See Table 4.1)

- No evidence of IVIG indication in controlled studies of patient with cystic fibrosis without immunodeficiencies

(Winnie et al. 1989; Balfour-Lynn et al. 2004; Smyth 2004)

4.10.2 *A, c** Asthma (*See Table 4.1)

- IVIG may be indicated as an adjuvant replacement treatment in immunodeficient patients with asthma and with chronic inflammations and respiratory symptoms.

(Schwartz and Berger 2002)

4.10.3 *A, c** CMV Pneumonitis (*See Table 4.1)

- IVIG or anti-CMV IVIG in combination with ganciclovir in relation to transplantation prolongs the survival of immunodeficient patients.

(Ljungman et al. 1992)

4.10.4 *B, a, b, d, f (A c)*[*] Solid Organ Transplantation ([*]See Table 4.1)

- Secondary immunodeficiency due to rituximab and other immunosuppressive regimens or due to antibody-mediated rejection of transplants are the rationale to administer IVIG.

(Burton et al. 2015)

4.10.5 *B, a, c*[*] Autoimmune Ophthalmopathy (Graves) ([*]See Table 4.1)

- Associated with hyperthyroiditis involving orbital tissues and autoantibodies.
- Main symptom: proptosis.
- Treatment: HD IVIG (6 courses, interval 3 weeks) versus corticosteroids demonstrated equal effects, but less adverse effects in the IVIG group.
- Recently, rituximab showed good responses in patients with severe disease.

(Kahaly et al. 1996)

4.10.6 *B, a, d, e, f*[*] Autoimmune Uveitis ([*]See Table 4.1)

- Inflammation of the vascular layers of the eye
- Ranges from visual impairment to blindness
- Treatment:
  - First line: corticosteroids or monoclonal.
  - In patients with refractory disease or with birdshot retinochorioidopathy, IVIG was successful in 50% of patients with visual improvement.

(Prete et al. 2016)

4.10.7 *B, a, b, d, e, f*[*] Autoimmune Liver Disease ([*]See Table 4.1)

- Pathology: chronic active autoimmune hepatitis with high serum liver enzymes, immune complexes, and periportal mononuclear infiltrates.
- HD IVIG improves the pathological findings with less adverse effects than with immunosuppressives (corticosteroids, rituximab).

(Vierling and Flores 2002)

4.10.8 *B, d*[*] Inflammatory Bowel Disease ([*]See Table 4.1)

- Inflammatory manifestation of the whole gastrointestinal tract of Crohn disease or of ulcerative colitis (lower colon).

- IVIG may be effective in immunosuppressiva refractory patients.

(Merkley et al. 2015)

4.10.9 *B, a, d, e, f** Acute Myocarditis (*See Table 4.1)

- HD IVIG improved cardiac function and decreased viral load in parvovirus B19-associated cardiomyopathy.

(Dennert et al. 2010)

4.10.10 *B, a, c** IgA Nephropathy (*See Table 4.1)

- A report of six patients demonstrated stabilization and delayed progression of loss of renal function after administration of IVIG.

(Rasche et al. 2006)

4.10.11 *B, a, b** Autoimmune Diabetes (*See Table 4.1)

A subgroup of patients with antibodies against islet cells responded to IVIG treatment with higher rates and longer duration of remission.

(Heinze 1996)

References

Adamski H, Bedane C, Bonnevalle A, Thomas P, Peyron JL, Rouchouse B, Cambazard F, Jeanmougin M, Viguier M. Solar urticaria treated with intravenous immunoglobulins. J Am Acad Dermatol. 2011;65(2):336–40.

Alabdali M, Barnett C, Katzberg H, Breiner A, Bril V. Intravenous immunoglobulin as treatment for myasthenia gravis: current evidence and outcomes. Expert Rev Clin Immunol. 2014;10(12):1659–65.

Alejandria MM, Lansang MA, Dans LF, Mantaring JB. Intravenous immunoglobulin for treating sepsis and septic shock. Cochrane Database Syst Rev. 2002;1:CD001090.

Alejandria MM, Lansang MA, Dans LF, Mantaring JB 3rd. Intravenous immunoglobulin for treating sepsis, severe sepsis and septic shock. Cochrane Database Syst Rev. 2013;9:CD001090. https://doi.org/10.1002/14651858.CD001090.pub2. Review.

Asano Y, Ihn H, Maekawa T, Kadono T, Tamaki K. High-dose intravenous immunoglobulin infusion in polyarteritis nodosa: report on one case and review of the literature. Clin Rheumatol. 2006;25(3):396–8.

Asherson RA, Cervera R, de Groot PG, Erkan D, Boffa MC, Piette JC, Khamashta MA, Shoenfeld Y, Catastrophic Antiphospholipid Syndrome Registry Project Group. Catastrophic antiphospholipid syndrome: international consensus statement on classification criteria and treatment guidelines. Lupus. 2003;12(7):530–4. Review.

Ata B, Tan SL, Shehata F, Holzer H, Buckett W. A systematic review of intravenous immunoglobulin for treatment of unexplained recurrent miscarriage. Fertil Steril. 2011;95(3):1080–5.e1-2. https://doi.org/10.1016/j.fertnstert.2010.12.021. Epub 2011 Jan 12. Review.
Balfour-Lynn IM, Mohan U, Bush A, Rosenthal M. Intravenous immunoglobulin for cystic fibrosis lung disease: a case series of 16 children. Arch Dis Child. 2004;89(4):315–9.
Berger M. Subcutaneous administration of IgG. Immunol Allergy Clin N Am. 2008;28(4): 779–802, viii.
Bidier M, Zschoche C, Gholam P, Enk AH, Hadaschik EN. Scleromyxoedema: clinical follow-up after successful treatment with high-dose immunoglobulins reveals different long-term outcomes. Acta Derm Venereol. 2012;92(4):408–9.
Billiau AD, Witters P, Ceulemans B, Kasran A, Wouters C, Lagae L. Intravenous immunoglobulins in refractory childhood-onset epilepsy: effects on seizure frequency, EEG activity, and cerebrospinal fluid cytokine profile. Epilepsia. 2007;48(9):1739–49. Epub 2007 May 23.
Boom V, Anton J, Lahdenne P, Quartier P, Ravelli A, Wulffraat NM, Vastert SJ. Evidence-based diagnosis and treatment of macrophage activation syndrome in systemic juvenile idiopathic arthritis. Pediatr Rheumatol. 2015;13:55. https://doi.org/10.1186/s12969-015-0055-3. Review.
Breda L, Franchini S, Marzetti V, Chiarelli F. Intravenous immunoglobulins for cutaneous polyarteritis nodosa resistant to conventional treatment. Scand J Rheumatol. 2016;45(2):169–70. https://doi.org/10.3109/03009742.2015.1092582. Epub 2015 Nov 3. No abstract available.
Breedveld FC, Brand A, van Aken WG. High dose intravenous gamma globulin for Felty's syndrome. J Rheumatol. 1985;12(4):700–2.
Burton SA, Amir N, Asbury A, Lange A, Hardinger KL. Treatment of antibody-mediated rejection in renal transplant patients: a clinical practice survey. Clin Transpl. 2015;29(2):118–23.
Cherin P, Belizna C, Cartry O, Lascu-Dubos G, de Jaeger C, Delain JC, Crave JC, Hachulla E. Long-term subcutaneous immunoglobulin use in inflammatory myopathies: a retrospective review of 19 cases. Autoimmun Rev. 2016;15(3):281–6. https://doi.org/10.1016/j.autrev.2015.12.003. Epub 2015 Dec 12. Review.
Cherqaoui B, Chausset A, Stephan JL, Merlin E. Intravenous immunoglobulins for severe gastrointestinal involvement in pediatric Henoch-Schönlein purpura: a French retrospective study. Arch Pediatr. 2016;23(6):584–90. https://doi.org/10.1016/j.arcped.2016.03.018. Epub 2016 Apr 26.
Crabol Y, Terrier B, Rozenberg F, Pestre V, Legendre C, Hermine O, Montagnier-Petrissans C, Guillevin L, Mouthon L, Groupe d'experts de l'Assistance Publique-Hôpitaux de Paris. Intravenous immunoglobulin therapy for pure red cell aplasia related to human parvovirus b19 infection: a retrospective study of 10 patients and review of the literature. Clin Infect Dis. 2013;56(7):968–77. https://doi.org/10.1093/cid/cis1046. Epub 2012 Dec 12. Review.
Crickx E, Machelart I, Lazaro E, Kahn JE, Cohen-Aubart F, Martin T, Mania A, Hatron PY, Hayem G, Blanchard-Delaunay C, de Moreuil C, Le Guenno G, Vandergheynst F, Maurier F, Crestani B, Dhote R, Silva NM, Ollivier Y, Mehdaoui A, Godeau B, Mariette X, Cadranel J, Cohen P, Puéchal X, Le Jeunne C, Mouthon L, Guillevin L, Terrier B, French Vasculitis Study Group. Intravenous immunoglobulin as an immunomodulating agent in antineutrophil cytoplasmic antibody-associated vasculitides: a French nationwide study of ninety-two patients. Arthritis Rheumatol. 2016;68(3):702–12. https://doi.org/10.1002/art.39472.
Crowley JC, Gropper MA. IV immunoglobulin: a useful tool for the severe pneumonia toolbox? Crit Care Med. 2016;44(1):250–1. https://doi.org/10.1097/CCM.0000000000001334. No abstract available.
Dalakas MC, Illa I, Dambrosia JM, Soueidan SA, Stein DP, Otero C, Dinsmore ST, McCrosky S. A controlled trial of high-dose intravenous immune globulin infusions as treatment for dermatomyositis. N Engl J Med. 1993;329(27):1993–2000.
Dalakas MC. Immunopathogenesis of inflammatory myopathies. Ann Neurol. 1995;37(Suppl 1):S74–86. Review.
Dalakas MC. The role of IVIg in the treatment of patients with stiff person syndrome and other neurological diseases associated with anti-GAD antibodies. J Neurol. 2005;252(Suppl 1):I19–25.
Dalakas MC, Medscape. Advances in the diagnosis, pathogenesis and treatment of CIDP. Nat Rev Neurol. 2011;7(9):507–17. https://doi.org/10.1038/nrneurol.2011.121. Review.
Dalakas MC. Inflammatory muscle diseases. N Engl J Med. 2015;372(18):1734–47. https://doi.org/10.1056/NEJMra1402225. Review. No abstract available.

Deener A, Mehra A, Bernstein L, Shliozberg J, Rubinstein A. Intravenous gammaglobulin treatment in HIV-1 infection. Immunol Allergy Clin N Am. 2008;28(4):851–9. https://doi.org/10.1016/j.iac.2008.06.001. Review.

Dennert R, Velthuis S, Schalla S, Eurlings L, van Suylen RJ, van Paassen P, Tervaert JW, Wolffs P, Goossens VJ, Bruggeman C, Waltenberger J, Crijns HJ, Heymans S. Intravenous immunoglobulin therapy for patients with idiopathic cardiomyopathy and endomyocardial biopsy-proven high PVB19 viral load. Antivir Ther. 2010;15(2):193–201.

Di Rosa R, Pietrosanti M, Luzi G, Salemi S, D'Amelio R. Polyclonal intravenous immunoglobulin: an important additional strategy in sepsis? Eur J Intern Med. 2014;25(6):511–6. https://doi.org/10.1016/j.ejim.2014.05.002. Epub 2014 May 27. Review.

Dodel R, Rominger A, Bartenstein P, Barkhof F, Blennow K, Förster S, Winter Y, Bach JP, Popp J, Alferink J, Wiltfang J, Buerger K, Otto M, Antuono P, Jacoby M, Richter R, Stevens J, Melamed I, Goldstein J, Haag S, Wietek S, Farlow M, Jessen F. Intravenous immunoglobulin for treatment of mild-to-moderate Alzheimer's disease: a phase 2, randomised, double-blind, placebo-controlled, dose-finding trial. Lancet Neurol. 2013;12(3):233–43.

Eftimov F, Winer JB, Vermeulen M, de Haan R, van Schaik IN. Intravenous immunoglobulin for chronic inflammatory demyelinating polyradiculoneuropathy. Cochrane Database Syst Rev. 2009;1:CD001797. https://doi.org/10.1002/14651858.CD001797.pub2. Review. Update in: Cochrane Database Syst Rev. 2013;12:CD001797.

Eleftheriou D, Brogan PA. Therapeutic advances in the treatment of vasculitis. Pediatr Rheumatol. 2016;14(1):26. https://doi.org/10.1186/s12969-016-0082-8. Review.

Enk A, Hadaschik E, Eming R, Fierlbeck G, French L, Girolomoni G, Hertl M, Jolles S, Karpati S, Steinbrink K, Stingl G, Volc-Platzer B, Zillikens D. European guidelines (S1) on the use of high-dose intravenous immunoglobulin in dermatology. J Dtsch Dermatol Ges. 2017;15(2):228–41. https://doi.org/10.1111/ddg.13013. Epub 2016 Dec 30.

Fagbemi AA, Torrente F, Hilson AJ, Thomson MA, Heuschkel RB, Murch SH. Massive gastrointestinal haemorrhage in isolated intestinal Henoch-Schonlein purpura with response to intravenous immunoglobulin infusion. Eur J Pediatr. 2007;166(9):915–9.

Fazekas F, Lublin FD, Li D, Freedman MS, Hartung HP, Rieckmann P, Sørensen PS, Maas-Enriquez M, Sommerauer B, Hanna K, PRIVIG Study Group; UBC MS/MRI Research Group. Intravenous immunoglobulin in relapsing-remitting multiple sclerosis: a dose-finding trial. Neurology. 2008;71(4):265–71. https://doi.org/10.1212/01.wnl.0000318281.98220.6f.

Gajdos P, Chevret S, Toyka KV. Intravenous immunoglobulin for myasthenia gravis. Cochrane Database Syst Rev. 2012;12:CD002277. https://doi.org/10.1002/14651858.CD002277.pub4. Review.

Hahn AF, Beydoun SR, Lawson V, IVIG in MMN Study Team, Oh M, Empson VG, Leibl H, Ngo LY, Gelmont D, Koski CL. A controlled trial of intravenous immunoglobulin in multifocal motor neuropathy. J Peripher Nerv Syst. 2013;18(4):321–30.

Harbo T, Andersen H, Jakobsen J. Long-term therapy with high doses of subcutaneous immunoglobulin in multifocal motor neuropathy. Neurology. 2010;75(15):1377–80.

Hart YM, Cortez M, Andermann F, Hwang P, Fish DR, Dulac O, Silver K, Fejerman N, Cross H, Sherwin A, et al. Medical treatment of Rasmussen's syndrome (chronic encephalitis and epilepsy): effect of high-dose steroids or immunoglobulins in 19 patients. Neurology. 1994;44(6):1030–6.

Heinze E. Immunoglobulins in children with autoimmune diabetes mellitus. Clin Exp Rheumatol. 1996;14(Suppl 15):S99–102. Review.

Huang YC, Li YC, Chen TJ. The efficacy of intravenous immunoglobulin for the treatment of toxic epidermal necrolysis: a systematic review and meta-analysis. Br J Dermatol. 2012;167(2):424–32. https://doi.org/10.1111/j.1365-2133.2012.10965.x. Review.

Hughes RA, Donofrio P, Bril V, Dalakas MC, Deng C, Hanna K, Hartung HP, Latov N, Merkies IS, van Doorn PA, ICE Study Group. Intravenous immune globulin (10% caprylate-chromatography purified) for the treatment of chronic inflammatory demyelinating polyradiculoneuropathy (ICE study): a randomised placebo-controlled trial. Lancet Neurol. 2008;7(2):136–44. https://doi.org/10.1016/S1474-4422(07)70329-0. Erratum in: Lancet Neurol. 2008 Sep;7(9):771.

Hughes RA, Swan AV, Raphaël JC, Annane D, van Koningsveld R, van Doorn PA. Immunotherapy for Guillain-Barré syndrome: a systematic review. Brain. 2007;130(Pt 9):2245–57.

Hughes RA, Swan AV, van Doorn PA. Intravenous immunoglobulin for Guillain-Barré syndrome. Cochrane Database Syst Rev. 2014;9:CD002063.

Imbach P, Lazarus AH, Kühne T. Intravenous immunoglobulins induce potentially synergistic immunomodulations in autoimmune disorders. Vox Sang. 2010;98(3 Pt 2):385–94. Review.

Jayne DR, Esnault VL, Lockwood CM. ANCA anti-idiotype antibodies and the treatment of systemic vasculitis with intravenous immunoglobulin. J Autoimmun. 1993;6(2):207–19. Review.

Jee SJ, Kim JH, Baek HS, Lee HB, Oh JW. Long-term efficacy of intravenous immunoglobulin therapy for moderate to severe childhood atopic dermatitis. Allergy Asthma Immunol Res. 2011;3(2):89–95.

Jolles S, Hughes J. Use of IGIV in the treatment of atopic dermatitis, urticaria, scleromyxedema, pyoderma gangrenosum, psoriasis, and pretibial myxedema. Int Immunopharmacol. 2006;6(4):579–91. Epub 2005 Dec 13. Review.

Kahaly G, Pitz S, Müller-Forell W, Hommel G. Randomized trial of intravenous immunoglobulins versus prednisolone in Graves' ophthalmopathy. Clin Exp Immunol. 1996;106(2):197–202.

Kerr JR, Cunniffe VS, Kelleher P, Bernstein RM, Bruce IN. Successful intravenous immunoglobulin therapy in 3 cases of parvovirus B19-associated chronic fatigue syndrome. Clin Infect Dis. 2003;36(9):e100–6.

Kobayashi T, Saji T, Otani T, Takeuchi K, Nakamura T, Arakawa H, Kato T, Hara T, Hamaoka K, Ogawa S, Miura M, Nomura Y, Fuse S, Ichida F, Seki M, Fukazawa R, Ogawa C, Furuno K, Tokunaga H, Takatsuki S, Hara S, Morikawa A, RAISE study group investigators. Efficacy of immunoglobulin plus prednisolone for prevention of coronary artery abnormalities in severe Kawasaki disease (RAISE study): a randomised, open-label, blinded-endpoints trial. Lancet. 2012;379(9826):1613–20.

Léger JM, Chassande B, Musset L, Meininger V, Bouche P, Baumann N. Intravenous immunoglobulin therapy in multifocal motor neuropathy: a double-blind, placebo-controlled study. Brain. 2001;124(Pt 1):145–53.

Levy Y, George J, Fabbrizzi F, Rotman P, Paz Y, Shoenfeld Y. Marked improvement of Churg-Strauss vasculitis with intravenous gammaglobulins. South Med J. 1999;92(4):412–4.

Liebman HA, Weitz IC. Autoimmune hemolytic anemia. Med Clin North Am. 2017;101(2):351–9. https://doi.org/10.1016/j.mcna.2016.09.007. Epub 2016 Dec 14. Review.

Ljungman P, Engelhard D, Link H, Biron P, Brandt L, Brunet S, Cordonnier C, Debusscher L, de Laurenzi A, Kolb HJ, et al. Treatment of interstitial pneumonitis due to cytomegalovirus with ganciclovir and intravenous immune globulin: experience of European Bone Marrow Transplant Group. Clin Infect Dis. 1992;14(4):831–5.

Lünemann JD, Nimmerjahn F, Dalakas MC. Intravenous immunoglobulin in neurology—mode of action and clinical efficacy. Nat Rev Neurol. 2015;11(2):80–9. https://doi.org/10.1038/nrneurol.2014.253. Epub 2015 Jan 6. Review.

Magraner MJ, Coret F, Casanova B. The effect of intravenous immunoglobulin on neuromyelitis optica. Neurologia. 2013;28(2):65–72. https://doi.org/10.1016/j.nrl.2012.03.014. Epub 2012 Jul 28. English, Spanish.

Mariotti J, Caberlon S, Bertinato E, Podda G, Pugliano MT, Cattaneo M. Primary autoimmune neutropenia in adults: case report and review of the literature. Transfusion. 2014;54(11):2906–10. https://doi.org/10.1111/trf.12711. Epub 2014 May 15. Review.

McCrindle BW, Rowley AH, Newburger JW, Burns JC, Bolger AF, Gewitz M, Baker AL, Jackson MA, Takahashi M, Shah PB, Kobayashi T, Wu MH, Saji TT, Pahl E, American Heart Association Rheumatic Fever, Endocarditis, and Kawasaki Disease Committee of the Council on Cardiovascular Disease in the Young; Council on Cardiovascular and Stroke Nursing; Council on Cardiovascular Surgery and Anesthesia; and Council on Epidemiology and Prevention. Diagnosis, treatment, and long-term management of Kawasaki disease: a scientific statement for health professionals from the American Heart Association. Circulation. 2017;135(17):e927–99. https://doi.org/10.1161/CIR.0000000000000484. Epub 2017 Mar 29. Review.

McGhee SA, Kaska B, Liebhaber M, Stiehm ER. Persistent parvovirus-associated chronic fatigue treated with high dose intravenous immunoglobulin. Pediatr Infect Dis J. 2005;24(3):272–4. Review.

Merkley SA, et al. Use of intravenous immunoglobulin for patients with inflammatory bowel disease with contraindications or who are unresponsive to conventional treatments. Inflamm Bowel Dis. 2015;21(8):1854–9.

Mitzel-Kaoukhov H, Staubach P, Müller-Brenne T. Effect of high-dose intravenous immunoglobulin treatment in therapy-resistant chronic spontaneous urticaria. Ann Allergy Asthma Immunol. 2010;104(3):253–8.

Mo L, Bao GC. Acquired factor VIII deficiency: two case reports and a review of literature. Exp Hematol Oncol. 2017;6:8. https://doi.org/10.1186/s40164-017-0068-3. eCollection 2017.

Moore JC, Arnold DM, Leber BF, Clare R, Molnar GJ, Kelton JG. Intravenous immunoglobulin as an adjunct to plasma exchange for the treatment of chronic thrombotic thrombocytopenic purpura. Vox Sang. 2007;93(2):173–5.

Mueller-Eckhardt C, Kiefel V. High-dose IgG for post-transfusion purpura-revisited. Blut. 1988;57(4):163–7. Review.

Newburger JW, Takahashi M, Beiser AS, Burns JC, Bastian J, Chung KJ, Colan SD, Duffy CE, Fulton DR, Glode MP, et al. A single intravenous infusion of gamma globulin as compared with four infusions in the treatment of acute Kawasaki syndrome. N Engl J Med. 1991;324(23):1633–9.

Nosadini M, Mohammad SS, Ramanathan S, Brilot F, Dale RC. Immune therapy in autoimmune encephalitis: a systematic review. Expert Rev Neurother. 2015;15(12):1391–419.

Perez EE, Orange JS, Bonilla F, Chinen J, Chinn IK, Dorsey M, El-Gamal Y, Harville TO, Hossny E, Mazer B, Nelson R, Secord E, Jordan SC, Stiehm ER, Vo AA, Ballow M. **Update** on the use of immunoglobulin in human disease: a review of evidence. J Allergy Clin Immunol. 2017;139(3S):S1–S46. https://doi.org/10.1016/j.jaci.2016.09.023. Epub 2016 Dec 29.

Prete M, Dammacco R, Fatone MC, Racanelli V. Autoimmune uveitis: clinical, pathogenetic, and therapeutic features. Clin Exp Med. 2016;16(2):125–36.

Rasche FM, Keller F, Lepper PM, Aymanns C, Karges W, Sailer LC, Müller LV, Czock D. High-dose intravenous immunoglobulin pulse therapy in patients with progressive immunoglobulin A nephropathy: a long-term follow-up. Clin Exp Immunol. 2006;146(1):47–53.

Rayment R, Brunskill SJ, Stanworth S, Soothill PW, Roberts DJ, Murphy MF. Antenatal interventions for fetomaternal alloimmune thrombocytopenia. Cochrane Database Syst Rev. 2005;1:CD004226. Review. Update in: Cochrane Database Syst Rev. 2011;(5):CD004226.

Relkin NR, Thomas RG, Rissman RA, Brewer JB, Rafii MS, van Dyck CH, Jack CR, Sano M, Knopman DS, Raman R, Szabo P, Gelmont DM, Fritsch S, Aisen PS, Alzheimer's Disease Cooperative Study. A phase 3 trial of IV immunoglobulin for Alzheimer disease. Neurology. 2017;88(18):1768–75. https://doi.org/10.1212/WNL.0000000000003904. Epub 2017 Apr 5.

Rübo J, Albrecht K, Lasch P, Laufkötter E, Leititis J, Marsan D, Niemeyer B, Roesler J, Roll C, Roth B, et al. High-dose intravenous immune globulin therapy for hyperbilirubinemia caused by Rh hemolytic disease. J Pediatr. 1992;121(1):93–7.

Sakthiswary R, D'Cruz D. Intravenous immunoglobulin in the therapeutic armamentarium of systemic lupus erythematosus: a systematic review and meta-analysis. Medicine (Baltimore). 2014;93(16):e86. https://doi.org/10.1097/MD.0000000000000086. Review.

Sallam MM, Abou-Aisha K, El-Azizi M. A novel combination approach of human polyclonal IVIG and antibiotics against multidrug-resistant Gram-positive bacteria. Infect Drug Resist. 2016;9:301–11. eCollection 2016.

Schwartz HJ, Berger M. Intravenous gamma-globulin therapy in bronchial asthma. Allergy Asthma Proc. 2002;23(1):15–8. Review.

Skeie GO, Apostolski S, Evoli A, Gilhus NE, Illa I, Harms L, Hilton-Jones D, Melms A, Verschuuren J, Horge HW, European Federation of Neurological Societies. Guidelines for treatment of autoimmune neuromuscular transmission disorders. Eur J Neurol. 2010;17(7):893–902.

Smyth RL. Intravenous immunoglobulin for cystic fibrosis lung disease. Arch Dis Child. 2004;89(4):298–9. No abstract available.

Sorensen PS, Fazekas F, Lee M. Intravenous immunoglobulin G for the treatment of relapsing-remitting multiple sclerosis: a meta-analysis. Eur J Neurol. 2002;9(6):557–63.

Stéphan JL, Koné-Paut I, Galambrun C, Mouy R, Bader-Meunier B, Prieur AM. Reactive haemophagocytic syndrome in children with inflammatory disorders. A retrospective study of 24 patients. Rheumatology (Oxford). 2001;40(11):1285–92.

Sunderkötter C, Nast A, Worm M, Dengler R, Dörner T, Ganter H, Hohlfeld R, Melms A, Melzer N, Rösler K, Schmidt J, Sinnreich M, Walter MC, Wanschitz J, Wiendl H. Guidelines on dermatomyositis—excerpt from the interdisciplinary S2k guidelines on myositis syndromes by the German Society of Neurology. J Dtsch Dermatol Ges. 2016;14(3):321–38. https://doi.org/10.1111/ddg.12909.

Tenti S, Cheleschi S, Guidelli GM, Galeazzi M, Fioravanti A. Intravenous immunoglobulins and antiphospholipid syndrome: how, when and why? A review of the literature. Autoimmun Rev. 2016;15(3):226–35. https://doi.org/10.1016/j.autrev.2015.11.009. Epub 2015 Dec 1. Review.

Twisk FN. The status of and future research into Myalgic encephalomyelitis and chronic fatigue syndrome: the need of accurate diagnosis, objective assessment, and acknowledging biological and clinical subgroups. Front Physiol. 2014;5:109.

van Doorn PA, Kuitwaard K, Walgaard C, van Koningsveld R, Ruts L, Jacobs BC. IVIG treatment and prognosis in Guillain-Barré syndrome. J Clin Immunol. 2010;30(Suppl 1):S74–8. https://doi.org/10.1007/s10875-010-9407-4. Review.

van Koningsveld R, Schmitz PI, Meché FG, Visser LH, Meulstee J, van Doorn PA, Dutch GBS study group. Effect of methylprednisolone when added to standard treatment with intravenous immunoglobulin for Guillain-Barré syndrome: randomised trial. Lancet. 2004;363(9404):192–6.

Viard I, Wehrli P, Bullani R, Schneider P, Holler N, Salomon D, Hunziker T, Saurat JH, Tschopp J, French LE. Inhibition of toxic epidermal necrolysis by blockade of CD95 with human intravenous immunoglobulin. Science. 1998;282(5388):490–3.

Vierling JM, Flores PA. Evolving new therapies of autoimmune hepatitis. Clin Liver Dis. 2002;6(3):825–50, ix. Review.

Voss LM, Wilson NJ, Neutze JM, Whitlock RM, Ameratunga RV, Cairns LM, Lennon DR. Intravenous immunoglobulin in acute rheumatic fever: a randomized controlled trial. Circulation. 2001;103(3):401–6.

Williams KA, Swedo SE, Farmer CA, Grantz H, Grant PJ, D'Souza P, Hommer R, Katsovich L, King RA, Leckman JF. Randomized, controlled trial of intravenous immunoglobulin for pediatric autoimmune neuropsychiatric disorders associated with streptococcal infections. J Am Acad Child Adolesc Psychiatry. 2016;55(10):860–867.e2. https://doi.org/10.1016/j.jaac.2016.06.017. Epub 2016 Aug 3.

Winkelhorst D, Murphy MF, Greinacher A, Shehata N, Bakchoul T, Massey E, Baker J, Lieberman L, Tanael S, Hume H, Arnold DM, Baidya S, Bertrand G, Bussel J, Kjaer M, Kaplan C, Kjeldsen-Kragh J, Oepkes D, Ryan G. Antenatal management in fetal and neonatal alloimmune thrombocytopenia: a systematic review. Blood. 2017;129(11):1538–47. https://doi.org/10.1182/blood-2016-10-739656. Epub 2017 Jan 27.

Winnie GB, Cowan RG, Wade NA. Intravenous immune globulin treatment of pulmonary exacerbations in cystic fibrosis. J Pediatr. 1989;114(2):309–14.

Wolfe GI, Barohn RJ, Foster BM, Jackson CE, Kissel JT, Day JW, Thornton CA, Nations SP, Bryan WW, Amato AA, Freimer ML, Parry GJ, Myasthenia Gravis-IVIG Study Group. Randomized, controlled trial of intravenous immunoglobulin in myasthenia gravis. Muscle Nerve. 2002;26(4):549–52.

Yamamoto K, Takamatsu J, Saito H. Intravenous immunoglobulin therapy for acquired coagulation inhibitors: a critical review. Int J Hematol. 2007;85(4):287–93. Review.

5 Anti-D: A Type of IVIg

Ramsha Khan and Alan H. Lazarus

5.1 Introduction

5.1.1 Anti-D as an IVIg

Rh immune globulin (anti-D) is a polyclonal IgG antibody directed against the Rhesus D (RhD) factor present on red blood cells (RBCs). It is a type of intravenous immunoglobulin (IVIg, which contains antibodies of the IgG isotype) isolated from the pooled plasma donated by two types of alloimmunized donors:

1. Rhesus D-negative (RhD−) male donors who have been intentionally immunized with RhD+ RBCs (Crow and Lazarus 2008; Semple 2010)
2. RhD− female donors who have been naturally immunized by Pregnancy with an RhD+ fetus (Semple 2010)

It is worth noting that although anti-D may be the desired antibody present in the preparation isolated from plasma, a variety of other antibodies will invariably also be included in the final solution, as will be discussed later (Crow and Lazarus 2008).

R. Khan, HBSc
Department of Laboratory Medicine and Pathobiology, Faculty of Medicine, University of Toronto, Toronto, ON, Canada

Keenan Research Centre of the Li Ka Shing Knowledge Institute at St. Michael's Hospital, Toronto, ON, Canada

A.H. Lazarus, PhD (✉)
Keenan Research Centre of the Li Ka Shing Knowledge Institute at St. Michael's Hospital, Toronto, ON, Canada

Centre for Innovation at The Canadian Blood Services, Ottawa, ON, Canada

Departments of Medicine and Laboratory Medicine & Pathobiology, Faculty of Medicine, University of Toronto, Toronto, ON, Canada
e-mail: LAZARUSA@smh.ca

P. Imbach (ed.), *Antibody Therapy*, https://doi.org/10.1007/978-3-319-68038-5_5

Being a donor-derived product, anti-D is available in limited quantities and carries a theoretical risk of transferring emerging pathogens and infectious diseases (Brinc and Lazarus 2009). Ethical concerns also stem from intentionally immunizing a large number of RhD− men (as only 15–20% are responders) with the RhD+ cells for the sole purpose of manufacturing anti-D.

5.1.2 Clinical Uses of Anti-D

Currently anti-D is used clinically to prevent hemolytic disease of the fetus and newborn (HDFN) and to treat immune thrombocytopenia (ITP) (Lazarus 2013; Semple 2010). It may also be used to clear RhD+ RBCs from the bloodstream when they have accidentally been transfused to RhD− individuals.

Hemolytic disease of the fetus and newborn (HDFN) occurs when alloimmunization causes the maternal immune system to destroy fetal RBCs expressing different, and thus, foreign, antigens when compared to the mother's RBCs (Hendrickson and Delaney 2016). The most predominant antigen causing HDFN is the D antigen (others include the Kell antigen and the Duffy antigen). RhD− mothers can be exposed to RhD+ RBCs, either through blood transfusions or from previous pregnancies with an RhD+ fetus (Hendrickson and Delaney 2016). Once the mother has been sensitized, subsequent pregnancies with an RhD+ fetus may be at risk of HDFN as the anti-D produced by the maternal immune system can potentially cross the placenta and destroy the fetal RBCs (Urbaniak and Greiss 2000). Currently, only prophylactic anti-D injections are able to prevent HDFN from occurring, and in many countries, the priority is to conserve it for HDFN prophylaxis instead of utilizing it to ameliorate ITP as discussed below (Lazarus 2013).

ITP is an autoimmune disorder characterized by low platelet levels primarily due to clearance mediated by platelet-reactive autoantibodies (Lazarus 2013). These antibodies are predominantly of the IgG1 and IgG3 isotypes although IgM and IgA subtypes may also be present (Semple 2010). In severe cases, ITP patients may experience lower energy levels and are at an increased risk of life-threatening bleeding. Some of the therapies for ITP include steroids, IVIg, and anti-D. First shown by Imbach et al. in 1981, high doses of IVIg are able to significantly raise platelet levels in ITP patients (Imbach et al. 1981). However the mechanism(s) through which IVIg is able to ameliorate ITP remains unclear even today. Anti-D is considered to be a first-line treatment for ITP and is able to ameliorate ITP at approximately 5-log fold lower dose than IVIg—50–75 ug/kg of anti-D is generally as effective as 1–2 g/kg of IVIg administered to ITP patients (Eghbali et al. 2016). Moreover, compared to other monoclonal antibodies that are used to modulate autoimmune diseases like ITP (such as anti-CD20; Rituximab), anti-D is administered at an approximately 2-log fold lower dose for a similar therapeutic response (Rosman et al. 2013; Nair and Jacob 2016). Nevertheless, like IVIg, the mechanism through which anti-D is able to ameliorate ITP also remains unclear. Research has proposed a few potential mechanisms which will be discussed later. If the first-line treatments are unsuccessful, other therapies involving anti-CD20, thrombopoietin, splenectomy and others may be considered (Semple 2010).

5.1.3 Black Box Warning on Anti-D Usage by the FDA

In 1995, the food and drug administration (FDA) granted approval for utilizing anti-D as a therapeutic for ITP patients. However in 2010 the FDA issued a black box warning for all anti-D products used in ITP. This mandated warning, to be printed on the package insert, is used to signify an increased risk of intravascular hemolysis associated with anti-D usage. It cautions about the increased risk of developing anemia, acute renal insufficiency, renal failure, disseminated intravascular coagulation (DIC), multisystem organ failure including acute respiratory distress syndrome (ARDS), and death. The warning also provides physicians with guidelines on how to proceed in the care of patients that had been injected with anti-D (FDA, 2009).

In response to the FDA-mandated warning, a working group was assembled at the instigation of Cangene bioPharma to evaluate the safety of anti-D. This panel of researchers, consisting of physicians and some scientists affiliated with the biotechnology industry, evaluated the safety data provided by Cangene and concluded that the safety profile of anti-D in ITP is not significantly different than that of other therapies, such as IVIg (Despotovic et al. 2012). The researchers also indicated that the adverse side effects can be prevented through careful selection of patients (e.g., excluding patients with predisposing conditions that may lead to an increased risk of DIC and ARDS) (Despotovic et al. 2012).

5.2 Potential Mechanisms of Action of Anti-D in ITP

The underlying mechanism(s) through which anti-D acts to ameliorate ITP remains unclear. Previous and ongoing work has allowed researchers to propose a number of mechanisms that may be at play—these include mononuclear phagocytic system (MPS) blockade, cytokine modulation, and the presence of anti-idiotype antibodies (Semple 2010; Crow and Lazarus 2008).

Much of the research related to mechanisms of anti-RBC antibodies in ITP has used mice as a model system. In the murine model of passive ITP, mice are injected with an antiplatelet antibody, such as MWReg30 which binds the glycoprotein IIb/IIIa (also known as αIIbβ3 or CD41/CD61) complex present on the surface of platelets and leads to the development of thrombocytopenia. However the D antigen on murine RBC is not immunogenic, and thus, other RBC antigens (and the corresponding antibodies) are used as surrogates to mimic the anti-D effect. One of the most common antibodies used in lieu of anti-D is TER-119. TER-119 binds the glycophorin-A (GPA)-associated protein on murine RBCs and has been shown previously to work successfully in murine models of ITP (Crow and Lazarus 2008; Deng and Balthasar 2007).

5.2.1 Mononuclear Phagocytic System (MPS) Blockade

The mononuclear phagocytic system (MPS) is a part of the immune system that includes macrophages. Macrophages are a major phagocytic cell population in the immune system and are found in most body tissues (Hume 2006). Macrophages express Fc receptors (FcRs) on their cell surface that bind the Fc portion of an antibody. These Fc receptors can be classified based on the type of antibody they bind—the most important ones for mediating phagocytosis of opsonized particles (such as RBCs and platelets) are the Fc-gamma receptors (FcγR) that bind IgG antibodies (Semple 2010). The human FcγR family includes several activating members (such as FcγRI, FcγRIIA, and FcγRIII) and an inhibitory member (FcγRIIB) that differ in their affinity to bind different molecular structures of IgG and in their ability to potentiate or inhibit immune responses (Bruhns and Jönsson 2015).

Salama et al. (1984) were the first to demonstrate the efficacy of anti-D in ameliorating ITP. Although the mechanism was not elucidated, they had postulated that anti-D was exerting its therapeutic effects through MPS blockade. The MPS blockage theory hypothesizes that since the RBCs are present in a much larger quantity than platelets, anti-D-opsonized RBCs competitively inhibit platelet phagocytosis by binding free FcγRs on macrophages, (Fig. 5.1) particularly those that are present in the spleen which is a primary site of MPS activity (Salama et al. 1983, 1984; Crow and Lazarus 2008). Over the years, MPS blockade was indirectly supported by various studies as the mechanism of action of anti-D in ITP (Becker et al. 1986; Bussel et al. 1991; Ware and Zimmerman 1998; Ambriz-Fernández et al. 2002). Evidence supporting this theory includes the therapeutic inefficacy of anti-D in ITP patients that are RhD− (Boughton 1991; Oksenhendler et al. 1988). However, of these RhD− patients, those who were positive for the Rh c antigen (on RBCs) did respond to anti-c therapy, and an increase in platelet counts was observed (Oksenhendler et al. 1988). This suggested that anti-RBC antibody (against the c, D, or presumably any other Rh antigen present on the surface of RBCs) sensitized red blood cells and blocked MPS consequently preventing platelet phagocytosis. More evidence supporting MPS blockade as the mechanism of action of anti-D stems from the observation that ITP patients who have previously had a splenectomy do not respond well to anti-D therapy (Bussel et al. 1991); however it has also been found that two splenectomized ITP patients did in fact respond to anti-D therapy (Ramadan and El-Agnaf 2005). Thus, more work is required to clearly determine whether or not anti-D functions (at least partially) through MPS blockade and how the presence and absence of a spleen affects that function.

5.2.2 FcγRs

As indicated previously, macrophages can bind antibodies through FcγRs expressed on the cell surface. These receptors may be involved in activating phagocytosis, such as FcγRIIIA, or inhibiting it, such as FcγRIIB. To our knowledge, no reports have actually observed macrophage FcγR-mediated phagocytosis of anti-D-opsonized RBCs. However much work has been done regarding the role of FcγRs in murine models of ITP using surrogate antibodies (such as TER-119).

It was recently shown that the Fc portion of the anti-RBC antibody TER-119 is required for ITP amelioration in a murine model (Yu et al. 2015). The results show that although the $F(ab')_2$ region of TER-119 alone is able to bind to the RBCs, it is unable to mediate phagocytosis. The $F(ab')_2$ region of TER-119 was unable to increase platelet levels in an ITP model or cause significant anemia. The same results were observed for TER-119 with a deglycosylated Fc region (Yu et al. 2015) demonstrating that both the Fc domain of TER-119 and Fc glycosylation are required for ITP amelioration and for inducing anemia. On the other hand, an earlier study done with TER-119 but with a murine model of autoimmune hemolytic anemia (AHA) lacking FcRr chains (the signaling component of activating FcrRs in mice) chains had concluded that FcγR-mediated mechanisms are not required by TER-119 to cause anemia (Chen et al. 2014). These seemingly differing results indicate that TER-119 may be inducing anemia through multiple different mechanisms in ITP and AHA and that in the ITP model, the native glycosylated Fc domains of the antibody are essential for disease amelioration.

The above results indicated that at least in murine passive ITP, FcγR binding is required for amelioration. Earlier work had attempted to determine which FcγRs might be involved. In 2005 Song et al. established a correlational relationship between anti-RBC antibody-mediated increase in platelet levels and the downregulation of FcγRIIIA on splenic macrophages in a murine model of ITP (Song et al. 2005). FcγRIIIA is an activating receptor found on the surface of macrophages, and based on the results of this study, it is likely that these anti-RBC antibodies modulate, inactivate, or neutralize FcγRIIIA or the FcγRIIIA pathway (Lazarus 2013). This, in turn, suggests that inhibition of MPS is, at the very least, a partial contributor to the mechanism of action of the anti-RBC antibodies used.

It was also shown that anti-RBC antibodies are able to ameliorate ITP in mice lacking FcγRIIB (Song et al. 2005). FcγRIIB is considered to be an inhibitory receptor present on macrophages, and when activated, it has been suggested to downregulate the phagocytic activity of the macrophage. Later research performed by Yu et al. in 2015 again found that TER-119 was able to ameliorate ITP in mice lacking inhibitory this receptor ($Fc\gamma RIIb^{-/-}$) indicating that these receptors are not required by the anti-RBC antibodies used to perform their function in ITP (Yu et al. 2015).

The research thus far had shown anti-RBC antibodies might be dependent on FcγR-mediated mechanisms to ameliorate ITP (e.g., by neutralizing FcγRIIIA function) and that the inhibitory receptor FcγRIIB was probably not an essential component of this mechanism. Building on this, further work showed that mice treated with the Fab region of a monoclonal antibody 2.4G2, an inhibitor of both FcγRIIB and FcγRIIIA, and with antiplatelet antibody (to induce ITP) developed a similar degree of anemia as the control group when treated with TER-119. This indicated that these receptors might not be required by the TER-119 anti-RBC antibody to cause anemia—however in vitro assays showed partial inhibition of RBC phagocytosis by RAW264.7 macrophages treated with 2.4G2. Combining this with the earlier results, at least two possibilities emerge:

1. That the anemia-inducing effects of an anti-RBC antibody may not be necessary for ameliorating ITP
2. That the in vivo vs in vitro role of FcγRs related to anti-RBC-mediated effects differs (Yu et al. 2015).

Taken together, some potential concepts advanced by the various studies include:

1. That IgG Fc domains and IgG Fc glycosylation of anti-RBC antibodies may be required for murine ITP amelioration
2. That anti-RBC antibodies may potentially interact with multiple FcγRs to initiate their ameliorative effects
3. That FcγRIIB expression is not required by anti-RBC antibodies to ameliorate murine ITP
4. That anti-RBC antibodies may modulate or inactivate the FcγRIIIA pathway

5.2.3 Cytokine Modulation

Numerous groups have documented the ability of anti-D to induce cytokine modulation. In 1994, Davenport et al. demonstrated in in vitro experiments that anti-D-opsonized red blood cells stimulated peripheral blood mononuclear cells (PBMCs) to secrete interleukin-1 receptor antagonist (IL-1Ra) (Davenport et al. 1994). IL-1Ra is structurally similar to IL-1 and can bind its receptor with equal affinity but is unable to induce signal transduction—thus IL-1Ra acts as a competitive inhibitor of IL-1 (Dripps et al. 1991).

Semple et al. followed up on this observation with a study in children with chronic ITP and demonstrated that along with IL-1Ra, several other pro- and anti-inflammatory cytokines and chemokines were present at increased levels. These included IL-6, GM-CSF, MCP-1α, TNF-α, and MCP-1 (Semple et al. 2002). Notably, IL-1Ra levels in serum were approximately 60-fold higher than baseline within 3 h of anti-D administration but returned to baseline by day 8 (along with the other cytokines and chemokines that were also observed to be elevated).

The researchers further went on to show that early increases in IL-1Ra levels were correlated with decreased platelet phagocytosis. An in vitro assay demonstrated that IL-1Ra directly inhibited the phagocytosis of anti-D-sensitized RBC by monocytes and granulocytes (Coopamah et al. 2003). However Crow et al. (2007) demonstrated in a murine model that while TER-119 was able to increase IL-1Ra levels, it was also able to ameliorate ITP in mice lacking the IL-1R receptor, the receptor for IL-1 and IL-1Ra. This indicated that at least in mice, IL-1R may not be essential for amelioration of ITP. This difference in the human and murine studies performed by Semple et al. and Crow et al., respectively, may be attributed to several reasons including the differences between species and methodologies (Semple 2010). It may also be because of differences between the antibodies used—TER-119 is able to mimic anti-D effectively in murine models, but it is in fact a surrogate antibody which may potentially account for some of the differences observed.

Further research is needed to help clarify the role and significance of IL-1Ra modulation in anti-RBC antibody-mediated ITP amelioration.

Other groups have also supported Semple et al.'s finding of increased levels of certain chemokines and cytokines (Malinowska et al. 2001; Branch et al. 2006; Cooper et al. 2004). Specifically, Cooper et al. found that 2 h after the anti-D treatment, there were increased levels of IL-6, IL-10, TNF-α, and MCP-1. This is in contrast with IVIg which induced an increase only in IL-10 levels 2 h posttreatment, suggesting that IVIg and anti-D may be exerting their therapeutic effects via differing mechanisms (Cooper et al. 2004).

Researchers have also shown that anti-D-induced cytokine changes in vitro can lead to a rapid (within 10–30 min) but transient increase in the production of reactive oxygen species, ROS, by human macrophages (Coopamah et al. 2003; Branch et al. 2006). This production of ROS induced by anti-D administration may be activating the MPS by providing "danger" signals (Semple 2010). The significance of these anti-RBC antibody-mediated changes in cytokine levels still remains to be elucidated fully.

5.2.4 Anti-idiotype Antibodies

An idiotype is composed of a collection of different antigenic determinants, known as idiotopes, in the variable region of the antibody. Anti-idiotype antibodies recognize and bind these antigenic determinants on other antibodies. Anti-idiotype antibodies play a role in immune system development and regulation, as proposed by Niels Kaj Jerne in his Nobel Prize winning immune network theory [reviewed in Semple (2010)].

Since anti-D is a polyclonal IgG enriched from donated plasma, it is expected that this preparation will contain various anti-idiotype antibodies. Boughton et al. showed that ITP patients that responded to anti-D treatment had a concomitant decrease in the platelet-associated autoantibodies directed against cell surface glycoproteins IIb/IIIa (Boughton et al. 1994). This finding supports the fact that anti-D contains neutralizing anti-idiotype antibodies that bind platelet autoantibodies and thus prevents them from inducing thrombocytopenia.

On the other hand, a commercial blend of 25 different monoclonal antibodies against the RhD antigen on human RBCs, rozrolimupab, was found to significantly elevate platelet levels in adult human patients with ITP at high doses (Lazarus 2013). Rozrolimupab would not be expected to contain anti-idiotype antibodies, indicating that these anti-idiotype antibodies are probably not essential for anti-D-mediated ITP amelioration. It has also been shown that murine monoclonal anti-RBC antibodies that mimic anti-D (and do not contain any anti-idiotype antibodies) are able to efficaciously increase platelet levels in murine models of ITP (Song et al. 2003). The efficacy of both rozrolimupab and monoclonal murine anti-RBC antibodies in ITP suggests that anti-idiotype antibodies are likely not the primary mechanism of action of anti-D although more research is required to confirm and assert this conclusion.

5.3 Replacement Strategies

Monoclonal replacements for anti-D have been tested in HDFN with mixed results—many were observed to decrease RBC immunization as desired although to a lesser extent than polyclonal anti-D, while others actually worsened the immune response (Kumpel 2007).

For ITP, one single monoclonal antibody was tested in seven adult patients in the late 1990s but led to disappointing results. It was found to bind RBCs and cause a similar degree of anemia as anti-D. However, there was little to no increase observed in platelet counts for six patients, while the seventh patient with mild ITP showed a transient response (Godeau et al. 1996). This study hinted at the possibility that perhaps monoclonal anti-D therapy is not efficacious for ITP patients. Following the publication of the results of this study, many researchers worked on murine models of ITP using various monoclonal antibodies (such as TER-119) to determine their efficacy and underlying mechanism (Lazarus 2013).

5.3.1 Rozrolimupab

In 2013, Symphogen (a Danish biotechnology company) manufactured a new therapeutic product as a potential replacement for anti-D. This therapeutic product, known as rozrolimupab, consists of 25 different monoclonal antibodies directed against the D antigen. A monoclonal blend, rozrolimupab, is made up entirely of human IgG1 antibodies that recognize multiple epitopes on the RhD antigen. A Phase I/II dose-escalation study conducted across multiple centers with 61 adult, nonsplenectomized RhD+ patients with chronic ITP has demonstrated that rozrolimupab has an efficacy and safety profile similar to that of other plasma-derived immunoglobulins (Robak et al. 2012). These findings provide evidence that if not a single monoclonal antibody, at the very least a multiple monoclonal antibody blend is able to successfully ameliorate ITP. These results also indicated that the other IgG isotypes present in polyclonal anti-D may not be essential for ITP amelioration. Polyclonal anti-D consists primarily of IgG1 antibodies, as used in rozrolimupab, but it also contains a smaller fraction of IgG2, IgG3, and IgG4 antibodies. Although the results of the study indicated that IgG1 itself is sufficient for ITP amelioration, the potential effects of the addition of other isotypes of IgG to rozrolimupab are not known (Lazarus 2013).

There are several benefits for using rozrolimupab as opposed to polyclonal anti-D. Most importantly, unlike donor-derived anti-D, rozrolimupab can be manufactured in vitro without any anticipated shortage of quantity and with a significantly lower risk of potentially transferring pathogens between individuals (Lazarus 2013). The efficacy of rozrolimupab has only been demonstrated in one study so far, and responses observed in further studies will help decide its future implications in clinical use.

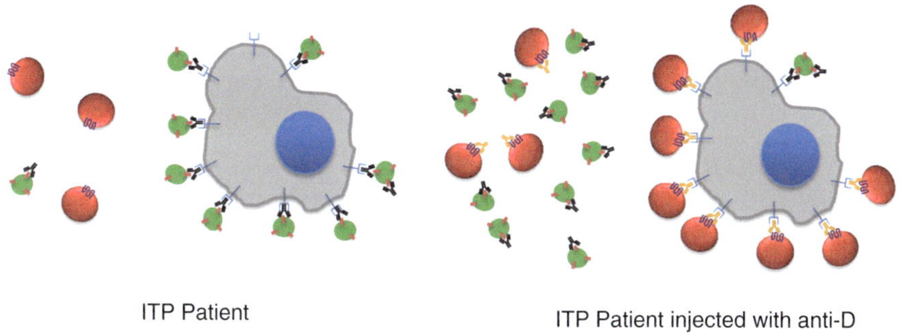

Fig. 5.1 Mononuclear phagocytic system blockade as a potential mechanism of action of anti-D in ITP. Left: In ITP, platelets are opsonized by anti-platelet antibody. Opsonized platelets then bind to FcγRs on macrophages leading to platelet phagocytosis thus decreasing platelet counts. Right: Anti-D binds to RhD+ RBCs and these opsonized RBCs outcompete opsonized platelets, thus sensitized RBCs occupy a greater number of FcγRs present on the surface of the macrophages (i.e. competitively inhibiting sensitized platelets from binding to the macrophage FcγRs). The macrophages phagocytose the bound RBCs leading to a decreased RBC count in some patients while platelet levels are elevated. Macrophages; FcγR; Platelet; Platelet surface antigen; RBC; RhD antigen; Anti-platelet antibody; Anti-D

Conclusion

Anti-D is a polyclonal immunoglobulin (IgG) directed against the D antigen present on human red blood cells and is used clinically to treat ITP and prevent HDFN. As a donor-derived product, it is present in limited quantities and carries the theoretical risk of potentially transferring pathogens. Coupled with the fact that the first priority for anti-D usage is in preventing HDFN, there is incentive present for developing a replacement to be utilized for ITP treatment. However the mechanism of action of anti-D in ITP remains unclear. To date, research has proposed MPS blockage, cytokine modulation, and the presence of idiotypic antibodies to contribute to the potential mechanisms. The discovery and efficacy of rozrolimupab, a monoclonal blend of anti-D, have provided support against idiotype antibodies as a potential mechanism of action and proved that it may be possible to replace polyclonal anti-D with a blend of multiple monoclonal recombinants. Building on the information already present, further research can help elucidate the mechanism of anti-RBC antibodies which can then be utilized to synthesize a replacement recombinant antibody for clinical use.

References

Ambriz-Fernández R, Martínez-Murillo C, Quintana-González S, Collazo-Jaloma J, Bautista-Juárez J. Fc receptor blockade in patients with refractory chronic immune thrombocytopenic purpura with anti-D IgG. Arch Med Res. 2002;33:536–40.

Becker T, Küenzlen E, Salama A, Mertens R, Kiefel V, Weiss H, Lampert F, Gaedicke G, Mueller-Eckhardt C. Treatment of childhood idiopathic thrombocytopenic purpura with rhesus antibodies (anti-D). Eur J Pediatr. 1986;145:166–9.

Boughton B. Anti-D Ig for treatment of immune thrombocytopenic purpura [letter; comment]. Blood. 1991;78:2157–8.

Boughton BJ, Cooke RM, Smith NA, Simpson AW. Autoimmune thrombocytopenia: anti-glycoprotein IIb/IIIa auto antibodies are reduced after human anti-D immunoglobulin treatment. Autoimmunity. 1994;18:141–4.

Branch DR, Shabani F, Lund N, Denomme GA. Antenatal administration of Rh-immune globulin causes significant increases in the immunomodulatory cytokines transforming growth factor-Beta and prostaglandin E2. Transfusion. 2006;46:1316–22.

Brinc D, Lazarus AH. Mechanisms of anti-D action in the prevention of hemolytic disease of the fetus and newborn. Hematology Am Soc Hematol Educ Program. 2009;2009(1):185–91.

Bruhns P, Jönsson F. Mouse and human FcR effector functions. Immunol Rev. 2015;268:25–51.

Bussel J, Graziano J, Kimberly R, Pahwa S, Aledort L. Intravenous anti-D treatment of immune thrombocytopenic purpura: analysis of efficacy, toxicity, and mechanism of effect [see comments]. Blood. 1991;77:1884–93.

Chen X, Ghaffar H, Jen CC, Lazarus AH. Antibody specific for the glycophorin A complex mediates intravenous immune globulin-resistant anemia in a murine model. Transfusion. 2014;54:655–64.

Coopamah MD, Freedman J, Semple JW. Anti-D initially stimulates an Fc-dependent leukocyte oxidative burst and subsequently suppresses erythrophagocytosis via interleukin-1 receptor antagonist. Blood. 2003;102:2862–7.

Cooper N, Heddle NM, Haas M, Reid ME, Lesser ML, Fleit HB, Woloski BM, Bussel JB. Intravenous (IV) anti-D and IV immunoglobulin achieve acute platelet increases by different mechanisms: modulation of cytokine and platelet responses to IV anti-D by FcgammaRIIa and FcgammaRIIIa polymorphisms. Br J Haematol. 2004;124:511–8.

Crow AR, Songs S, Semple JW, Freedman J, Lazarus AH. A role for IL-1 receptor antagonist or other cytokines in the acute therapevtic effects of ivlg?. Blood. 2007;22:109:155–8.

Crow AR, Lazarus AH. The mechanisms of action of intravenous immunoglobulin and polyclonal anti-D immunoglobulin in the amelioration of immune thrombocytopenic purpura: what do we really know? Transfus Med Rev. 2008;22:103–16.

Davenport RD, Burdick MD, Strieter RM, Kunkel SL. In vitro production of Interleukin-1 receptor antagonist in IgG-mediated red cell incompatibility. Transfusion. 1994;34:297–303.

Deng R, Balthasar JP. Comparison of the effects of antibody-coated liposomes, IVIG, and anti-RBC immunotherapy in a murine model of passive chronic immune thrombocytopenia. Blood. 2007;109(6):2470.

Despotovic JM, Lambert MP, Herman JH, Gernsheimer TB, Mccrae KR, Tarantino MD, Bussel JB. RhIG for the treatment of immune thrombocytopenia: consensus and controversy (CME). Transfusion. 2012;52:1126–36; Quiz 1125.

Dripps DJ, Brandhuber BJ, Thompson RC, Eisenberg SP. Interleukin-1 (IL-1) receptor antagonist binds to the 80-kDA IL-1 receptor but does not initiate IL-1 signal transduction. J Biol Chem. 1991;266:10331–6.

Eghbali A, Azadmanesh P, Bagheri B, Taherahmadi H, Sadeghi Sedeh B. Comparison between IV immune globulin (IVIG) and anti-D globulin for treatment of immune thrombocytopenia: a randomized open-label study. Fundam Clin Pharmacol. 2016;30:385–9.

FDA U. Warning - Rh(D) immune globulin intravenous (Human). In: Administration, F. A. D. editor. 2009.

Godeau B, Oksenhendler E, Brossard Y, Bartholeyns J, Leaute JB, Duedari N, Schaeffer A, Bierling P. Treatment of chronic autoimmune thrombocytopenic purpura with monoclonal anti-D. Transfusion. 1996;36:328–30.
Hendrickson JE, Delaney M. Hemolytic disease of the fetus and newborn: modern practice and future investigations. Transfus Med Rev. 2016;30:159–64.
Hume DA. The mononuclear phagocyte system. Curr Opin Immunol. 2006;18:49–53.
Imbach P, Barandun S, D'apuzzo V, Baumgartner C, Hirt A, Morell A, Rossi E, Schöni M, Vest M, Wagner HP. High-dose intravenous gammaglobulin for idiopathic thrombocytopenic purpura in childhood. Lancet. 1981;1:1228–31.
Kumpel BM. Efficacy of RhD monoclonal antibodies in clinical trials as replacement therapy for prophylactic anti-D immunoglobulin: more questions than answers. Vox Sang. 2007;93:99–111.
Lazarus AH. Monoclonal versus polyclonal anti-D in the treatment of ITP. Expert Opin Biol Ther. 2013;13:1353–6.
Malinowska I, Obitko-Płudowska A, Buescher ES, Wasik M, Rokicka-Milewska R. Release of cytokines and soluble cytokine receptors after intravenous anti-D treatment in children with chronic thrombocytopenic purpura. Hematol J. 2001;2:242–9.
Nair AB, Jacob S. A simple practice guide for dose conversion between animals and human. J Basic Clin Pharm. 2016;7:27–31.
Oksenhendler E, Bierling P, Brossard Y, Schenmetzler C, Girard PM, Seligmann M, Clauvel JP. Anti-RH immunoglobulin therapy for human immunodeficiency virus-related immune thrombocytopenic purpura. Blood. 1988;71:1499–502.
Ramadan KM, El-Agnaf M. Efficacy and response to intravenous anti-D immunoglobulin in chronic idiopathic thrombocytopenic purpura. Clin Lab Haematol. 2005;27:267–9.
Robak T, Windyga J, Trelinski J, Von Depka Prondzinski M, Giagounidis A, Doyen C, Janssens A, Alvarez-Román MT, Jarque I, Loscertales J, Rus GP, Hellmann A, Jêdrzejczak WW, Kuliczkowski K, Golubovic LM, Celeketic D, Cucuianu A, Gheorghita E, Lazaroiu M, Shpilberg O, Attias D, Karyagina E, Svetlana K, Vilchevska K, Cooper N, Talks K, Prabhu M, Sripada P, Bharadwaj TP, Næsted H, Skartved NJ, Frandsen TP, Flensburg MF, Andersen PS, Petersen J. Rozrolimupab, a mixture of 25 recombinant human monoclonal RhD antibodies, in the treatment of primary immune thrombocytopenia. Blood. 2012;120:3670–6.
Rosman Z, Shoenfeld Y, Zandman-Goddard G. Biologic therapy for autoimmune diseases: an update. BMC Med. 2013;11:88.
Salama A, Kiefel V, Amberg R, Mueller-Eckhardt C. Treatment of autoimmune thrombocytopenic purpura with rhesus antibodies anti-Rh0(D). Blut. 1984;49:29–35.
Salama A, Mueller-Eckhardt C, Kiefel V. Effect of intravenous immunoglobulin in immune thrombocytopenia. Lancet. 1983;2:193–5.
Semple JW. Anti-D: basic concepts and mechanisms of action in autoimmunity. In: Lazarus AH, Semple JW, editors. Immunoglobulin therapy. Bethesda: Aabb Press; 2010.
Semple JW, Allen D, Rutherford M, Woloski M, David M, Wakefield C, Butchart S, Freedman J, Blanchette V, Group, C. C. S. P. S. Anti-D (WinRho SD) treatment of children with chronic autoimmune thrombocytopenic purpura stimulates transient cytokine/chemokine production. Am J Hematol. 2002;69:225–7.
Song S, Crow AR, Freedman J, Lazarus AH. Monoclonal IgG can ameliorate immune thrombocytopenia in a murine model of ITP: an alternative to IVIG. Blood. 2003;101:3708–13.
Song S, Crow AR, Siragam V, Freedman J, Lazarus AH. Monoclonal antibodies that mimic the action of anti-D in the amelioration of murine ITP act by a mechanism distinct from that of IVIg. Blood. 2005;105:1546–8.
Urbaniak SJ, Greiss MA. RhD haemolytic disease of the fetus and the newborn. Blood Rev. 2000;14:44–61.
Ware RE, Zimmerman SA. Anti-D: mechanisms of action. Semin Hematol. 1998;35:14–22.
Yu X, Menard M, Seabright G, Crispin M, Lazarus AH. A monoclonal antibody with anti-D-like activity in murine immune thrombocytopenia requires Fc domain function for immune thrombocytopenia ameliorative effects. Transfusion. 2015;55:1501–11.

Mechanisms of Action and Immunomodulation by IVIg

6

Alan H. Lazarus

6.1 Introduction

Autoantibodies represent a significant presence in mediating tissue damage in a multitude of autoimmune syndromes. In many of these diseases, the autoantibodies exert their inflammatory effect through activating Fc receptors for IgG (FcγRs), a well-established class of immune cell surface receptors that interact with the Fc domain of IgG. There are four classes of activating FcγRs: FcγRI which binds non-complexed IgG with high affinity and FcγRIIA, FcγRIII, and FcγRIV which are known as low-affinity receptors and bind complexed IgG.

FcγRIIA is found in humans but not mice, while FcγRIV exists in mice but not humans. There is also an Fc receptor known as an inhibitory receptor (FcγRIIB) which exists in both mice and humans. Although this last receptor is known as an inhibitory receptor, it is nevertheless capable of mediating clearance of soluble immune complexes in the liver (Ganesan et al. 2012). Conversely although FcγRIII is well known as an activating receptor, it also can mediate inhibitory signalling controlling inflammatory responses (Aloulou et al. 2012). IVIg anti-inflammatory activity has been implicated in disease models where autoantibodies and Fc receptors play a pivotal role in the autoimmune pathophysiology.

IVIg was originally used as a replacement product for those deficient in IgG. However, with the appreciation that IVIg has immunomodulatory effects in autoimmunity, its use has greatly expanded. Some of the challenges with clearly

A.H. Lazarus, PhD
Centre for Innovation at The Canadian Blood Services, Ottawa, ON, Canada

Keenan Research Centre of the Li Ka Shing Knowledge Institute at St. Michael's Hospital, Toronto, ON, Canada

Departments of Medicine and Laboratory Medicine & Pathobiology, Faculty of Medicine, University of Toronto, Toronto, ON, Canada
e-mail: LAZARUSA@smh.ca

P. Imbach (ed.), *Antibody Therapy*, https://doi.org/10.1007/978-3-319-68038-5_6

understanding the mechanism of action of IVIg in autoimmunity are that we have an incomplete knowledge of autoimmune pathophysiology particularly in patients. Studies in animal models have predominated as tools in attempting to unravel the mechanisms of IVIg action. Even among well-studied murine models such as the krn model of rheumatoid arthritis (Kouskoff et al. 1996), the immune pathophysiology is often more complex than we originally anticipated. To appreciate the role of IVIg in ameliorating autoimmune disease activity, it becomes critically important to understand the pathophysiology which we are attempting to reverse with IVIg. For this reason, a passive model of immune thrombocytopenia (ITP) has been favoured for understanding IVIg action. Part of the reason for selecting murine ITP as a model to understand IVIg action is that it is clear that the majority of patients with ITP in fact benefit from IVIg therapy. This contrasts with other animal models often used to understand IVIg action including murine models of rheumatoid arthritis or multiple sclerosis where the corresponding human diseases do not fare as well or as consistently as IVIg responses in ITP.

One of the strengths of the passive murine ITP model include that we can control the antibody causing thrombocytopenia. Available are a variety of monoclonal antiplatelet antibodies which mediate thrombocytopenia in mice. Some of these antibodies mediate the thrombocytopenia in a manner dependent on activating Fc receptors (Li and Kimberly 2014). In fact some monoclonal antibodies can specifically cause thrombocytopenia through a selected activating Fc receptor such as via FcγRIII or via FcγRIV (Yu et al. 2016). In addition, monoclonal antiplatelet antibodies are available that cause thrombocytopenia independent of any activating Fc receptor (e.g. anti-GPIb), and in this case IVIg anti-inflammatory activity does not affect the thrombocytopenia (Webster et al. 2006; Li et al. 2015). There is further an available immune active model of murine ITP where we can control the thrombocytopenia mediated by either humoral immunity or T cell-mediated immunity. In the active ITP model, IVIg anti-inflammatory activity was evident when the thrombocytopenia was caused by humoral immunity but not by T cell-dependent active ITP (Chow et al. 2010). Thus the murine thrombocytopenia models have contributed greatly to our understanding of IVIg mechanisms.

6.2 Anti-idiotype Antibodies

Anti-idiotype antibodies are found in normal healthy individuals and are antibodies that can bind the antigen-combining region of pathogenic antibodies and neutralize them. One of the concepts in autoimmunity is that the normal repertoire of a patient's antibodies is dysregulated which contributes to autoimmune tissue destruction. Since a normal repertoire of anti-idiotype antibodies would be expected in IVIg, it was hypothesized that this could explain IVIg anti-inflammatory effects (Table 6.1). IVIg has been known to display anti-idiotype antibodies relevant to a number of diseases including lupus, pemphigus vulgaris, antiphospholipid syndrome and other diseases. Early work demonstrated that IVIg contains antibodies capable of neutralizing the activity of autoantibodies directed against the major platelet autoantigen,

Table 6.1 Selected potential mechanisms of IVIg immunomodulation in ITP and other diseases

Anti-idiotype antibodies
Mononuclear phagocytic system blockade
Cytokine modulation
Neonatal Fc receptor
IgG Fc region sialylation
Dendritic cell activity
T regulatory cell activity
Immune complex formation
Antibody dimers/multimers
Apoptosis
Complement
Effects on B cells
Other mechanisms

glycoprotein (GP) IIb/IIIa (Berchtold et al. 1989). Conversely, however, other work found IVIg to be ineffective in autoantibody neutralization in patients with ITP (Barbano et al. 1989). In murine and rat models of passive ITP, studies from two different groups showed that anti-idiotype antibodies were not necessary for disease amelioration (Crow et al. 2001; Hansen and Balthasar 2002).

Thus at least in ITP, the contribution of anti-idiotype antibodies to IVIg activity could be questionable.

It is important to note that IVIg has efficacy in a large number of different autoimmune diseases and inflammatory states. While it would be nice, or convenient, to consider that IVIg may have the same mechanism of action in all diseases, it is equally possible that IVIg works by different mechanisms in different diseases. Recent data in chronic inflammatory demyelinating polyneuropathy (CIDP) patients has shown that following IVIg administration, there is an increase in the measurable number of IgG dimer levels in some responding patients. Although it is certainly possible that the formation of these IgG dimers could mediate IVIg activity by mechanism not involving autoantibody neutralization (discussed in the immune complex section of this review), the IgG dimers formed in the patients after administration of IVIg actually contained antibodies with reactivity against peripheral nerve fibres (Ritter et al. 2015). These results allowed the authors to speculate that the immune complexes formed following IVIg administration in these patients likely included autoantibodies from the patients and anti-idiotype antibodies from the IVIg. Whether neutralization of the autoantibodies is the mechanism underlying IVIg anti-inflammatory effects in CIDP remains to be explored but is certainly a mechanism worthy of exploring further in this disease and perhaps others.

6.3 Mononuclear Phagocytic System (MPS) Blockade

In ITP, the site of platelet clearance is largely considered to be the spleen and liver which are organs that also host the MPS (previously referred to as the reticuloendothelial system). In patients with autoantibodies directed to the major platelet autoantigen (GPIIbIIIa), phagocytic platelet destruction by the MPS has long been considered to be the predominant mechanism contributing to the thrombocytopenia. Early direct experiments that MPS blockade by IVIg could rescue antibody-opsonized cells from phagocytosis were experiments by Fehr et al. (1982) who demonstrated that in patients with ITP who were not splenectomised, that IVIg treatment prolonged the in vivo clearance of antibody-opsonized erythrocytes. These results have been confirmed by others (reviewed in; Crow and Lazarus 2008).

The first report of the treatment of an autoimmune disease with IVIg was by Imbach et al. (1981) who demonstrated that IVIg improves ITP. Salama then noticed that IVIg caused anaemia and postulated that the success of IVIg in treating ITP was due to IVIg binding erythrocytes and competitively inhibiting macrophages in the MPS by the sensitized erythrocytes (Salama et al. 1983). One year later Salama and colleagues showed that anti-D could treat ITP in RhD-positive patients (Salama et al. 1984). This elegant hypothesis and clinical success firmly cemented in the concept that IVIg and anti-D both work by competitively blocking the MPS, and most ITP-treating physicians have used IVIg and anti-D interchangeably in RhD+ patients.

Clarkson and colleagues also showed that direct inactivation of the MPS using antibodies that bind and block activating Fc receptors were also able to ameliorate ITP (Clarkson et al. 1986). In the passive murine ITP model, recent work has shown that a monomeric antibody-fusion protein which binds and blocks activating Fc receptors was also able to ameliorate the thrombocytopenia (Yu et al. 2016).

Although MPS blockade is an accepted theory to explain the mechanisms of action of IVIg in ITP, some patients have responded to F(ab′)2 fragments of IVIg which essentially have no Fc receptor binding activity (Tovo et al. 1984; Burdach et al. 1986). The original concept behind MPS blockade was that MPS blockade is due to a direct competitive mechanism whereby opsonized platelets are competing with IVIg which bound to an antigen in a patient. However, this is not the only potential mechanism of MPS blockade; another possibility includes that IVIg-opsonized erythrocytes, once phagocytosed, poison the macrophage by the release of iron. Although it seems likely that inhibition of the MPS likely underlies at least some of the activity of IVIg, further work is needed.

6.4 Cytokine Modulation

A number of studies have examined patient’s pre-and post-IVIg administration to look for changes in cytokine levels commensurate with disease amelioration. Changes in interleukin (IL)- 6, IL- 8, tumour necrosis factor (TNF) α and IL-1 receptor antagonist were found increased after 1 h of IVIg administration (Aukrust et al. 1994). Increases in IL-10 2 h post-IVIg administration and monocyte chemotactic protein-1 (MCP-1) 7 days posttreatment were observed by Cooper et al. (2004). Work from the laboratory of Donald Branch and colleagues suggested that IL-11 may explain IVIg activity in experimental autoimmune encephalomyelitis (Figueiredo et al. 2014), while work from Ravetch and colleagues suggested that

IL-33 (Anthony et al. 2011) or CSF-1 (Bruhns et al. 2003) may explain IVIg activity in murine models of autoimmunity. Work from the author's laboratory using mice separately deficient for the IL-1 receptor, IL-4, IL-10, IL-12β, TNFα, interferon γ receptor and macrophage inflammatory protein (MIP)1α showed that IVIg could still ameliorate murine ITP demonstrating that the presence of these individual cytokines is not critical in the amelioration of thrombocytopenia (Crow et al. 2007). In addition IVIg worked normally in mice deficient for the common cytokine receptor γ chain (an immune signalling component required for signal transduction through the receptors for IL-2, IL-4, IL-7, IL-9, IL-15, and IL-21) in the same study. In addition, work from Aubin and colleagues showed that mice exposed to IVIg displayed no modulation of messenger RNA for 84 different cytokines, chemokines, or receptor messenger RNAs (Aubin et al. 2007). Recent data has shown that IVIg can upregulate the expression of the MiR-146a microRNA controlling cytokine signalling pathways in human monocytes affecting the expression of several cytokines (Loubaki et al. 2017).

A recent study performed in 11 patients with CIDP treated with IVIg interestingly showed decreases in mRNA from blood cells for three genes related to the TNFα receptor 1 (TNFR1) pathway in patients who responded to IVIg (Richard et al. 2016). In this study, the authors analysed pretreatment levels of each mRNA with responses 3 weeks after the initiation of IVIg therapy.

Some of the challenges with assessing the contribution of different cytokines to IVIg action include the time of cytokine analysis, whether cytokines are being examined from plasma or a cell fraction, and in mRNA studies whether these transcripts actually result in the release of the cytokine. In addition, there is always the possibility that changes in a mRNA from a particular cellular subset may be overshadowed by other subsets present in the sample. Again it cannot be overemphasized the additional possibility that IVIg works by different mechanisms in different diseases.

6.5 Neonatal Fc Receptor (FcRn)

IgG has a long half-life in serum, and this is largely contributed to by the activity of FcRn which binds IgG and protects it from intracellular degradation allowing it to be trafficked out of the cell (Roopenian and Akilesh 2007). IVIg has been shown to accelerate the clearance of pathogenic antibodies (Li et al. 2005). Because IVIg is given at a very high dosage, it has the capability of saturating the FcRn and accelerating the clearance of IgG molecules from the host. The accelerated clearance of IgG from the host would include all antibodies including those that are pathogenic as well as the IVIg itself.

To directly address the hypothesis of the contribution of FcRn activity to IVIg effects in ITP, we used two different models of FcRn genetically-deficient mice and clearly showed that IVIg ameliorated antiplatelet antibody-mediated thrombocytopenia in the absence of FcRn (Crow et al. 2011). These results demonstrated that IVIg is not dependent on FcRn expression for its ameliorative effect in acute murine passive ITP. Although it is possible that in other diseases there is a role for FcRn activity in IVIg action, this could be unlikely given our results in the ITP model. An additional complexity for FcRn in mediating the effects of IVIg in ITP is that IVIg effects can be seen in patients within 1 or 2 days, whereas the ability of FcRn to significantly deplete autoantibodies generally tends to take longer. For this reason we do not favour the FcRn hypothesis for explaining IVIg effects.

6.6 IgG Fc Region Sialylation and the Inhibitory Fc Receptor (FcγRIIB)

Perhaps one of the most controversial areas of IVIg mechanisms is in the area of IgG Fc region sialylation. IgG molecules have an asparagine amino acid corresponding to position 297 on the Fc region of IgG which is occupied by N-linked glycosylation. The glycan structure at this position generally determines the ability of the IgG to interact with Fc receptors as well as activate complement. Different glycan structures at this position can increase or decrease the ability of the IgG to interact with Fc receptors generating antibodies that can have altered inflammatory activities (Schwab and Nimmerjahn 2013). In the case of IVIg, it was hypothesized that an altered glycan structure could also mediate anti-inflammatory activity. This anti-inflammatory activity was shown to be mediated by the presence of a terminal sialic acid on the glycan structure. A number of high-impact papers published on this hypothesis have demonstrated a very specific anti-inflammatory pathway through which these sialic acid-containing IgG molecules mediate immunomodulatory effects in autoimmunity. The pathway was demonstrated to commence by the sialic acid expressing IgG Fc region interacting with a molecule on the surface of dendritic cells called dendritic cell-specific intercellular adhesion molecule-3-grabbing non-integrin (DC-SIGN) in humans. Stimulation of this pathway then led to the involvement of a number of intermediates including IL-33, basophils and the inhibitory Fc receptor (FcγRIIB) mediating anti-inflammatory activity. Although several investigators have shown support for this theory, a much larger number of investigators have addressed various aspects of this pathway and not found support for the hypothesis. For those who are interested, readers are referred to reviews which discuss this hypothesis from a positive perspective (Anthony and Ravetch 2010; Schwab and Nimmerjahn 2013) as well some which discuss the concept less favourably (von Gunten et al. 2014; Crow and Lazarus 2016).

6.7 Dendritic Cells (DC) and Immunomodulation

DC play a central role in the priming of adaptive immune responses, yet they can also tolerize peripheral CD4+ and CD8+ T cells, and DC have been viewed as promising targets for immunotherapy. IVIg has been known to inhibit T-cell proliferation and T-cell cytokine production, but the mechanism of how IVIg could mediate these effects was originally unknown. IVIg was then shown to inhibit the maturation of DC and modulate their activation and survival, possibly resulting in abrogation of T-cell activation and proliferation (reviewed in; Crow et al. 2009). DC involvement in IVIg activity at that time was poorly understood. Were the DC inflammatory or anti-inflammatory? How did IVIg affect these DC? Were DC involved directly or indirectly with IVIg? What was the active component within the IVIg preparation that affected these DC?

These questions were addressed when it was shown that IVIg action was likely the result of the formation of IgG immune complexes in the recipient (Siragam et al. 2005) and that these immune complexes likely bound to activating Fc receptors on the surface of DC triggering their anti-inflammatory activity (Siragam et al. 2006). An additional possibility was that there were IgG dimers in the IVIg product (Teeling et al. 2001) or that IVIg formed dimers or multimers soon after in vivo injection and that these perhaps bound activating Fc receptors on the DC. Although all of the downstream elements of this pathway have yet to be discovered, this pathway has been well supported by the work of others in several disease models (reviewed in; Crow et al. 2009).

DC are potent antigen presenting cells that are well-positioned to stimulate the production of T regulatory cells (Trinath et al. 2013) as well as initiate other anti-inflammatory pathways. In fact, a number of studies have shown that IVIg stimulates the production of T regulatory cells that have activity not just in ITP but also other disease models (Massoud et al. 2017). Although the complete linkage between DC and T regulatory cells has not yet been confirmed, IVIg induces the induction of a cyclooxygenase-2-dependent prostaglandin E2 pathway in DC (Trinath et al. 2013), and recent studies have shown that IVIg specifically induces an upregulation in tolerizing dendritic cells in the spleen (Kapur et al. 2016). Some of the other recent immunomodulatory effects downstream of IVIg administration include increases in the appearance of myeloid-derived suppressor cells which can also shed light on some of IVIgs immunomodulatory effects (Aslam et al. 2017).

6.8 Immune Complexes, IgG Multimers, and Potential Future Therapeutics

IVIg can potentially bind to a number of different particulate or soluble antigens, and different antibodies within IVIg may be responsible for different therapeutic effects through a variety of mechanisms. As indicated above, early work showed that IVIg could contain dimers or multimers which appeared to cause side effects in some patients. Later work then showed that the IgG dimers present in IVIg could potentially mediate IVIg activity in murine passive ITP (Teeling et al. 2001).

We speculated that perhaps IVIg, upon injection into a patient, could also form small molecular weight immune complexes which could bind and trigger anti-inflammatory activity through activating Fc receptors on dendritic cells. The first step in this process showed that IgG targeted to a soluble antigen could recapitulate the effects of IVIg in murine ITP (Siragam et al. 2005). We observed that antibodies forming immune complexes with an experimental antigen (ovalbumin) as well as endogenous mouse albumin or mouse transferrin could all mediate IVIg-like activity in both murine ITP and in a murine model of arthritis. Because these immune complexes worked at a 1000-fold lower dose than IVIg, this gave rise to the concept that IVIg could potentially be replaced with either an immune complex or a modified "synthetic immune complex". The advent of molecular engineering and the ability to create IgG Fc fusion proteins consisting of multiple Fc regions linked to each other has given rise to a number of different potential IVIg recombinant replacements.

Multimerized IgG Fc products fall into a number of different categories and have been recently discussed and compared in detail (Zuercher et al. 2016). One type of IgG multimer, called a Stradomer has used fusion of the human IgG2 hinge region to a human IgG1 Fc, allowing the IgG1 Fc fragment to form multimers. These Stradomers have protective effects in murine passive ITP, collagen-induced arthritis, a mouse model of myasthenia gravis and an experimental autoimmune neuritis model (Niknami et al. 2013). Hexa-Fc or HexaGard was selected to oligomerize monomeric Fc into well-defined hexameric oligomers capable of binding to high-affinity Fc receptors (Czajkowsky et al. 2015). Another molecule called SIF3 is a trimeric Fc molecule where the Fab portions of IgG have been substituted with human IgG Fc fragments and has anti-inflammatory activity in the passive murine ITP model and murine arthritis. In addition, a number of other similar strategies are available and have recently been discussed (Zuercher et al. 2016).

6.9 Other Mechanisms

In addition to the mechanisms and therapeutics discussed in this review, there are a number of other potential mechanisms of IVIg action including the ability of IVIg to affect programmed cell death or apoptosis and the ability of IVIg to mediate effects in conjunction with complement and effects on B cells. Although IVIg is used worldwide to treat a multitude of different autoimmune syndromes, its mechanism(s) of action remain unresolved. The push to replace IVIg with a monoclonal antibody will hopefully alleviate many of the problems with IVIg and give rise to a more effective product for patients.

References

Aloulou M, Ben Mkaddem S, Biarnes-Pelicot M, Boussetta T, Souchet H, Rossato E, Benhamou M, Crestani B, Zhu Z, Blank U, Launay P, Monteiro RC. IgG1 and IVIg induce inhibitory ITAM signaling through FcγRIII controlling inflammatory responses. Blood. 2012;119(13):3084–96.

Anthony RM, Ravetch JV. A novel role for the IgG Fc glycan: the anti-inflammatory activity of sialylated IgG Fcs. J Clin Immunol. 2010;30(S1):9–14.

Anthony RM, Kobayashi T, Wermeling F, Ravetch JV. Intravenous gammaglobulin suppresses inflammation through a novel TH2 pathway. Nature. 2011;475(7354):110–3.

Aslam R, Burack WR, Segel GB, McVey M, Spence SA, Semple JW. Intravenous immunoglobulin treatment of spleen cells from patients with immune thrombocytopenia significantly increases the percentage of myeloid-derived suppressor cells. Br J Haematol. 2017. [Epub ahead of print].

Aubin E, Lemieux R, Bazin R. Absence of cytokine modulation following therapeutic infusion of intravenous immunoglobulin or anti-red blood cell antibodies in a mouse model of immune thrombocytopenic purpura. Br J Haematol. 2007;136(6):837–43.

Aukrust P, Frøland SS, Liabakk NB, Müller F, Nordøy I, Haug C, Espevik T. Release of cytokines, soluble cytokine receptors, and interleukin-1 receptor antagonist after intravenous immunoglobulin administration in vivo. Blood. 1994;84(7):2136–43.

Barbano G, Saleh MN, Mori PG, LoBuglio AF, Shaw DR. Effect of intravenous gammaglobulin on circulating and platelet-bound antibody in immune thrombocytopenia. Blood. 1989;73(3):662–5.

Berchtold P, Dale GL, Tani P, McMillan R. Inhibition of autoantibody binding to platelet glycoprotein IIb/IIIa by anti-idiotypic antibodies in intravenous gammaglobulin. Blood. 1989;74(7):2414–7.

Bruhns P, Samuelsson A, Pollard JW, Ravetch JV. Colony-stimulating factor-1-dependent macrophages are responsible for IVIG protection in antibody-induced autoimmune disease. Immunity. 2003;18(4):573–81.

Burdach SE, Evers KG, Geursen RG. Treatment of acute idiopathic thrombocytopenic purpura of childhood with intravenous immunoglobulin G: comparative efficacy of 7S and 5S preparations. J Pediatr. 1986;109(5):770–5.

Chow L, Aslam R, Speck ER, Kim M, Cridland N, Webster ML, Chen P, Sahib K, Ni H, Lazarus AH, Garvey MB, Freedman J, Semple JW. A murine model of severe immune thrombocytopenia is induced by antibody- and CD8+ T cell-mediated responses that are differentially sensitive to therapy. Blood. 2010;115(6):1247–53.

Clarkson SB, Bussel JB, Kimberly RP, Valinsky JE, Nachman RL, Unkeless JC. Treatment of refractory immune thrombocytopenic purpura with an anti-Fc gamma-receptor antibody. N Engl J Med. 1986;314(19):1236–9.

Cooper N, Heddle NM, Haas M, Reid ME, Lesser ML, Fleit HB, Woloski BMR, Bussel JB. Intravenous (IV) anti-D and IV immunoglobulin achieve acute platelet increases by different mechanisms: modulation of cytokine and platelet responses to IV anti-D by FcgammaRIIa and FcgammaRIIIa polymorphisms. Br J Haematol. 2004;124(4):511–8.

Crow AR, Lazarus AH. The mechanisms of action of intravenous immunoglobulin and polyclonal anti-d immunoglobulin in the amelioration of immune thrombocytopenic purpura: what do we really know? Transfus Med Rev. 2008;22(2):103–16.

Crow AR, Lazarus AH. Mechanistic properties of intravenous immunoglobulin in murine immune thrombocytopenia: support for FcγRIIB falls by the wayside. Semin Hematol. 2016;53:S20–2.

Crow AR, Song S, Semple JW, Freedman J, Lazarus AH. IVIg inhibits reticuloendothelial system function and ameliorates murine passive-immune thrombocytopenia independent of anti-idiotype reactivity. Br J Haematol. 2001;115(3):679–86.

Crow AR, Song S, Semple JW, Freedman J, Lazarus AH. A role for IL-1 receptor antagonist or other cytokines in the acute therapeutic effects of IVIg? Blood. 2007;109(1):155–8.

Crow AR, Brinc D, Lazarus AH. New insight into the mechanism of action of IVIg: the role of dendritic cells. J Thromb Haemost. 2009;7:245–8.

Crow AR, Suppa SJ, Chen X, Mott PJ, Lazarus AH. The neonatal Fc receptor (FcRn) is not required for IVIg or anti-CD44 monoclonal antibody-mediated amelioration of murine immune thrombocytopenia. Blood. 2011;118(24):6403–6.

Czajkowsky DM, Andersen JT, Fuchs A, Wilson TJ, Mekhaiel D, Colonna M, He J, Shao Z, Mitchell DA, Wu G, Dell A, Haslam S, Lloyd KA, Moore SC, Sandlie I, Blundell PA, Pleass RJ. Developing the IVIG biomimetic, Hexa-Fc, for drug and vaccine applications. Sci Rep. 2015;5(u):9526.

Fehr J, Hofmann V, Kappeler U. Transient reversal of thrombocytopenia in idiopathic thrombocytopenic purpura by high-dose intravenous gamma globulin. N Engl J Med. 1982;306(21):1254–8.

Figueiredo CA, Drohomyrecky PC, McCarthy SDS, Leontyev D, Ma X-Z, Branch DR, Dunn SE. Optimal attenuation of experimental autoimmune encephalomyelitis by intravenous immunoglobulin requires an intact interleukin-11 receptor. PLoS One. 2014;9(7):e101947. Edited by O. Aktas.

Ganesan LP, Kim J, Wu Y, Mohanty S, Phillips GS, Birmingham DJ, Robinson JM, Anderson CL. FcγRIIb on liver sinusoidal endothelium clears small immune complexes. J Immunol. 2012;189(10):4981–8.

Hansen RJ, Balthasar JP. Effects of intravenous immunoglobulin on platelet count and antiplatelet antibody disposition in a rat model of immune thrombocytopenia. Blood. 2002;100(6):2087–93.

Imbach P, Barandun S, d'Apuzzo V, Baumgartner C, Hirt A, Morell A, Rossi E, Schöni M, Vest M, Wagner HP. High-dose intravenous gammaglobulin for idiopathic thrombocytopenic purpura in childhood. Lancet (Lond Engl). 1981;1(8232):1228–31.

Kapur R, Aslam R, Kim M, Guo L, Ni H, Segel GB, Semple JW. Thymic-derived tolerizing dendritic cells are upregulated in the spleen upon treatment with intravenous immunoglobulin in a murine model of immune thrombocytopenia. Platelets. 2016;28:1–4.

Kouskoff V, Korganow AS, Duchatelle V, Degott C, Benoist C, Mathis D. Organ-specific disease provoked by systemic autoimmunity. Cell. 1996;87(5):811–22.

Li X, Kimberly RP. Targeting the Fc receptor in autoimmune disease. Expert Opin Ther Targets. 2014;18(3):335–50.

Li N, Zhao M, Hilario-Vargas J, Prisayanh P, Warren S, Diaz LA, Roopenian DC, Liu Z. Complete FcRn dependence for intravenous Ig therapy in autoimmune skin blistering diseases. J Clin Invest. 2005;115(12):3440–50.

Li J, van der Wal DE, Zhu G, Xu M, Yougbare I, Ma L, Vadasz B, Carrim N, Grozovsky R, Ruan M, Zhu L, Zeng Q, Tao L, Zhai Z, Peng J, Hou M, Leytin V, Freedman J, Hoffmeister KM, Ni H. Desialylation is a mechanism of Fc-independent platelet clearance and a therapeutic target in immune thrombocytopenia. Nat Commun. 2015;6:7737.

Loubaki L, Chabot D, Paré I, Drouin M, Bazin R. MiR-146a potentially promotes IVIg-mediated inhibition of TLR4 signaling in LPS-activated human monocytes. Immunol Lett. 2017;185:64–73.

Massoud AH, Kaufman GN, Xue D, Béland M, Dembele M, Piccirillo CA, Mourad W, Mazer BD. Peripherally generated foxp3(+) regulatory T cells mediate the immunomodulatory effects of IVIg in allergic airways disease. J Immunol. 2017;198(7):2760–71.

Niknami M, Wang M-X, Nguyen T, Pollard JD. Beneficial effect of a multimerized immunoglobulin Fc in an animal model of inflammatory neuropathy (experimental autoimmune neuritis). J Peripher Nerv Syst. 2013;18(2):141–52.

Richard A, Corvol J-C, Debs R, Reach P, Tahiri K, Carpentier W, Gueguen J, Guillemot V, Labeyrie C, Adams D, Viala K, Cohen Aubart F. Transcriptome analysis of peripheral blood in chronic inflammatory demyelinating polyradiculoneuropathy patients identifies TNFR1 and TLR pathways in the IVIg response. Medicine. 2016;95(19):e3370.

Ritter C, Bobylev I, Lehmann HC. Chronic inflammatory demyelinating polyneuropathy (CIDP): change of serum IgG dimer levels during treatment with intravenous immunoglobulins. J Neuroinflammation. 2015;12(1):148.

Roopenian DC, Akilesh S. FcRn: the neonatal Fc receptor comes of age. Nat Rev Immunol. 2007;7(9):715–25.

Salama A, Mueller-Eckhardt C, Kiefel V. Effect of intravenous immunoglobulin in immune thrombocytopenia. Lancet (Lond Engl). 1983;2(8343):193–5.

Salama A, Kiefel V, Amberg R, Mueller-Eckhardt C. Treatment of autoimmune thrombocytopenic purpura with rhesus antibodies (anti-Rh0(D)). Blut. 1984;49(1):29–35.

Schwab I, Nimmerjahn F. Intravenous immunoglobulin therapy: how does IgG modulate the immune system? Nat Rev Immunol. 2013;13(3):176–89.

Siragam V, Brinc D, Crow AR, Song S, Freedman J, Lazarus AH. Can antibodies with specificity for soluble antigens mimic the therapeutic effects of intravenous IgG in the treatment of autoimmune disease? J Clin Invest. 2005;115(1):155–60.

Siragam V, Crow AR, Brinc D, Song S, Freedman J, Lazarus AH. Intravenous immunoglobulin ameliorates ITP via activating Fc gamma receptors on dendritic cells. Nat Med. 2006;12(6):688–92.

Teeling JL, Jansen-Hendriks T, Kuijpers TW, de Haas M, van de Winkel JG, Hack CE, Bleeker WK. Therapeutic efficacy of intravenous immunoglobulin preparations depends on the

immunoglobulin G dimers: studies in experimental immune thrombocytopenia. Blood. 2001;98(4):1095–9.
Tovo PA, Miniero R, Fiandino G, Saracco P, Messina M. Fc-depleted vs intact intravenous immunoglobulin in chronic ITP. J Pediatr. 1984;105(4):676–7.
Trinath J, Hegde P, Sharma M, Maddur MS, Rabin M, Vallat J-M, Magy L, Balaji KN, Kaveri SV, Bayry J. Intravenous immunoglobulin expands regulatory T cells via induction of cyclooxygenase-2-dependent prostaglandin E2 in human dendritic cells. Blood. 2013;122(8):1419–27.
von Gunten S, Shoenfeld Y, Blank M, Branch DR, Vassilev T, Käsermann F, Bayry J, Kaveri S, Simon H-U. IVIG pluripotency and the concept of Fc-sialylation: challenges to the scientist. Nat Rev Immunol. 2014;14(5):349.
Webster ML, Sayeh E, Crow M, Chen P, Nieswandt B, Freedman J, Ni H. Relative efficacy of intravenous immunoglobulin G in ameliorating thrombocytopenia induced by antiplatelet GPIIbIIIa versus GPIbalpha antibodies. Blood. 2006;108(3):943–6.
Yu X, Menard M, Prechl J, Bhakta V, Sheffield WP, Lazarus AH. Monovalent Fc receptor blockade by an anti-Fc receptor/albumin fusion protein ameliorates murine ITP with abrogated toxicity. Blood. 2016;127(1):132–8.
Zuercher AW, Spirig R, Baz Morelli A, Käsermann F. IVIG in autoimmune disease - potential next generation biologics. Autoimmun Rev. 2016;15(8):781–5.

7 Immunomodulatory Drugs and Monoclonal Antibodies

Howard A. Liebman

7.1 Immunity: Recognition of Nonself

The traditional classification of the human immune system divides the host response to external pathogens and transformed cells into innate immunity and adaptive immunity (Parkin and Cohen 2001). The innate immune system is comprised of neutrophils, monocytes, macrophages, dendritic cells, NK lymphocytes, and the plasma complement proteins. More recent definitions have expanded the innate immune system to include platelets, endothelium, and the coagulation cascade (Parkin and Cohen 2001; Blumberg et al. 2009; Mantovani et al. 1997; Loof et al. 2011). The innate immune system represents the first line of host defense against foreign pathogens. Innate immunity performs its immune surveillance function via Toll-like receptors which recognize conserved pathogen-associated molecular patterns (PAMPS) but also pattern-recognition receptors (PRRs) and NK receptors (Kawai and Akira 2011). The initial response of the innate immune systems feeds into and directs the subsequent responses of adaptive immunity by antigen processing and cytokine production (Parkin and Cohen 2001).

Adaptive immunity involves the expression of a targeted lymphoid response against foreign pathogens involving thymic (T) lymphocytes and antibody-producing B lymphocytes. The targeted responses of the adaptive immune system can further recruit and amplify the cellular responses of the innate immune system (Parkin and Cohen 2001). This is performed in large part by antibody-mediated pathogen clearance. Antibodies can also mediate complement lysis of pathogens in

H.A. Liebman, MA, MD
Jane Anne Nohl Division of Hematology and Center for the Study of Blood Diseases, Keck School of Medicine of the University of Southern California, Los Angeles, CA, USA

Norris Cancer Center, 1441 Eastlake Ave, Rm 3466, Los Angeles, CA 90033, USA
e-mail: Liebman@usc.edu; liebman_h@med.usc.edu

P. Imbach (ed.), *Antibody Therapy*, https://doi.org/10.1007/978-3-319-68038-5_7

addition to Fc-receptor phagocytosis of pathogens by neutrophils, monocytes, macrophages, and hepatic Kupffer cells. Also cytokines and immune-modulatory molecules produced by lymphocytes can activate and upregulate innate immune responses by activation of subtypes of monocytes and macrophages (Gordon and Taylor 2005). Cellular immune responses of the cytotoxic (CD8+) T lymphocytes can clear viral infected and transformed cells. Both antibody and cellular immune responses are regulated by antigen-specific helper/inducer (CD4+) T lymphocytes. The CD4 lymphocyte can also function as an effector cell, enhancing the intracellular macrophage killing of pathogens by the production of interferon-γ (Gordon and Taylor 2005).

7.2 Autoimmunity: Loss of Self-Tolerance

During the development of mature B and T cells, lymphoid precursors highly attracted to self-antigens are eliminated. Lymphocytes in the bone marrow will become B cells and those that enter the thymus will become T cells. As they are maturing, those cells that are self-reactive will undergo apoptosis, in a process that is called central tolerance. Most of the deletion of strongly self-reactive T lymphocytes occurs in the thymus (Palmer 2003; Sakaguchi 2004).

Most of the lymphocytes that recognize nonself (foreign) antigens will, therefore, enter the peripheral circulation occupying lymph nodes, spleen, and bone marrow where they will expand when they meet antigen. A few self-recognizing lymphocytes with low reactivity to self will also enter the peripheral circulation, where they will either remain inactive or be deleted when activated in order to prevent disease. This is called peripheral tolerance (Sakaguchi 2004; Takahashi and Nomura 2003). Peripheral tolerance is mediated in large part by natural and inducible T regulatory cells (T_{reg}) (Gordon and Taylor 2005; Palmer 2003; Sakaguchi 2004; Takahashi and Nomura 2003).

The existence of families with multiple individuals with autoimmune disorders, an increased risk of autoimmune disorders in siblings, and the pronounced increased risk of such disorders in identical twins strongly speaks to a genetic propensity for autoimmune diseases (Kuchroo et al. 2012; Gregersen and Behrens 2006). Murine and human genome-wide studies have found a number of genes associated with an increased risk of autoimmunity. While some genes are well known to be associated with immune regulation, genes in the major histocompatibility complex (MHC) region account for the greatest number of genetic associations with autoimmune disease (Rioux et al. 2009). Such changes in the MHC genes may account for the failure to delete some lower affinity self-reacting lymphocytes which can escape central deletion.

Environmental factors undoubtedly contribute to the development of autoimmunity. Even in identical twins, the incidence of autoimmune disorders is only 40–50% of the monozygotic sibling (Selmi et al. 2004). There are a number of environmental factors that have been shown capable of inducing autoimmune responses in genetically susceptible individuals. Epidemiologic studies have found associations between acute and chronic viral or bacterial infections, immunizations, environmental toxins, certain drugs, smoking, vitamin D deficiency, and even changes in the intestinal microbiome to potentially induce autoimmune disorders (Kuchroo et al. 2012; Gregersen and Behrens 2006; Kosiewicz et al. 2014).

The innate immune system also plays an important role in maintaining self-tolerance. However, an aberrant innate immune response to pathogens, drugs, toxins, or commensal microbiota can induce a severe inflammatory state presenting the adaptive immune system with autoantigens derived from damaged tissues and inducing an adaptive T- and B-lymphocyte autoimmune reaction. Under such circumstances the presence of inflammatory-induced co-stimulatory cytokines such as interleukin 6 (IL-6) and tumor necrosis factor-α (TNF-α) further drives the adaptive immune response by inhibiting T_{reg} suppressor function leading to a chronic autoimmune state (Kuchroo et al. 2012; Gregersen and Behrens 2006; Dissanayake et al. 2011).

In susceptible individuals, the induction of autoimmunity pushes the T-lymphocyte repertoire toward a pro-inflammatory state defined by a pattern of cytokines expressed by the subsets of thymic lymphocytes (Kuchroo et al. 2012; Gregersen and Behrens 2006). The inflammatory T_H1 CD4+ helper lymphocyte repertoire is defined by the production of interferon-γ, interleukin 2 (IL-2), and TNF. The T_H17 lymphocyte repertoire is defined by the secretion of IL-17 and IL-22. A third pro-inflammatory repertoire termed T_{FH} lymphocytes expresses the CD4+ inducible T-cell co-stimulator receptor and the C-X-C chemokine 5 receptor and secretes IL-21. T_{FH} lymphocytes support the expansion of autoantibody production. A T_H2 repertoire expresses the anti-inflammatory cytokine Il-10, along with IL-4, IL-5, IL-6, IL-9, and IL-13, which can invoke strong antibody responses and inhibit some neutrophil and macrophage effector functions (Del Prete 1998). Suppression of the pro-inflammatory lymphocyte repertoires requires reconstitution of T_{reg} suppressor function (Kuchroo et al. 2012; Gregersen and Behrens 2006; Sakaguchi et al. 2006).

The challenge for the clinician is to modulate the immune system in patients with autoimmune disease resulting in a therapeutic induced self-tolerance without inducing significant immune suppression, therefore, diminishing the patient's immune response to foreign pathogens and transformed cells. The heterogeneity of the underlying pathophysiology may account for the variable responses to many treatment regimens. In addition, the process of immunomodulation can in and of itself result in further disruption of immune tolerance resulting in the emergence on new autoimmune disorders. This can occur with immune suppression in patients with bone marrow or solid organ transplants (Minchinton and Waters 1985; Taylor et al. 2006). The recent use of the cytotoxic anti-CD52 monoclonal antibody, alemtuzumab, in multiple sclerosis has resulted in a surprisingly high incidence of autoimmune disorders suggesting that imbalance in T-lymphocyte recovery after significant lymphocyte depletion can lead to a loss of self-tolerance (Cuker et al. 2011; Daniels et al. 2014; Von Kutzleben et al. 2016; Jones et al. 2013).

7.3 Therapeutic Approaches to Immune Modulation

The development of immune-modulating therapies for induction of self-tolerance with transplantation and treatment of autoimmune disorders has progressed rapidly since the first reports by Schwartz and Dameshek on the induction of immune tolerance in rabbits with 6-mercaptopurine (Schwartz and Dameshek 1959, 1960). Only 4 years after their initial reports, they subsequently reported on the use of the drug for treatment of patients with autoimmune hemolytic anemia (Schwartz and Dameshek 1962). Most often designated as immunosuppress drugs, subsequent therapeutic agents have been developed that target one or more components of the immune system. They can be broadly defined as inhibitors of T-lymphocyte activation and proliferation, inhibitors of B-lymphocyte activation and proliferation, inhibitors of the innate immunity, inhibitors of immune cell trafficking, cytokine inhibitors, and drugs that deplete T or B lymphocytes or both (Table 7.1). In addition they can also be classified as cytotoxic drugs used to deplete broad or specific

Table 7.1 Targets of immune-modulating agents

T lymphocyte	B lymphocyte	Monocyte, macrophage	Inhibitors of cell trafficking	Cytokine and cytokine receptor inhibitors
Corticosteroids	Corticosteroids	Corticosteroids	Corticosteroids	Corticosteroids
6-Mercaptopurine	IVIG	IVIG	IVIG	IVIG
Azathioprine	6-Mercaptopurine	6-Mercaptopurine	Natalizumab	*TNF inhibitors*
Mycophenolate	Azathioprine	Azathioprine	Crizanlizumab[a]	Infliximab
Cyclophosphamide	Mycophenolate	Mycophenolate	GMI1070[b]	Adalimumab
Alemtuzumab	Cyclophosphamide	Cyclophosphamide		Golimumab
Cyclosporine	Alemtuzumab	Fostamatinib[c]		Certolizumab
Tacrolimus	Rituximab			*IL-1 inhibitors*
Sirolimus	Ofatumumab			Anakinra
Everolimus	Veltuzumab			Canakinumab
BI655064[d]	Ocrelizumab			Rilonacept
BMS98004[d]				*IL-12/23 inhibitors*
				Ustekinumab
				IL-6 inhibitors
				Tocilizumab
				IL-17 inhibitors
				Secukinumab
				Ixekizumab
				Brodalumab
				BAFF inhibitors
				Belimumab

[a]Crizanlizumab is a P selectin inhibitor in trial
[b]GMI 1070 is an E-selectin inhibitor in trial
[c]Fostamatinib is a Syk inhibitor in clinical trial
[d]BI655064 and BMS986004 are CD40 ligand inhibitors in clinical trial

cellular populations or agents that inhibit signaling pathways which can mediate their effect by blocking extracellular or intracellular targets. The contemporary repertoire of immune-modulating agents has expanded from such cytotoxic chemotherapeutic agents as cyclophosphamide, methotrexate, and 6-mercaptopurine to now include humanized monoclonal antibodies that either are lymphocyte cytotoxic, cytokine inhibitory, and cytokine receptor inhibitory or block important trafficking molecules for neutrophils, monocytes, or lymphocytes. In addition, there are an expanding number of small molecules that inhibit important intracellular signaling pathways in lymphocytes. These can be cytotoxic for selected lymphocyte cellular populations or downregulate lymphocyte cellular responses to activating signals.

7.4 Glucocorticosteroids

Glucocorticosteroids (GC) were the first (Hench et al. 1949) and remain one of the most important agents for the treatment of autoimmune disorders with the broadest spectrum of immune-modulatory effects (Van der Goes et al. 2014). The spectrum of their biologic effects can change with increasing doses. At low doses they affect immune cell trafficking, downregulate FcR expression on macrophages and neutrophils, and modulate cell signaling. With higher doses they can induce apoptosis of eosinophils and mast cells, inhibit dendritic cell differentiation, and suppress cytokine production from T lymphocytes, macrophages, endothelial cells, and smooth muscle cells. At very high doses, they can induce apoptosis of plasma cells and T and B lymphocytes. Corticosteroids can inhibit B-lymphocyte differentiation into plasma cells (Yan et al. 2015). Long-lived T-lymphocyte memory cells appear to be resistant to the cytotoxic effect of corticosteroids. A recently described subset of T lymphocytes termed IL-17 producing CD4/CD8 double-negative T lymphocytes were described in patients with Sjogren's syndrome. When studied this subpopulation of thymic lymphocytes was resistant to dexamethasone treatment when compared to CD4+ and CD8+ thymic lymphocytes (Alunno et al. 2013). This and other studies show that different subsets of T lymphocytes may have significant differences in their sensitivity to corticosteroids.

Compared to other immune-modulating agents, the onset of action by glucocorticoids can be very rapid. Upon binding to the glucocorticoid receptor (GR), the complex of the receptor with the glucocorticoid (GR/GC) is rapidly transported to the nucleus where it binds to the glucocorticoid binding sites for transcription of specific genes. Among such gene products are other transcription factors which work with the GR to induce transcription of additional gene products in what is termed a feed-forward gene regulatory loop (Meijsing et al. 2009; Psarra and Sekeris 2009; Sasse et al. 2013). In addition to its role in gene transcription, the GR/GC complex has direct and indirect effects on mitochondrial function and as yet unexplained cytoplasmic cellular effects.

7.5 Intravenous Immunoglobulin

Intravenous immunoglobulin (IVIG) was first shown to have immunomodulatory effects in the treatment of immune thrombocytopenia (Imbach et al. 1981; Newland et al. 1983). While most responses as a single agent are of short duration, longer duration responses were reported in an early trial on the treatment of ITP with repeated infusions for patients not candidates for splenectomy (Bussel et al. 1988). A number of possible mechanisms for the immune-modulatory effects of IVIG have been proposed using murine experimental models and translational studies of treated patients (Imbach et al. 2010). It is reasonable to assume that there are several different immune-modulatory mechanisms mediated by this complex mixture of antibodies, inclusive of immune complexes, anti-idiotypic antibodies, cytokines, and cellular receptors that can affect the underlying immunopathology for a variety of autoimmune disorders (Seite et al. 2008; Blasczyk et al. 1993). Its toxicities have been well characterized and maybe related to the patients' age, comorbidities, the rate of IVIG infusion, and the dose of IVIG used (Hamrock 2006). However, the lack of uniformity in most IVIG preparations could also explain the variability in therapeutic response. It is notable that when given in a 24-h continuous infusion combined with platelet transfusions, it induced sustained increases in platelet counts for refractory patients who previously failed to respond to IVIG (Chandramouli and Rodgers 2000; Olson et al. 2016). Other chapters in this volume will cover, in greater detail, the biologic and immune-modulatory effects of IVIG. However, it could be generalized that IVIG, after corticosteroids, is the broadest immunomodulatory agent affecting both the innate and adaptive immune system (Imbach et al. 2010).

IVIG has often been combined with other immunomodulatory agents. Not cytotoxic, IVIG immune-modulatory effects spare bone marrow function. It is often combined with corticosteroids in regimens for refractory ITP and autoimmune hemolytic anemia (Bussel et al. 1988; Boruchov et al. 2007; Barcellini et al. 2014). When combined with corticosteroids, the combination also appears to reduce the incidence and severity of unwanted IVIG toxicities such as infusion-associated reactions and aseptic meningitis. In the treatment of chronic ataxic neuropathy, IVIG has also been combined with rituximab (Loscher et al. 2013). Combination therapy for refractory ITP patients has also incorporated vincristine and azathioprine (Boruchov et al. 2007).

7.6 Cytotoxic Chemotherapeutic Agents

Cytotoxic agents such as cyclophosphamide (CTX), methotrexate (MTX), azathioprine (AZA), 6-mercaptopurine (6-MP), and mycophenolate mofetil (MMF) all demonstrate a broad spectrum of cellular cytotoxicity that can deplete T and B lymphocytes along with general bone marrow suppression. They also, in a dose-dependent manner, inhibit bone marrow production of important effectors of the innate immune system, neutrophils, and macrophages.

7.6.1 Cyclophosphamide

The immunologic effects of cyclophosphamide have been most extensively studied and have documented significant dose-related immune-modulating effects. Low doses of CTX can transiently suppress $CD4^{+}FOXP3^{+}$ T regulatory cells, shifting the CD4 T-lymphocyte repertoire toward a $T_{H}1$ inflammatory pattern (Ghiringhelli et al. 2007). Higher doses have a broader depletion of T and B lymphocytes. With higher doses the $FOXP3^{+}$regulatory T lymphocytes and hematopoietic stem cells are much more resistant to cyclophosphamide due to their increased expression of aldehyde dehydrogenase (Kanakry et al. 2013). Clinically, the superiority of high-dose intravenous CTX versus low-dose oral CTX for the treatment of autoimmune disorders has been clearly demonstrated in clinical trials on its use for the treatment of vasculitic disorders (de Groot et al. 2009). Complete remission was obtained with low doses of CTX when given as intravenous pulses (de Groot et al. 2009).

7.6.2 Methotrexate

Methotrexate, a dihydrofolate reductase inhibitor, was initially developed as an anti-neoplastic agent but is often used today as an immune modulator in rheumatoid arthritis and other autoimmune disorders. It rapidly induces apoptosis of activated lymphocytes. Lymphocytes in G0 or G1 phase of the cell cycle are resistant to the drugs cytotoxic effect (Genestier et al. 1998). This selective deletion of activated T lymphocytes may partially explain how MTX therapy in juvenile rheumatoid arthritis predominantly suppresses T effector cell activity but spares T regulatory cells (Calasan et al. 2015). Methotrexate is now most often used in combination therapy of rheumatoid arthritis but contributes to higher response which is associated with suppression of Th1/Th2 and Th17 phenotype with increase in T_{reg} number and function (Lina et al. 2011).

7.6.3 Azathioprine, 6-Mercaptopurine, and Mycophenolate

Less is known about the dose-related immunologic effects of 6-MP, AZA, and MMF on T-lymphocyte subsets. AZA, 6-MP, and MMF influence purine synthesis by inhibiting the proliferative response of lymphocytes to activating stimuli. AZA and 6-MP inhibit the first step of de novo purine synthesis suppressing both T and B lymphocytes. The antiproliferative effect is nonselective and can result in significant neutropenia from bone marrow suppression at higher doses (Maltzman and Koretzky 2003). MMF is more selective for lymphocyte suppression by both inhibiting purine synthesis and by competitive inhibition of inosine monophosphate dehydrogenase (IMPDH). Activated lymphocytes are highly dependent on the IMPDH salvage pathway for purine synthesis (Allison and Eugui 1996). Therefore, there is less direct bone morrow suppression and greater lymphocyte selectivity (Sollinger 1995).

In randomized trials to evaluate the efficacy of AZA and MMF in prevention of acute graft rejection after kidney transplantation, MMF has shown higher efficacy (Merion et al. 2000). However, there is no comparative data on the use of these agents in the treatment of autoimmune disease. Using these agents, response to treatment may require several months of therapy. A study on the treatment of immune thrombocytopenia (ITP) with AZA, response in some patients took up to 4 months (Quiquandon et al. 1990).

7.7 Monoclonal Antibodies

Monoclonal antibodies, targeting specific antigens on lymphocyte subsets, have proven to be important therapeutic agents for the treatment of various autoimmune disorders. The contemporary repertoire of therapeutic immune-modulating humanized monoclonal antibodies can be classified as either cytotoxic for subsets of lymphocytes or inhibitory of important cytokines or chemokines, their receptors, and important cellular trafficking molecules.

7.7.1 Cytotoxic Monoclonal Antibodies

The B-lymphocyte antigen, CD20, was the first target for the development of a humanized monoclonal antibody. This was antigen originally selected as a potential target for treatment of B-cell lymphomas. Rituximab, the first of these humanized monoclonal antibodies to target the CD20 antigen on B lymphocytes, has been successfully utilized in the treatment of a number of autoimmune disorders. There are case reports and Phase II clinical trials on its use in patients with autoimmune hemolytic anemia, immune thrombocytopenia, coagulation factor VIII inhibitors, thrombotic thrombocytopenic purpura, rheumatoid arthritis, vasculitis, cryoglobulinemia, multiple sclerosis, and neuromyelitis optica (Dierickx et al. 2015; Patel et al. 2012; Franchini and Lippi 2008; Coca and Sanz 2012; Cacoub et al. 2012; Rubenstein et al. 2006). However, in the United States, rituximab is only FDA approved for the treatment of rheumatoid arthritis in combination with methotrexate. It is frequently combined with corticosteroids and other immune-modulating agents when used to treat autoimmune disorders (Bussel et al. 2014; Gupta et al. 2002). What is notable in regard to these antibody-mediated disorders is that the pathogenic antibodies are IgG immunoglobulins, produced primarily by plasma cells which show minimal CD20 expression. Despite this, treatment responses, depending upon the specific immunopathic disorder, range from 20 to 80%. In ITP, studies by Stasi and colleagues found that specific changes in the T-lymphocyte repertoire best define those patients who obtain a complete response to rituximab treatment compared to patients who failed to respond (Stasi et al. 2007, 2008). Increases in $CD4^{+}FOXP3^{+}$ T regulatory cells number and function are seen in the patients who obtain long-term complete remissions (Stasi et al. 2007, 2008). This effect may be due to modulation or B- and T-lymphocyte cross talk or depletion of

B lymphocytes as antigen-presenting cells. The later mechanism may be favored since anti-CD20 therapy given to adult ITP patients in the first year after diagnosis appears to be associated with a higher rate of complete response. This was further supported by a Phase II trial of a subcutaneous anti-CD20 humanized monoclonal antibody, veltuzumab, which showed a higher response to patients treated in the first year (Liebman et al. 2013). The anti-CD20 humanized monoclonal antibody, ocrelizumab, has recently been FDA approved for the treatment of primary progressive multiple sclerosis, becoming only the second humanized B-cell-depleting monoclonal to be FDA approved to treat nonmalignant autoimmune disorders (Montalban et al. 2017).

Alemtuzumab is a humanized monoclonal antibody that binds to the CD52 antigen present on most mature lymphocytes. It rapidly depletes both T and B lymphocytes and was originally approved in the United States for the treatment of refractory chronic lymphocytic leukemia. A number of case reports and small clinical trials have documented its use in several autoimmune disorders (Ru and Liebman 2003; Gomez-Almaguer et al. 2010). Recently, alemtuzumab was approved in the United States and Europe for the treatment of relapsing-remitting multiple sclerosis with significant clinical superiority over β-interferon 1a (Cohen et al. 2012). However, an unexpected late complication of this highly effective therapy has been the development of a variety of autoimmune disorders. Over a third of patients develop immune thyroid disease, most often Grave's disease, which is distinctly different from the pattern of thyroid disease that develops in the general population (Daniels et al. 2014; Weetman 2014). Also cases of immunopathic renal disease have been observed which include membranous glomerulonephritis and anti-GBM antibody disease (Goodpasture's disease) (Clatworthy et al. 2008). In 2% of patients treated in the clinical trials, acute decreases in platelet counts consistent with ITP were observed, beginning 14–36 months after the last injection of alemtuzumab (Cuker et al. 2011). These ITP cases all responded to standard ITP first-line therapies and all appeared to develop unmaintained remissions similar to pediatric ITP patients. The occurrence of the late development of other autoimmune disorders, despite effective control of the patients' multiple sclerosis, suggests that the potent lymphoid depletion by alemtuzumab results in a prolonged and significant defect in peripheral immune tolerance that can persist for years after treatment.

7.7.2 Noncytotoxic Immune-Modulating Monoclonal Antibodies

A number of humanized monoclonal antibodies have been developed to bind to and inhibit inflammatory cytokines or their receptors. The first initial therapeutic target was tumor necrosis factor-alpha (TNF-α). TNF is a broad family of potent cytokines central to systemic inflammation (Aggarwal 2003). It is produced by activated cells of the innate immune system including macrophages, neutrophils, eosinophils, NK cells, and mast cells. Inappropriate expression has been linked to a number of inflammatory autoimmune disorders such as rheumatoid arthritis, Crohn's disease, ulcerative colitis, and psoriasis (Rutgeerts et al. 2005). The first of these antibodies, infliximab, which targets TNFα, has documented efficacy in inflammatory bowel disease, rheumatoid arthritis, psoriasis, and ankylosing spondylitis (Aggarwal 2003; Rutgeerts et al. 2005; Sands et al. 2004; Maini et al. 1999; Fong et al. 2016). Golimumab, adalimumab, and certolizumab are the second, third, and fourth anti-TNF-α inhibitory antibodies with the same general clinical indications as infliximab (Hibi et al. 2017; Colombel et al. 2007; Weinblatt et al. 2017). Adalimumab was the first totally humanized monoclonal therapeutic antibody, but except for this structural difference, there appear to be no significant therapeutic advantages to this antibody over the other two approved TNF-α inhibitory antibodies. A TNF receptor fusion protein, etanercept, acts as a competitive inhibitor of TNF binding to its receptor and is a therapeutic alternative to direct TNF inhibition.

The next generation of inhibitory antibodies targeted interleukin 1 (IL-1). IL-1 is produced by cells of the innate immune system, macrophages, monocytes, fibroblasts, and dendritic cells. It may also be produced by endothelial cells, NK cells, and B lymphocytes. There are 11 members of the IL-1 cytokine family, with IL-1 alpha and IL-1 beta being the most often studied (Garlanda et al. 2013). IL-1 is a central mediator of the inflammatory response of the body against infection. It induces expression of adhesion molecules on endothelial cells which results in neutrophil and monocyte adhesion to the vessel wall, rolling, and diapedesis into tissues. It is also the major inducer of TNF and the febrile response to infection. Canakinumab was the first FDA-approved humanized monoclonal directed against IL-1 beta to treat auto-inflammatory syndromes such as cryopyrin-associated periodic syndromes and more recently to treat juvenile rheumatoid arthritis (Kuemmerle-Deschner et al. 2016; Orrock and Ilowite 2016). The antibody also has documented efficacy in familial Mediterranean fever and other rare inflammatory syndrome (Kucuksahin et al. 2017; Gattorno et al. 2017). Similar to the TNF receptor competitive inhibitor, etanercept, interleukin 1 receptor competitive inhibitors, anakinra and rilonacept, have also demonstrated activity in the treatment of rheumatoid arthritis and other inflammatory disorders.

Therapeutic inhibitory humanized monoclonal antibodies inhibitory of interleukin 6 (IL-6), tocilizumab; inhibitory of interleukin 17 (IL-17), secukinumab, ixekizumab, and brodalumab; inhibitory of the interleukin 12/23 complex (IL12/23), ustekinumab; and inhibitory of B-cell-activating factor (BAFF), belimumab, are now approved for various immunopathic disorders.

Tocilizumab has demonstrated therapeutic efficacy in rheumatoid arthritis (Teitsma et al. 2016) and giant cell arteritis (Ostrowsk et al. 2014). Secukinumab, ixekizumab, and brodalumab have FDA approval and efficacy in the treatment of refractory psoriasis and psoriatic arthritis (Mease 2015; Mease et al. 2016, 2017). Ustekinumab by inhibition of IL12/23 downregulates the production of IL17 (Mease 2015). Therefore, it is not surprising that it has similar efficacy in the treatment of psoriasis and psoriatic arthritis (Kavanaugh et al. 2016). Belimumab is the first immune-modulating therapy approved for the treatment of systemic lupus erythematosus (Lutalo and D'Cruz 2014). The antibody also shows promise in the treatment of primary Sjogren's disease (Mariette et al. 2015).

7.8 Inhibitory Drugs of T-Lymphocyte Function

Calcineurin inhibitors, cyclosporine and tacrolimus, inhibit the calcineurin-mediated dephosphorylation the transcription factor nuclear factor of activated T cells (NF-AT), which is necessary for interleukin (IL)-2 transcription and T-cell activation. The potent T-lymphocyte suppression has made these drugs the primary therapeutic agents for preventing graft rejection for solid organ and bone marrow transplants (Wiederrecht et al. 1993). They have been used in a number of small studies for the treatment of autoimmune disorders, but their toxicities and inability to induce long-term remissions in most patients have limited their use. In refractory ITP low-dose cyclosporine (2–3 mg/kg) in several small case series could induce remissions in 40–50% of patients treated (Gesundheit et al. 2001; Kappers-Klunne and van't Veer 2001; Choi et al. 2015). However, approximately 70% of patients relapse after drug withdrawal. The addition of cyclosporine to combination regimens appears to enhance responsiveness in patients with refractory ITP (Choi et al. 2015).

Sirolimus and everolimus are inhibitors of the mTOR pathway through which a number of cytokines induce cell proliferation. Sirolimus blocks the T-lymphocyte proliferative stimulus of Il-2. However, the drug has a differential effect on T-lymphocyte subsets and appears to have little suppressive effects on the in $CD4^+FOXP3^+$ T regulatory cells (Shan et al. 2014). This may be an important role of the drug in its use for the treatment of graft versus host disease following allogeneic bone marrow transplant. Only a few case reports and case series have been published on the use of sirolimus for autoimmune disorders, the majority in pediatric disorders (Miano et al. 2014; Chatrath et al. 2014). However, a recent report has suggested an important role for the mTOR pathway in the pathophysiology of the antiphospholipid antibody syndrome (Canaud et al. 2014).

7.9 Summary

The increasing number of therapeutic agents for autoimmune disorders has significantly improved the outcomes for many patients but has resulted in only a small number of sustained unmaintained remissions. The variability of treatment outcomes to individual agents has clearly heterogeneous. As suggested by Cines and colleagues, many autoimmune disorders, like immune thrombocytopenia, should best be termed a syndrome and not a disease (Cines et al. 2009). Unraveling the heterogeneity of the various autoimmune disorders should result in better selection of therapeutic agents for the treatment of such patients.

References

Aggarwal BB. Signalling pathways of the TNF superfamily: a double-edged sword. Nat Rev Immunol. 2003;3:745–56.

Allison AC, Eugui EM. Purine metabolism and immunosuppressive effects of mycophenolate mofetil (MMF). Clin Transpl. 1996;10:77–84.

Alunno A, Bistoni O, Bartoloni E, Catebi S, Bigerna B, et al. Il-17 producing CD4⁻CD8⁻ cells are expanded in peripheral blood, infiltrate salivary glands and are resistant to corticosteroids in patients with primary Sjogren's syndrome. Ann Rheum Dis. 2013;72:2865–292.

Barcellini W, Fattizzo B, Zaninoni A, Radice T, Nichele I, et al. Clinical heterogeneity and predictors of outcome in primary autoimmune hemolytic anemia: a GIMEMA study of 308 patients. Blood. 2014;124:2930–6.

Blasczyk R, Westhoff U, Grosse-Wilde H. Soluble CD4, Cd8, and HLA molecules in commercial immunoglobulin preparations. Lancet. 1993;341:789–90.

Blumberg N, Spinelli SL, Francis CW, Taubman MB, Phipps RP. The platelet as an immune cell. CD40 ligand and transfusion immunomodulation. Immunol Res. 2009;45:251–60.

Boruchov DM, Gururangan S, Dirscoll MC, Bussel JB. Multiagent induction and maintenance therapy for patients with refractory immune thrombocytopenic purpura (ITP). Blood. 2007;110:3526–31.

Bussel JB, Pharm LC, Aledort L, Nachman R. Maintenance treatment of adults with chronic refractory immune thrombocytopenic purpura using repeated intravenous infusions of gammaglobulin. Blood. 1988;72:121–7.

Bussel JB, Lee CS, Seery C, Lmahiyerobo AA, Thompson MV, et al. Rituximab and three dexamethasone cycles provide responses similar to splenectomy in women with immune thrombocytopenia of less than two years. Haematologica. 2014;99:1264–71.

Cacoub P, Comarmond C, Domont F, Savey L, Saadoun D. Cryoglobulinemia Vasculitis. Am J Med. 2012;128:950–5.

Calasan MB, Vastert SJ, Scholman RC, Verweij F, Klein M, et al. Methrotrexate treatment affects effector but not regulatory T cells in juvenile idiopathic arthritis. Rheumatology. 2015;54:1724–34.

Canaud G, Bienaime F, Tabarin F, Bataillon G, Seilhean D, Noel LH, et al. Inhibition of the mTORC pathway in the antiphospholipid syndrome. N Engl J Med. 2014;371:303–12.

Chandramouli NB, Rodgers GM. Prolonged immunoglobulin and platelet infusion for treatment of immune thrombocytopenia. Am J Hematol. 2000;65:85–6.

Chatrath H, Allen L, Boyer TD. Use of sirolimus in the treatment of refractory autoimmune hepatitis. Am J Med. 2014;127:1128–31.

Choi PY, Roncolato F, Badoux X, Ramanathan S, Ho SJ, Chong BH. A novel triple therapy for ITP using high-dose dexamethasone, low-dose rituximab, and cyclosporine (TT4). Blood. 2015;126:500–3.

Cines DB, Bussel JB, Liebman HA, Luning Prak ET. The ITP syndrome: a diverse set of disorders with different immune mechanisms. Blood. 2009;113:6511–21.

Clatworthy MR, Wallin EF, Jayne DR. Antiglomerular basement membrane disease after alemtuzumab. N Engl J Med. 2008;359:768–9.

Coca A, Sanz I. Updates on B-cell immunotherapies for systemic lupus erythematosus and Sjogren's syndrome. Curr Opin Rheumtol. 2012;24:451–6.

Cohen JA, Coles AJ, Arnold DL, Confavreux C, Fox EJ, et al. Alemtuzumab for patients with relapsing multiple sclerosis after disease-modifying therapy: a randomised controlled phase 3 trial. Lancet. 2012;380:1819–28.

Colombel JF, Sandborn WJ, Rutgeerts P, et al. Adalimumab for maintenance of clinical response and remission in patients with Crohn's disease: the CHARM trial. Gastroenterology. 2007;132:52–65.

Cuker A, Coles AJ, Sullivan H, Fox E, Goldberg M, et al. A distinctive form of immune thrombocytopenia in a phase 2 study of alemtuzumab for the treatment of relapsing-remitting multiple sclerosis. Blood. 2011;118:6299–305.

Daniels GH, Vladic A, Brinar V, Zavalishin I, Valente W, et al. Alemtuzumab-related thyroid dysfunction in a phase 2 trial of patients with relapsing-remitting multiple sclerosis. J Clin Endocrinol Metab. 2014;99:80–9.

de Groot K, Harper L, Jayne DR, Flores Suarez LF, Gregorini G, Gross WL, et al. Pulse versus daily oral cyclophosphamide for induction of remission in antineutrophil cytoplasmic antibody-associated vasculitis: a randomized trial. Ann Intern Med. 2009;150:670–80.

Del Prete G. The concept of type-1 and type-2 helper T cells and their cytokines in humans. Int Rev Immunol. 1998;16:427–55.

Dierickx D, Kentos A, Delannoy A. The role of rituximab in adults with warm antibody autoimmune hemolytic anemia. Blood. 2015;125:3223–9.

Dissanayake D, Hall H, Brown NB, Elford AR, Hamilton SR, Murakami K, et al. Nuclear factor-κB1 controls the functional maturation of dendritic cells and prevents the activation of autoreactive T cells. Nat Med. 2011;17:1663–7.

Fong W, Holroyd C, Davidson B, Armstrong R, Harvey N, et al. The effectiveness of a real life dose reduction strategy for tumour necrosis factor inhibitors in ankylosing spondylitis and psoriatic arthritis. Rheumatology. 2016;55:1837–42.

Franchini M, Lippi G. Acquired factor VIII inhibitors. Blood. 2008;112:250–5.

Garlanda C, Dinarello CA, Mantovani A. The interleukin-1 family: back to the future. Immunity. 2013;39:1003–18.

Gattorno M, Obici L, Cattalini M, Tormey V, Abrams K, et al. Canakinumab reverses overexpression of inflammatory response genes in tumour necrosis factor receptor-associated periodic syndrome. Ann Rheum Dis. 2017;76:303–9.

Genestier L, Paillot R, Bonnefoy-Bernard N, Meffre G, Flacher M, et al. Immunosuppressive properties of methotrexate: apoptosis and clonal deletion of activated peripheral T cells. J Clin Invest. 1998;102:322–8.

Gesundheit B, Cividalli G, Freeman A, Yatziv S, Koren G, Baruchel S. Cyclosporin A in the treatment of refractory immune thrombocytopenia purpura in children. Eur J Haematol. 2001;66:347–51.

Ghiringhelli F, Menard C, Puig PE, Ladoire S, Roux S, Martin F, Solary E, et al. Metronomic cyclophosphamide regimen selectively depletes CD4+CD25+ regulatory T cells and restores T and NK effector functions in end stage cancer patients. Cancer Immunol Immunother. 2007;56:641–8.

Gomez-Almaguer D, Solano-Genesta M, Tarin-Arzaga L, Herrera-Garza JL, Cantu-Rodriguez OG, et al. Low dose rituximab and alemtuzumab combination therapy for patient with steroid-refractory autoimmune cytopenias. Blood. 2010;116:4783–5.

Gordon S, Taylor PR. Monocyte and macrophage heterogeneity. Nat Rev Immunol. 2005;5:953–64.

Gregersen PK, Behrens TW. Genetics of autoimmune diseases-disorders of immune homeostasis. Nat Rev Genet. 2006;7:917–28.

Gupta N, Kavuru S, Patel D, Janson D, Driscoll N, et al. Rituximab-based chemotherapy for steroid-refractory autoimmune hemolytic anemia of chronic lymphocytic leukemia. Leukemia. 2002;16:2092–5.

Hamrock DJ. Adverse events associated with intravenous immunoglobulin therapy. Int Immunopharamacol. 2006;6:535–42.

Hench PS, Kendall EC, Slocumb CH, Polley HF. The effect of a hormone of the adrenal cortex (17-hydroxy-11-dehydrocorterone compound E) and pituitary adrenocorticotropic hormone on rheumatoid arthritis. Mayo Clin Proc. 1949;24:181–97.

Hibi T, Imai Y, Senoo A, Ohta K, Ukyo Y. Efficacy and safety of golimumab 52-week maintenance therapy in Japanese patients with moderate to severely active ulcerative colitis: a phase 3, double-blind, randomized, placebo-controlled study-(PURSUIT-J study*)*. J Gastroenterol. 2017;03:21.

Imbach P, Barandun S, d'Apuzzo V, Baumgartner C, Hirt A, et al. High-dose intravenous immunoglobulin for idiopathic thrombocytopenic purpura in childhood. Lancet. 1981;1:1228–31.

Imbach P, Lazarus AH, Kuhne T. Intravenous immunoglobulins induce potentially synergistic immunomodulations in autoimmune disorders. Vox Sang. 2010;98:385–94.

Jones JL, Thompson SAJ, Loh P, Davies JL, Tuohy OC, et al. Human autoimmunity after lymphocyte depletion is causes by homeostatic T-cell proliferation. PNAS. 2013;110:20200–5.

Kanakry DG, Ganguly S, Zhurak M, Bolanos-Meade J, Thoburn C, et al. Aldehyde dehydrogenase expression drives human regulatory T cell resistance to posttransplantation cyclophosphamide. Sci Transl Med. 2013;5:211ra157.

Kappers-Klunne MC, van't Veer MB. Cyclosporin A for the treatment of patients with chronic idiopathic thrombocytopenic purpura refractory to corticosteroids or splenectomy. Br J Haematol. 2001;114:121–5.

Kavanaugh A, Puig L, Gottlieb AB, Ritchlin C, You Y, et al. Efficacy and safety of ustekinumab in psoriatic arthritis patients with peripheral arthritis and physician-reported spondylitis: post-hoc analyses from two phase III, multicentre, double-blind, placebo-controlled studies (PSUMMIT-1/PSUMMIT-2). Ann Rheum Dis. 2016;75:1984–8.

Kawai T, Akira S. Toll-like receptors and their crosstalk with other innate receptors in infection and immunity. Immunity. 2011;34:637–50.

Kosiewicz MM, Dryden GW, Chhabra A, Alard P. Relationship between gut microbiota and development of T cell associated disease. FEBS Lett. 2014;588:4195–206.

Kuchroo V, Ohashi PS, Sartor RB, Vinuesa CG. Dysregulation of immune homeostasis in autoimmune disease. Nat Med. 2012;18:42–7.

Kucuksahin O, Yildizgoren MT, Ilgen U, Ates A, Kinikli G, et al. Anti-interleukin-1 treatment in 26 patients with refractory familial mediterranean fever. Mod Rheumatol. 2017;27:350–5.

Kuemmerle-Deschner JB, Hofer F, Endres T, Kortus-Goetze B, Blank N, Weisbarth-Riedel E, et al. Real-life effectiveness of canakinumab in cryopyrin-associated periodic syndrome. Rheumatology. 2016;55:689–96.

Liebman HA, Saleh MN, Bussel JB, Negrea OG, Horne H, Wegener WA, Goldenberg DM. Low-dose anti-CD20 veltuzumab given intravenously or subcutaneously is active in relapsed immune thrombocytopenia: a phase I study. Br J Haematol. 2013;162:693–701.

Lina C, Conghua W, Nan L, Ping Z. Combined treatment of etanercept and MTX reverses Th1/Th2, Th17/Treg imbalance in patients with rheumatoid arthritis. J Clin Immunol. 2011;31:596–605.

Loof TG, Morgelin M, Johansson L, Oehmcke S, Olin AI, Dickneite G, et al. Coagulation, an ancestral serine protease cascade, exerts a novel function in early immune defense. Blood. 2011;118:2589–98.

Loscher WN, Woertz A, Wallnofer M, Wanschitz JV, Luef G. Successful treatment of CANOMAD with IVIg and rituximab. J Neurol. 2013;260:1168–70.

Lutalo PM, D'Cruz DP. Update on belimumab for the management of systemic lupus erythematosus. Expert Opin Biol Ther. 2014;14:1701–8.

Maini R, St Clair EW, Breedveld F, et al. Infliximab (chimeric anti-tumour necrosis factor alpha monoclonal antibody) versus placebo in rheumatoid arthritis patients receiving concomitant methotrexate: a randomised phase III trial. ATTRACT Study Group. Lancet. 1999;354:1932–9.

Maltzman JS, Koretzky GA. Azathioprine: old drug, new actions. J Clin Invest. 2003;111:1122–4.

Mantovani A, Bussolino M, Introna M. Cytokine regulation of endothelial function: from molecular level to the bedside. Immunol Today. 1997;18:231–40.

Mariette X, Seror R, Quartuccio L, Baron G, Salvin S, et al. Efficacy and safety of belimumab in primary Sjogren's syndrome: results of the BELISS open-label phase II study. Ann Rheum Dis. 2015;74:526–31.

Mease PJ. Inhibition of interleukin-17, interleukin-23 and the TH17 cell pathway in the treatment of psoriatic arthritis and psoriasis. Curr Opin Rheumatol. 2015;27:127–33.

Mease PJ, Genovese MC, Mutebi A, Viswanathan HN, Chau D, et al. Improvement in psoriasis signs and symptoms assessed by the psoriasis symptom inventory with brodalumab treatment in patients with psoriatic arthritis. J Rheumatol. 2016;43:343–9.

Mease PJ, van der Heijde D, Ritchlin CT, Okada M, Cuchacovich RS, et al. Ixekizumab, an interleukin-17A specific monoclonal antibody, for the treatment of biologic-naïve patients with active psoriatic arthritis: results from the 24-week randomised, double-blind, placebo-controlled and active (adalimumab)-controlled period of the phase III trial SPIRIT-P1. Ann Rheum Dis. 2017;76:79–87.

Meijsing SH, Pufall MA, So AY, Bates DL, Chen L, Yamamoto KR. DNA binding site sequence directs glucocorticoid receptor structure and activity. Science. 2009;324:407–10.

Merion RM, Henry ML, Melzer JS, Sollinger H, et al. Randomized, prospective trial of mycophenolate mofetil versus azathioprine for prevention of acute renal allograft rejection after simultaneous kidney-pancreas transplantation. Transplantation. 2000;70:105–11.

Miano M, Calvillo M, Palmisani E, Fioredda F, Micalizzi C, Svahn J, et al. Sirolimus for the treatment of multi-resistant autoimmune haemolytic anaemia in children. Br J Haematol. 2014;167:571–4.

Minchinton RM, Waters AH. Autoimmune thrombocytopenia and neutropenia after bone marrow transplantation. Blood. 1985;66:752–3.
Montalban X, Hauser SL, Kappos L, Arnold DL, Bar-Or A, et al. Ocrelizumab versus placebo in primary progressive multiple sclerosis. N Engl J Med. 2017;376:209–20.
Newland AC, Trealeaven JG, Minchinton RM, Waters AH. High-dose intravenous IgG in adults with autoimmune thrombocytopenia. Lancet. 1983;1:84–7.
Olson SR, Chu C, Shatzel JJ, Deloughery TG. The platelet "boilermaker": a treatment protocol to rapidly increase platelets in patients with immune thrombocytopenia. Am J Hematol. 2016. https://doi.org/10.1002/ajh.24409.
Orrock JE, Ilowite NT. Canakinumab for the treatment of active systemic juvenile idiopathic arthritis. Expert Rev Clin Pharmacol. 2016;9:1015–24.
Ostrowsk RA, Bussey MR, Tehrani R, Jay W. Biologic therapy for therapy for the treatment of giant cell arteritis. Neuro-Ophthalmology. 2014;38:107–12.
Palmer E. Negative selection—clearing out the bad apples from the T-cell repertoire. Nat Rev Immunol. 2003;3:383–91.
Parkin J, Cohen B. An overview of the immune system. Lancet. 2001;357:1777–89.
Patel VL, Mahevas M, Lee SY, Stasi R, Cunningham-Rundles S, Godeau B, et al. Outcomes 5 years after response to rituximab therapy in children and adults with immune thrombocytopenia. Blood. 2012;119:5989–95.
Psarra AMG, Sekeris CE. Glucocorticoid receptors and other nuclear transcription factors in mitochondria and possible functions. Biochim Biophys Acta. 2009;1787:431–6.
Quiquandon I, Fenaux P, Caulier MT, Pagniez D, Huart JJ, Bauters F. Re-evaluation of the role of azathioprine in the treatment of adult chronic idiopathic thrombocytopenic purpura: a report on 53 cases. Br J Haematol. 1990;74:223–8.
Rioux JC, Goyette P, Vyse TJ, Hammarström L, Fernando MMA, Green T, et al. Mapping of multiple susceptibility variants within the MHC region for 7 immune-mediated diseases. Proc Natl Acad Sci U S A. 2009;106:18680–5.
Ru J, Liebman HA. Successful treatment of refractory pure red cell aplasia associated with lymphoproliferative disorders with the anti-CD52 monoclonal antibody alemtuzumab (CAMPATH-1H). Br J Haematol. 2003;123:278–81.
Rubenstein E, Arkfeld DG, Metyas S, Shinada S, Liebman HA. Rituximab treatment for resistant antiphospholipid syndrome. J Rheumatol. 2006;33:355–7.
Rutgeerts P, Sandborn WJ, Feagan BG, et al. Infliximab for induction and maintenance therapy for ulcerative colitis. N Engl J Med. 2005;353:2462–76.
Sakaguchi S. Naturally arising CD4+ regulatory T cells for immunologic self-tolerance and negative control of immune responses. Annu Rev Immunol. 2004;22:531–62.
Sakaguchi S, Ono M, Setoguchi R, Yagi H, Hori S, Fehervari Z, et al. Foxp3^{+}CD25^{+} CD4^{+} natural regulatory cells in dominant self-tolerance and autoimmune disease. Immunol Rev. 2006;212:8–27.
Sands BE, Anderson FH, Bernstein CN, et al. Infliximab maintenance therapy for fistulizing Crohn's disease. N Engl J Med. 2004;350:876–85.
Sasse SK, Mailloux CM, Barczak AJ, Wang Q, Altonsy MO, Jain MK, et al. The glucocorticoid receptor and KLF15 regulate gene expression dynamics and integrate signals through feed-forward circuitry. Mol Cell Biol. 2013;33:2104–15.
Schwartz R, Dameshek W. Drug-induced immune tolerance. Nature. 1959;183:1682–3.
Schwartz R, Dameshek W. The effect of 6-mercaptopurine on homograft reactions. J Clin Invest. 1960;39:952–9588.
Schwartz R, Dameshek W. Treatment of autoimmune hemolytic anemia with 6-mercaptopurine and thioguanine. Blood. 1962;19:483–500.
Seite JF, Shoenfeld Y, Youinou P, Hillion S. What is the content of the magic draft IVIg? Autoimmun Rev. 2008;7:432–9.
Selmi C, Mayo MJ, Bach N, Ishibashi H, Invernizzi P, Gish RG, et al. Primary biliary cirrhosis in monozygotic and dizygotic twins: genetics, epigenetics, and environment. Gastroenterology. 2004;127:485–92.

Shan J, Feng L, Li Y, Sun G, Chen X, Chen P. The effects of rapamycin on regulatory T cells: its potential time-dependent role in inducing transplant tolerance. Immunol Lett. 2014;182:74–86.
Sollinger HW, For the U.S. Renal Transplant Mycophenolate Mofetil Study Group. Mycophenolate mofetil for the prevention of acute rejection in primary cadaveric renal allograft recipients. Transplantation. 1995;60:225–35.
Stasi R, Del Poeta G, Stipa E, Evangelista ML, Trawinska MM, Cooper N, et al. Response to B-cell depleting therapy with rituximab reverts the abnormalities of T-cell subsets in patients with idiopathic thrombocytopenic purpura. Blood. 2007;110:2924–30.
Stasi R, Cooper N, Del Poeta G, Stipa E, Laura Evangelista M, Abruzzese E, et al. Analysis of regulatory T-cell changes in patients with idiopathic thrombocytopenic purpura receiving B cell-depleting therapy with rituximab. Blood. 2008;112:1147–50.
Takahashi T, Nomura T. Foxp3+CD25+CD4+ natural regulatory T cells in dominant self-tolerance and autoimmune disease. Immunol Rev. 2003;212:8–27.
Taylor RM, Bockenstedt P, Su GL, Marrero JA, Pelliter SM, et al. Immune thrombocytopenic purpura following liver transplantation: a case series and review of the literature. Liver Transpl. 2006;12:781–91.
Teitsma XM, Marijnissen AKA, Bijlsma JWJ, Lafeber FPJ, Jacobs JWG. Tocilizumab as monotherapy or combination therapy for treating active rheumatoid arthritis: a meta-analysis of efficacy and safety reported in randomized controlled trials. Arthritis Res Ther. 2016;18:211–24.
Van der Goes MC, Jacobs JW, Bijlsma JW. The value of glucocorticoid co-therapy in different rheumatic diseases-positive and adverse effects. Arthritis Res Ther. 2014;16(Suppl 2):1–13.
Von Kutzleben S, Pryce G, Giovannoni G, Baker D. Depletion of CD52-positive cells inhibits the development of central nervous system autoimmune disease, but depletes an immune-tolerance promoting CD8 T-cell population. Implications for secondary autoimmunity of alemtuzumab in multiple sclerosis. Immunology. 2016;150:444–55.
Weetman AP. Graves' disease following immune reconstitution or immunomodulatory treatment: should we manage it any differently? Clin Endocrinol. 2014;80:629–32.
Weinblatt ME, Bingham CO 3rd, Burmester G-R, Bykerk VP, Furst DE, et al. A phase 3 study evaluating continuation, tapering, and withdrawal of certolizumab pegol after 1 year of therapy in early rheumatoid arthritis patients. Arthritis Rheumatol. 2017. (print online).
Wiederrecht G, Lam E, Hung S, Martin M, Sigal N. The mechanism of action of FK-506 and cyclosporin A. Ann N Y Acad Sci. 1993;696:9–19.
Yan S, Xigo-mei D, Wang Q-T, Sun X-J, Wei W. Prednisone treatment inhibits the differentiation of B lymphocytes into plasma cells in MRL/MpSlac lpr mice. Acta Pharmacol Sin. 2015;36:1367–1376.

Use of Intravenous Immunoglobulin in Neurology

8

Marinos C. Dalakas

8.1 Introduction

Intravenous immunoglobulin (IVIG), a pooled of polyclonal IgG from the serum of thousands of donors, has been used as an anti-inflammatory and immunomodulating agent for the treatment of several autoimmune diseases. It has played a fundamental role in the treatment of several autoimmune neurological disorders with at least three indications approved by regulatory agencies and with established efficacy in additional neurological diseases based on controlled studies. The first indication was in 2008, for chronic inflammatory demyelinating polyneuropathy (CIDP), followed by Guillain-Barre syndrome (in Europe and Asia) and then multifocal motor neuropathy (MMN) (Lunneman et al. 2015a, b; Hughes et al. 2009). In this review, I will provide a summary on the current use of IVIG in neurological diseases based on controlled studies, highlight the autoimmune rationale for using IVIg based on the underlying pathophysiology, and briefly mention some of the ongoing studies.

The clear and sometimes dramatic benefit exerted by IVIg in certain neurological disorders has inevitably led to a rather liberal use of the drug even for diseases where the data is weak or not evidence based, generating difficulties with insurance carriers even for diseases with clear indications. Most importantly, we are now witnessing the continuous use of IVIg for patients who may not anymore need it because the disease has been put into remission or in a chronic stability status after several monthly IVIg infusions. Until biomarkers of disease activity are identified,

M.C. Dalakas, MD, FAAN
Department of Neurology, Thomas Jefferson University, Philadelphia, PA, USA

Neuroimmunology Unit, Department of Pathophysiology, National and Kapodistrian University of Athens Medical School, Athens, Greece
e-mail: marinos.dalakas@jefferson.edu; mdalakas@med.uoa.gr

P. Imbach (ed.), *Antibody Therapy*, https://doi.org/10.1007/978-3-319-68038-5_8

periodic assessments are now advocated for these patients to establish their need for continuous immunotherapy, by tapering the IVIg dose or temporarily stopping IVIg to ensure its judicious use for continuous chronic long-term therapy (Lunneman et al. 2015a, b).

8.2 Evidence from Controlled Trials

8.2.1 Guillain-Barre Syndrome (GBS)

8.2.1.1 Definition and Pathophysiology

This is an acute demyelinating polyneuropathy that causes weakness or paralysis of the limbs and respiratory muscles within 2–4 weeks from onset. Although the exact target antigen is still unknown, molecular mimicry, antiglycolipid antibodies, T cell sensitization, activated macrophages, and complement are the main immunopathological features of the disease (Lunneman et al. 2015a, b; Hughes et al. 2009; Dalakas 2004; Gold et al. 2007; Yuki and Hartung 2012). In addition to the classic demyelinating form of GBS, there are GBS variants, such as the acute axonal motor or motorsensory forms, the Miller-Fisher syndrome or acute dysautonomia (Yuki and Hartung 2012). Although IVIG appears to be also helpful in these patient subsets, controlled studies have been conducted only in the classic sensorimotor demyelinating form.

8.2.1.2 Management

Based on at least two randomized trials, one dose of IVIG (5-day regimen of 0.4 g/kg/d) was comparable to plasmapheresis (PE) in outcome measures including time to unaided walking and discontinuation of ventilation [class I evidence] (Sandoglobulin Guillain-Barré Syndrome Trial Group 1997). Combining IVIG with PE or with 500 mg intravenous methylprednisolone produced no incremental response (Lunneman et al. 2015a, b; Sandoglobulin Guillain-Barré Syndrome Trial Group 1997). IVIg also remains the treatment of choice in childhood GBS, based on observations attesting to a faster recovery and reduced morbidity, but controlled studies are not available and may not be ever conducted.

GBS is a monophasic disease, but many patients remain with significant weakness within the first month of the disease, in spite of the early initiation of IVIg therapy. Whether a second IVIg infusion may add more benefit when improvement has not occurred or it is inadequate 3 weeks after the first infusion remains unclear in spite of anecdotal evidence. A controlled study assessing the benefit of a second IVIG infusion is currently ongoing in the Netherlands. This is immunologically justified because a small increase in serum IgG level, 2 weeks after one IVIg infusion, was independently associated with significantly slower recovery and more disability at 6 months (Kuitwaard et al. 2009). It is anticipated that this study will provide credence to the observation that a low DeltaIgG 2 weeks after the initial infusion may be a sign that a higher dosage or a second infusion might be helpful for patients who exhibit poor outcome.

8.2.2 Chronic Inflammatory Demyelinating Polyneuropathy (CIDP)

8.2.2.1 Definition and Pathophysiology

Chronic inflammatory demyelinating polyneuropathy (CIDP) is characterized by slow onset (over weeks to months) weakness, areflexia, and impaired sensation. Antibodies, activated T cells, and complement have been implicated in the cause of the disease (Dalakas 2011). A subset of patients, accounting for 10% of total CIDP, has IgG4 antibodies against two nodal antigens, neurofascin-155 and contactin; this subset is important in discussing IVIg effectiveness because most of these antibody-positive CIDP patients respond poorly to IVIg (Dalakas and Gooch 2016).

8.2.2.2 Management

Controlled studies have shown that steroids, plasmapheresis, and IVIG are equally effective on a short-term basis (Dalakas 2011). The ICE trial, the largest ever conducted in CIDP, has showed that IVIG is safe and effective not only for short-term but also for long-term leading to the first FDA-approved indication for a brand of IVIG (class I evidence) (Hughes et al. 2008). A strong and positive effect on quality of life and improvement in some electrophysiological measurements were also noted. In most patients, IVIG becomes clearly effective after 6 weeks, necessitating the need for at least 2–3 infusions before concluding that it is ineffective. Although IVIg is generally considered as first-line therapy based on the ICE trial, the choice of how best to initiate therapy (choosing between prednisone, IVIg, or plasmapheresis which are all effective) is judged against cost, long-term side effects, patient age, venous access, disease severity, and concurrent illnesses. Clinically, patients more likely to respond to IVIG therapy are those with disease duration of less than a year, a relapsing course, no difference in strength between arms and legs, and electrophysiological signs of demyelination with conduction block (Lunneman et al. 2015a, b). FcγRIIB expression was reported to be decreased in treatment-naïve CIDP patients and upregulated upon clinically effective IVIG therapy suggesting that the effect on FcγRIIB may be a factor predicting the patients more likely to respond to IVIG (Lunneman et al. 2015a, b). Increased Fc glycosylation seems also associated with disease remission and response to IVIg, but the evidence is not yet strong enough to serve as a disease biomarker.

IVIg is not effective in patients who have a demyelinating neuropathy, resembling CIDP, accompanied by an IgM monoclonal gammopathy with antibodies to myelin-associated glycoprotein, based on a controlled study (Dalakas et al. 1996).

8.2.3 Multifocal Motor Neuropathy

8.2.3.1 Definition and Pathophysiology

Multifocal motor neuropathy (MMN) presents with a slow onset weakness and muscular atrophy in the distal upper extremities, areflexia, preserved sensation, and conduction block of the motor axons. IgM antibodies to GM1 ganglioside are seen in up to 50% of these patients (Federico et al. 2000; Hahn et al. 2013).

8.2.3.2 Management

Unlike CIDP and GBS, MMN does not respond to steroids or plasmapheresis but responds only to IVIG. Efficacy has been established with a number of controlled trials, and IVIg is now FDA-approved for MMN (Hahn et al. 2013). The improvement lasts from 3 to 6 weeks, requiring a new reinfusion at almost predictable time periods. As symptoms diminish, the electrophysiologic conduction block may resolve. Therapy starts with 2 g/kg, but the response can be maintained with a 1 g/kg, a pattern also followed for CIDP.

8.2.4 Myasthenia Gravis

8.2.4.1 Definition and Pathophysiology

Myasthenia gravis (MG) is characterized by fluctuating weakness or fatigability of the extraocular, bulbar, respiratory, and limb muscles. It is the prototypic autoimmune disease mediated by pathogenic antibodies to the acetylcholine receptors (AChR); up to 5–7% of patients are seronegative, while another 5% have anti MuSK antibodies (Vincent 2002).

8.2.4.2 Management

Patients with MG respond fairly well to the available therapies, such as anticholinesterases, steroids, or immunosuppressants. Plasmapheresis is effective for crises or severe exacerbations. The use of IVIG in MG has been examined in randomized trials for treating exacerbations in lieu of plasmapheresis. In two randomized trials, IVIG was as effective as plasmapheresis at day 15 (Gajdos et al. 1997). In one of the studies, there was no difference between patients randomized to 1 g/kg for 1 day versus 2 g/kg for 2 days (Gajdos et al. 2005). IVIG was also superior to placebo, 14 days after therapy, in patients with moderate to severe MG and "worsening weakness" (Lunneman et al. 2015a, b; Gajdos et al. 2012). Although IVIG may be effective on a short-term basis, its role in the chronic management of the disease or as a steroid-sparing drug has not yet been established, but two currently ongoing trials are precisely aimed to address these questions. At present, IVIG may be justified in lieu of plasmapheresis for acutely worsening disease to prevent or minimize impending bulbar or respiratory failure or prepare a weak patient for thymectomy. IVIG may be also effective in Lambert-Eaton Myasthenic Syndrome, based on a small placebo-controlled study, that showed a statistically significant increase in muscle strength compared to placebo, 2–4 weeks after therapy (Bain et al. 1996).

8.2.5 Inflammatory Myopathies

8.2.5.1 Definition and Pathophysiology

The main subsets in this large family of diseases include: dermatomyositis (DM), polymyositis (PM), necrotizing autoimmune (NAM), and inclusion body myositis (IBM) (Dalakas 2004a; Dalakas 2015). Dermatomyositis causes proximal muscle weakness and a violaceous rash on the face and extremities. Early deposition of membranolytic attack complex (MAC) on the endomysial capillaries leads to capillary destruction, muscle ischemia, and inflammation. Polymyositis is a rare T-cell-mediated disease T cell Receptor clonality (O'Hanlon et al 1994), causing subacute onset of muscle weakness; NAM is a macrophage-mediated, and possibly-antibody-fixing, process, directed against muscle fibers that cause more severe, and often acute, muscle weakness. IBM is a chronic disease with slowly progressive proximal and distal weakness along with muscle atrophy caused by a combination of T-cell-mediated cytotoxicity along with a degenerative process associated with protein misfolding (Dalakas 2015).

8.2.5.2 Management

In a double-blind, placebo-controlled study, IVIg was effective in dermatomyositis patients resulting in significant improvement of strength and muscle function, compared to placebo, and a marked improvement of the active skin rash as shown in Fig. 8.1 (Dalakas et al. 1993). Repeat muscle biopsies demonstrated significant improvement in the muscle cytoarchitecture including increased muscle fiber diameter, as shown in Fig. 8.2, revascularization, reduction of inflammation, interception of complement deposition, resolution of immunopathology, and downregulation of inflammatory mediators at the protein, mRNA, and gene level (Raju et al. 2005;

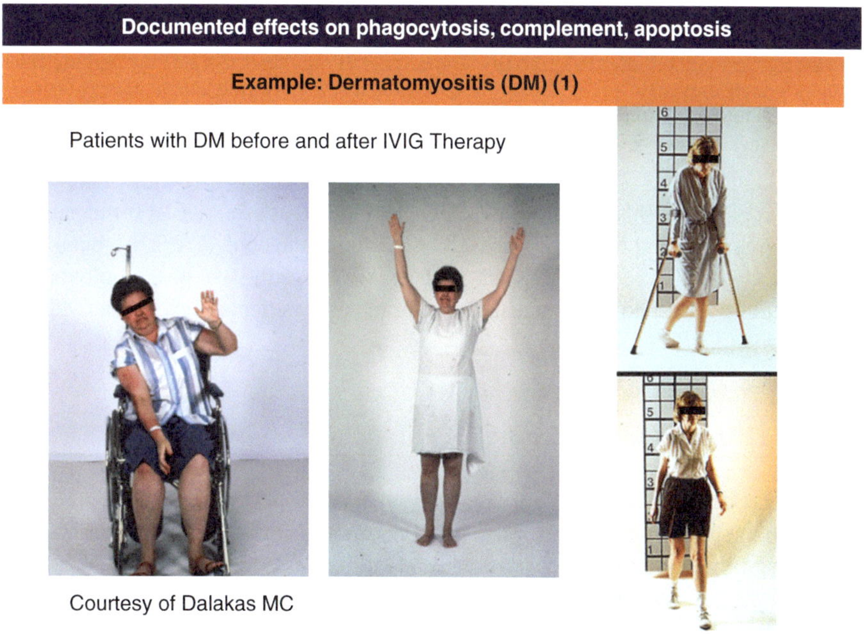

Fig. 8.1 Two patients with refractory Dermatomyositis participating in the controlled study (Dalakas at al 1993) after 3 months of IVIg therapy show a dramatic imrprovement in muscle strength

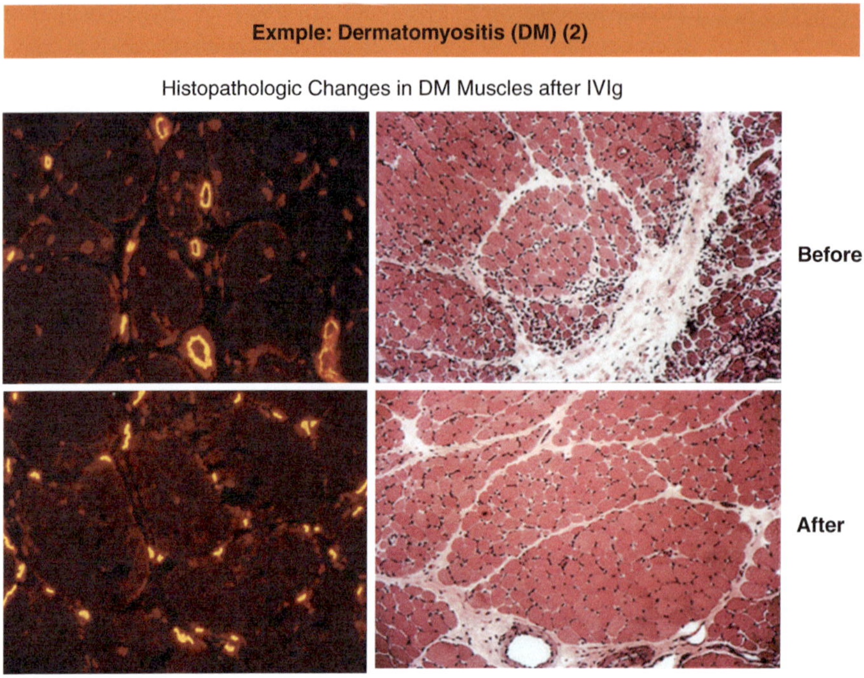

Fig. 8.2 Muscle biopsy specimens from the same patient taken from the left arm (*before*) IVIg and the right arm (*after*) after IVIg therapy. The number of capillaries (*left*)and the perifascicular atrophy with inflammation before therapy have been completely resolved after therapy coinciding with the resolution of muscle strength. The number of capilaries with the dilated lumen (*left*) were also normalized due to neovascularization

Dalakas et al. 1993; Basta and Dalakas 1994). IVIg seems effective in some patients with polymyositis and NAM (Dalakas 2004b; Lunneman et al. 2015a, b), but a controlled study has not been performed. IVIg is ineffective in IBM based on two controlled studies; it did however statistically improve the patients' dysphagia (Dalakas et al. 1997).

8.2.6 Stiff-Person Syndrome

8.2.6.1 Definition and Pathophysiology

Stiff-person syndrome (SPS) is a disabling autoimmune disorder characterized by muscle rigidity, episodic muscle spasms, and antibodies to glutamic acid decarboxylase (GAD65).

8.2.6.2 Management

In a placebo-controlled, crossover study, IVIG significantly decreased stiffness scores, and substantially increased walking and functions of daily activities (Dalakas et al. 2001). The study concluded that IVIG is effective as supplementary therapy in patients with SPS who do not adequately respond to first line drugs, such as diazepam, baclofen, and other GABA-enhancing drugs.

8.2.7 Novel, Promising, or Ongoing Applications

8.2.7.1 Alzheimer Disease (AD)

In AD the amyloid-β (Aβ) peptide, derived from amyloid precursor protein, is viewed as a major pathogenic element in the formation of plaques in the patients' brains. Naturally occurring antibodies against Aβ have been detected in the serum and CSF of healthy subjects, and IVIG has been shown to contain autoantibodies against Aß, suggesting that it may have a therapeutic role via an immune-mediated Aβ-degrading pathway. In an open-label pilot study of 8 patients, IVIG after 6 months of therapy, increased the level of Aβ peptide in the serum, decreased its levels in the CSF, and resulted in improved cognitive function prompting a phase II placebo-controlled study. In 24 AD patients with mild-to-moderate disease IVIG infusions, either 0.4 or 0.8 g/kg/month after 6 months of therapy, significantly increased the anti-Aβ antibody and Aβ 40/42 peptides in plasma and decreased Aβ 40/42 peptides in the CSF resulting in significant stabilization of cerebral glucose uptake measured by PET-18-fluorodeoxyglucose scanning (Dodel et al. 2004). These results prompted a large phase III trial that randomized 390 patients for 18 months. The results, which were just published, showed that IVIg was not effective (Relkin et al. 2017).

8.2.7.2 Post-polio Syndrome

This is a chronic degenerative condition clinically characterized by new muscular weakness, fatigue, and pain that develop many years after an initial attack of acute paralytic poliomyelitis. Although it is thought to be due to attrition of the surviving motor neurons (Dalakas 1986), immune activation has been observed consisting of lymphocytic infiltrates in the patient's spinal cords and even the patients' muscles (Dalakas 1988) observed even 30 years after the original infection, and upregulation of RNA for tumor necrosis factor (TNF), IFN-γ, interleukin (IL)-4, and IL-10 cytokines in the CSF, suggesting the possibility of a persistent smoldering inflammatory response. Following IVIG treatment, IFN-γ and TNF mRNA levels were reduced in the CSF prompting a controlled trial performed in 135 patients. The results, although underwhelming and of uncertain clinical importance, did show certain significant differences in some physical activity and quality of life scores (Gonzalez et al. 2006). These results prompted a phase III FDA-approved international clinical trial that is currently ongoing.

8.2.7.3 Subcutaneous IgG and Therapeutic Perspectives in Neurology

Subcutaneous IgG, not for replacement therapy but for immunomodulation, is becoming attractive as immunotherapy in several autoimmune neurological diseases. After the efficacy of subcutaneous IgG has been documented in uncontrolled studies in CIDP, MMN, and dermatomyositis, a number of multicenter,

FDA-approved trials are currently ongoing to establish efficacy of IgG as chronic therapy given subcutaneously in lieu of the intravenous route.

8.2.7.4 Surrogate Biomarkers of Efficacy

As with other immunomodulatory agents, a subset of the neurological patients does not benefit from IVIG therapy, and, at present, we are unable to predict which are those patients more likely to respond to IVIg. Although surrogate parameters that predict response to therapy from the outset are needed, they have not yet been fully developed or validated. The potential role of molecules such as FcγRIIB and sialylated Fc and changes in regulatory genes have been explored, but the results, based on small series, are not adequate to reliably identify those neurological patient subsets that may be resistant or not adequately responding to IVIg.

References

Bain PG, Motomura M, Newsom-Davis J, et al. Effects of intravenous immunoglobulin on muscle weakness and calciumchannel autoantibodies in the Lambert–Eaton myasthenic syndrome. Neurology. 1996;47:678–68.

Basta M, Dalakas MC. High-dose intravenous immunoglobulin exerts its beneficial effect in patients with dermatomyositis by blocking endomysial deposition of activated complement fragments. J Clin Invest. 1994;94:1729–35. https://doi.org/10.1172/JCI117520.

Dalakas MC, Elder G, Hallett M, et al. A long term follow-up study of patients with postpoliomyelitis neuromuscular symptoms. N Engl J Med. 1986;314:959–63.

Dalakas MC. Morphological changes in the muscles of patients with post-poliomyelitis neuromuscular symptoms. Neurology. 1988;38:99–104.

Dalakas MC. The use of intravenous immunoglobulin in the treatment of autoimmune neurological disorders: evidence-based indications and safety profile. Pharmacol Ther. 2004a;102:177–93.

Dalakas MC. Inflammatory disorders of muscle: progress in polymyositis, dermatomyositis and inclusion body myositis. Curr Opin Neurol. 2004b;17(5):561–7.

Dalakas MC. Intravenous immunoglobulin in autoimmune neuromuscular diseases. JAMA. 2004;291:2367–75. https://doi.org/10.1001/jama.291.19.2367.

Dalakas MC. Advances in the diagnosis, pathogenesis and treatment of CIDP. Nat Rev Neurol. 2011;7:507–17. https://doi.org/10.1038/nrneurol.2011.121.

Dalakas MC. Inflammatory myopathies. N Engl J Med. 2015;372:1734–47.

Dalakas MC, Gooch C. Close to the node but far enough: what nodal antibodies tell us about CIDP and its therapies. Neurology. 2016;86:1–2.

Dalakas MC, et al. A controlled trial of high-dose intravenous immune globulin infusions as treatment for dermatomyositis. N Engl J Med. 1993;329:1993–2000. https://doi.org/10.1056/NEJM199312303292704.

Dalakas MC, et al. A controlled study of intravenous immunoglobulin in demyelinating neuropathy with IgM gammopathy. Ann Neurol. 1996;40:792–5. https://doi.org/10.1002/ana.410400516.

Dalakas MC, et al. Treatment of inclusion-body myositis with IVIg: a double-blind, placebo-controlled study. Neurology. 1997;48:712–6.

Dalakas MC, et al. High-dose intravenous immune globulin for stiff-person syndrome. N Engl J Med. 2001;345:1870–6. https://doi.org/10.1056/NEJMoa01167.

Dodel RC, et al. Intravenous immunoglobulins containing antibodies against beta-amyloid for the treatment of Alzheimer's disease. J Neurol Neurosurg Psychiatry. 2004;75:1472–4. https://doi.org/10.1136/jnnp.2003.033399.

Federico P, Zochodne DW, Hahn AF, Brown WF, Feasby TE. Multifocal motor neuropathy improved by IVIg: randomized, double-blind, placebo-controlled study. Neurology. 2000;55:1256–62.

Gajdos P, Chevret S, Clair B, Tranchant C, Chastang C. Clinical trial of plasma exchange and high-dose intravenous immunoglobulin in myasthenia gravis. Myasthenia Gravis Clinical Study Group. Ann Neurol. 1997;41:789–96. https://doi.org/10.1002/ana.410410615.
Gajdos P, et al. Treatment of myasthenia gravis exacerbation with intravenous immunoglobulin: a randomized double-blind clinical trial. Arch Neurol. 2005;62:1689–93. https://doi.org/10.1001/archneur.62.11.1689.
Gajdos P, Chevret S, Toyka KV. Intravenous immunoglobulin for myasthenia gravis. Cochrane Database Syst Rev. 2012;12:CD002277. https://doi.org/10.1002/14651858.CD002277.pub4.
Gold R, Stangel M, Dalakas MC. Drug insight: the use of intravenous immunoglobulin in neurology—therapeutic considerations and practical issues. Nat Clin Pract Neurol. 2007;3:36–44. https://doi.org/10.1038/ncpneuro0376.
Gonzalez H, et al. Intravenous immunoglobulin for post-polio syndrome: a randomised controlled trial. Lancet Neurol. 2006;5:493–500. https://doi.org/10.1016/S1474-4422(06)70447-1.
Hahn AF, Beydoun SR, Lawson V, et al. A controlled trial of IVIG in multifocal motor neuropathy. J Peripher Nerv Syst. 2013;18:321–30.
Hughes RA, et al. Intravenous immune globulin (10% caprylate-chromatography purified) for the treatment of chronic inflammatory demyelinating polyradiculoneuropathy (ICE study): a randomised placebo-controlled trial. Lancet Neurol. 2008;7:136–44. https://doi.org/10.1016/S1474-4422(07)70329-0.
Hughes RA, Dalakas MC, Cornblath DR, et al. Clinical applications of intravenous immunoglobulin in neurology. Clin Exp Immunol. 2009;158(Suppl 1):34–2.
Kuitwaard K, et al. Pharmacokinetics of intravenous immunoglobulin and outcome in Guillain-Barre syndrome. Ann Neurol. 2009;66:597–603. https://doi.org/10.1002/ana.21737.
Lunneman JD, Quast I, Dalakas MC. Efficacy of intravenous immunoglobulin in neurological diseases. Neurotherapeutics. 2015a;13:34–46.
Lunneman JD, Nimmerjahn F, Dalakas MC. Intravenous immunoglobulin in neurology: mode of action and clinical efficacy. Nat Rev Neurol. 2015b;11:80–9.
O'Hanlon TP, Dalakas MC, Plotz PH, Miller FW. Predominant α/β T cell receptor variable and joining gene expression by muscle-infiltrating lymphocytes in the idiopathic inflammatory myopathies. J Immunol. 1994;152:2569–76.
Raju R, Dalakas MC. Gene expression profile in the muscles of patients with inflammatory myopathies: effect of therapy with IVIg and biologic validation of clinical relevant genes. Brain. 2005;128:1887–96.
Relkin NR, Thomas RG, Rissman RA, et al. A phase 3 trial of IV immunoglobulin for Alzheimer disease. Neurology. 2017;88:1–8.
Sandoglobulin Guillain-Barré Syndrome Trial Group. Randomised trial of plasma exchange, intravenous immunoglobulin, and combined treatments in Guillain-Barre syndrome. Plasma Exchange/Sandoglobulin Guillain-Barre Syndrome Trial Group. Lancet. 1997;349:225–30.
Vincent A. Unravelling the pathogenesis of myasthenia gravis. Nat Rev Immunol. 2002;2:797–804. https://doi.org/10.1038/nri916.
Yuki N, Hartung HP. Guillain-Barre syndrome. N Engl J Med. 2012;366:2294–304. https://doi.org/10.1056/NEJMra1114525.

9 Use of Intravenous Immunoglobulin in Dermatology

Jochen H.O. Hoffmann and Alexander H. Enk

9.1 Expert Review and Update in Dermatology

Good clinical evidence on the effective use of intravenous immunoglobulin (IVIg) in dermatological conditions can be found as early as 1984 and 1986, when Furusho et al. (1984) and Newburger et al. (1986), respectively, reported the successful application of IVIg in Kawasaki syndrome. Seven years later, Dalakas et al. (1993) reported the first successful randomized controlled trial of IVIg in the treatment of dermatomyositis. Ever since, IVIg has evolved as an important second- and third-line treatment option for severe dermatological conditions like autoimmune blistering diseases and scleromyxedema. Other dermatological conditions that may respond to IVIg treatment include vasculitis and toxic epidermal necrolysis (Table 9.1). Still, IVIg treatment is off-label for most dermatological indications. The most current guidelines on the use of IVIg in dermatology were provided by the European Dermatology Forum in 2016 (Enk et al. 2016). Other comprehensive guidelines on the use of IVIg exist for the United Kingdom (Provan et al. 2008) and Australia (Group NICRW 2012).

9.2 Autoimmune Blistering Diseases

Autoimmune blistering diseases encompass dermatological conditions in which the immune system launches a mainly humoral immune response against self-antigens involved in keratinocyte cell-cell adhesion (pemphigus group) or the connection

J.H.O. Hoffmann (✉) • A.H. Enk
Department of Dermatology, University of Heidelberg, Heidelberg, Germany
e-mail: Jochen.Hoffmann@med.uni-heidelberg.de; Alexander.Enk@med.uni-heidelberg.de

P. Imbach (ed.), *Antibody Therapy*, https://doi.org/10.1007/978-3-319-68038-5_9

Table 9.1 Dermatological indications for the use of IVIg

Condition	Line of treatment	Level of evidence
Pemphigus vulgaris and foliaceus	Second or third	RCT (Amagai et al. 2009), CS, CR
Bullous pemphigoid	Third	RCT (Amagai et al. 2017), CS, CR
Mucous membrane pemphigoid, epidermolysis bullosa acquisita	Second or third	CS, CR
Dermatomyositis	Second or third	RCT (Dalakas et al. 1993), CS, CR
Systemic lupus erythematosus	Selected cases	RCT (Boletis et al. 1999; Perricone et al. 2008), CS, CR
Scleromyxedema	First or second	CS, CR
Kawasaki syndrome	First	CS, CR
ANCA-associated vasculitis	Third	RCT (Jayne et al. 2000), CS, CR
Toxic epidermal necrolysis	First[a]	CS, CR

RCT randomized controlled trial, *CR* case report, *CS* case series
[a]This indication is highly controversial

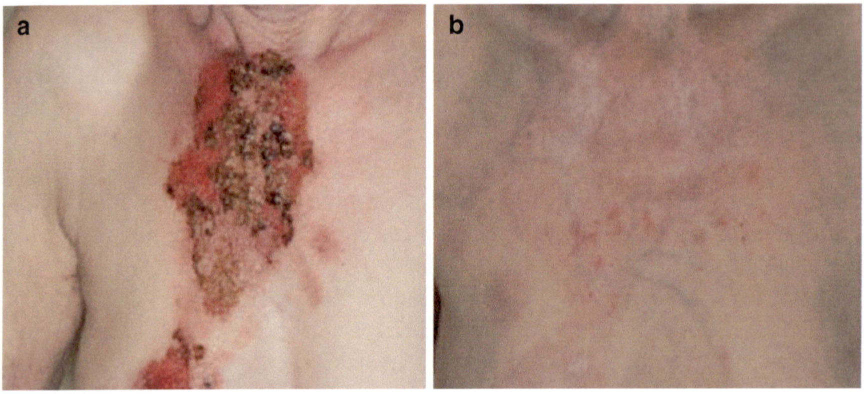

Fig. 9.1 Pemphigus vulgaris. Images of the chest area of a patient with severe mucocutaneous pemphigus vulgaris resistant to treatment with oral prednisolone (up to 3 mg/kg body weight), mycophenolate mofetil (3 g/day), and hemolysis in response to dapsone (**a**). We initiated concomitant treatment with IVIg (2 g/kg body weight) over a course of 2 days every 4 weeks. Under the combined immunosuppression, disease activity finally subsided. The dosage of prednisolone and mycophenolate mofetil could be reduced stepwise. The patient is still in remission after 4 years (**b**)

between epidermis and dermis (pemphigoid group, epidermolysis bullosa acquisita). The resultant clinical picture is dominated by blisters (especially pemphigoid group, epidermolysis bullosa acquisita) and erosions (especially pemphigus group) on the skin and adjacent mucous membranes. Before the advent of immunosuppressive therapy, autoimmune blistering diseases often took a lethal course due to cachexia and superinfection.

Very convincing clinical evidence from two randomized controlled trials exists for the use of IVIg in pemphigus vulgaris, pemphigus foliaceus, and bullous pemphigoid (Amagai et al. 2017, 2009). Figure 9.1 shows images of a patient with severe pemphigus vulgaris of the skin and mucous membranes who responded to

Table 9.2 IVIg in autoimmune bullous disease

Indication	Second or third line, in combination with systemic steroids and steroid-sparing immunosuppressants
Dosage	2 g/kg body weight over a period of 2–5 days
Intervals	4 weeks

IVIg treatment. Several case series highlight the effectiveness of IVIg in mucous membrane pemphigoid and epidermolysis bullosa acquisita. Furthermore, based on analogy and case reports, the use of IVIg is advocated in severe and treatment-resistant cases of other autoimmune blistering diseases with a similar pathophysiology. IVIg is recommended as an adjuvant second- or third-line treatment after unsuccessful application of a conventional immunosuppressive combination therapy including a systemic steroid and, most commonly, mycophenolate mofetil or azathioprine (Eming et al. 2015; Enk et al. 2016; Feliciani et al. 2015; Venning et al. 2012). The initiation of IVIg is usually flanked with high-dose oral corticosteroids (prednisolone 1–2 mg/kg body weight) to initiate remission. Usually, 2 g/kg body weight of IVIg distributed over the course of 2–5 days is infused every 4 weeks (Table 9.2). If no sustained response is observed after four to six treatment cycles, temporary escalation with the anti-CD20 antibody rituximab can be considered (Ahmed et al. 2006). In case of a response, the systemic steroid is tapered to 5 mg/day prednisolone, followed by a taper and discontinuation of the steroid sparing conventional immunosuppressive. Subsequently, the intervals of IVIg treatment are extended to 6 weeks, and, finally, IVIg treatment is discontinued.

9.3 Dermatomyositis

Dermatomyositis is an idiopathic inflammatory myositis and a member of the ill-defined group of collagen vascular diseases. Complement-mediated small vessel damage is thought to contribute to disease pathogenesis; however, no single pathogenic model is ubiquitously accepted to date. Apart from mostly proximal muscle weakness, dermatomyositis presents with photo-distributed erythema and poikiloderma, "Gottron" papules over the extensor aspects of the knuckles, and, usually, prominent alterations of the nail fold capillaries. Due to the involvement of the heart and lung, and the occurrence of dermatomyositis as a paraneoplastic syndrome, the mortality in adult patients is considerably high with reported 5-year survival rates down to 65%. Overlap syndromes, in particular with scleroderma, are not uncommon.

Systemic steroids are the mainstay of dermatomyositis treatment. The beneficial effect of adjuvant IVIg on dermatomyositis, in particular on neuromuscular symptoms, was convincingly demonstrated in a randomized controlled trial (Dalakas et al. 1993) and multiple case series and reports. The current European IVIg guideline recommends the addition of IVIg after failure of systemic steroid monotherapy (Enk et al. 2016). The introduction of a steroid-sparing immunosuppressant, most commonly azathioprine or

Table 9.3 IVIg in dermatomyositis

Indication	Second or third line, in combination with systemic steroids; 1st line in severe cases in combination with systemic steroids
Dosage	2 g/kg body weight over a period of 2–5 days
Intervals	4 weeks

mycophenolate mofetil, can be regarded as an alternative second-line approach (Sunderkotter et al. 2016). Simultaneous first-line application of systemic steroids and IVIg may be justified in severe cases (Enk et al. 2016). Usually, systemic steroids are recommended at high initial doses (prednisolone 1–2 mg/kg body weight). The recommended dosage of IVIg is 2 g/kg body weight over a period of 2–5 days. Treatment intervals are commonly 4 weeks (Table 9.3). The authors tend to flank initiation of IVIg treatment with high-dose oral corticosteroids. Response to treatment is usually fast, and effects can be expected after the third to fourth treatment cycle at the latest. If patients respond to treatment, systemic steroids can be slowly tapered to 5 mg/day. Subsequently, IVIg intervals can be extended to 6 weeks, and, finally, IVIg treatment can be discontinued.

9.4 Systemic Lupus Erythematosus

Systemic lupus erythematosus (SLE) is a protean multisystem autoimmune disease, which is prominently associated with the production of antinuclear, in particular, anti-double-stranded DNA autoantibodies. Specific cutaneous manifestations range from the idiosyncratic butterfly rash to UV-induced hyperkeratotic plaques with atrophic scarring. Systemic manifestations are manifold and potentially life-threatening, including lupus nephritis, encephalitis, and arthritis.

Randomized controlled trials highlight the use of IVIg in lupus nephritis, where it was shown to be equally effective as cyclophosphamide over a course of 18 months (Boletis et al. 1999), and in pregnant patients with SLE and recurrent spontaneous abortions, where IVIg reduced lupus activity scores and pregnancy loss (Perricone et al. 2008). However, the duration of the former study was criticized, as differences in the efficiency of treatments may not manifest for up to 5 years in SLE (Mulhearn and Bruce 2015). Several small case series and reports document beneficial effects of IVIg treatment in a broad range of SLE manifestations. Depending on the involved organs, current treatment recommendations include systemic corticosteroids, antimalarials, non-steroidal anti-inflammatory drugs, methotrexate, azathioprine, mycophenolate mofetil, cyclophosphamide, and rituximab (Hahn et al. 2012; Tunnicliffe et al. 2015). Based on the available data, IVIg may be considered as maintenance treatment in selected cases of lupus nephritis refractory to more established treatment options. Other manifestations of SLE that may prompt consideration of IVIg include neuropsychiatric lupus, in particular, Guillain-Barré syndrome associated with SLE, lupus-associated immune thrombocytopenia, and SLE in pregnancy (Mulhearn and Bruce 2015). In SLE, IVIg is usually administered at doses ranging from 400 mg to 2 g/kg body weight over 2–5 days in 4-week intervals (Table 9.4).

Table 9.4 IVIg in systemic lupus erythematosus

Indication	Selected cases if other established treatment options failed or are contraindicated
Dosage	400 mg to 2 g/kg body weight over a period of 2–5 days
Intervals	Usually 4 weeks

Table 9.5 IVIg in scleromyxedema

Indication	First or second line
Dosage	2 g/kg body weight over a period of 2–5 days
Intervals	4 weeks

9.5 Scleromyxedema

Scleromyxedema is a chronic disease of unknown etiology that results in the dermal deposition of mucin and dermal fibrosis. It is usually associated with a monoclonal gammopathy. Clinically, patients develop symmetric waxy papules and indurated plaques mainly on the trunk, face, and upper extremities. Apart from disfigurement, dermatogenic contractures can severely impair mobility. Internal organ and in particular neurological involvements are feared and potentially lethal complications.

Successful application of IVIg in scleromyxedema was reported in several case series and reports. Furthermore, given the frequent association of scleromyxedema with paraproteinemia, there is a pathophysiologic rationale for beneficial effects of IVIg. Due to the low effectiveness and potential side effects of other therapeutic strategies, e.g., chemotherapeutic agents, the current European IVIg guideline supports the use of IVIg first line in severe cases (Enk et al. 2016). It is recommended at a dosage of 2 g/kg body weight over a period of 2–5 days in 4-week intervals (Table 9.5). If the treatment is not effective after 6 months, it should be discontinued. If the patient responds, the treatment intervals can be extended to 6 weeks, and, finally, treatment can be discontinued. However, relapses after treatment cessation are not unusual, and long-term treatment may be necessary.

9.6 Kawasaki Disease

Kawasaki disease designates an acute generalized vasculitis that mainly affects children. It was hypothesized that the disease might be triggered by an unknown infectious agent in genetically predisposed individuals. Clinically, Kawasaki disease starts with high fever (>40 °C), which is accompanied by unilateral cervical lymphadenopathy in most cases. Subsequently, a pronounced erythema of the tongue and oral cavity, conjunctival injection, and morbilliform, scarlatiniform, or purpuric exanthema usually ensue. The disease can be complicated by myocardial, coronary, neurological, and gastrointestinal involvements, which are mainly responsible for mortality and residual functional impairment.

Table 9.6 IVIg in Kawasaki disease

Indication	First line in combination with acetylsalicylic acid
Dosage	2 g/kg body weight over 12 h
Intervals	Single cycle, may be repeated if standard treatment fails

The mainstay of treatment of Kawasaki disease is the application of 2 g/kg body weight IVIg over 12 h in combination with acetylsalicylic acid (Table 9.6). If the standard treatment fails, a second dose of IVIg is usually recommended (Neudorf and Lilienthal 2013; Newburger et al. 2004). Kawasaki disease is currently the only dermatological condition for which IVIg use is officially approved by the European drug agency and US food and drug administration.

9.7 ANCA-Associated Vasculitis

The group of anti-neutrophil cytoplasmic antibody (ANCA) associated vasculitis encompasses granulomatosis with polyangiitis (GPA, Wegener's disease), eosinophilic granulomatosis with polyangiitis (EGPA, Churg-Strauss syndrome), and microscopic polyangiitis (MPA). Pathophysiologically, ANCA antibodies are thought to cause neutrophil granulocyte degranulation within small-to-medium size vessels and subsequent organ damage. Forty to fifty percent of patients experience skin symptoms, mainly inflammatory nodules, palpable and retiform purpura, and ulceration, at some point during their disease course. Organ involvement includes potentially fatal cardiac, pulmonary, and renal damage.

A randomized controlled trial conducted in the year 2000 found a beneficial effect of adjuvant IVIg in ANCA-associated vasculitis (Jayne et al. 2000). However, only a single dose of IVIg was used, and the observation period was short (3 months). Apart from this study, several smaller case series document favorable results under IVIg treatment. Still, a recent Cochrane review concluded that insufficient evidence exists for the use of IVIg in GPA (Fortin et al. 2013). According to the current European IVIg guideline, IVIg remains a valid adjuvant treatment option for selected refractory vasculitis patients if other, more established treatments failed or are contraindicated (Enk et al. 2016). IVIg was used at 2 g/kg body weight over a period of 2–5 days in most published studies. Given the experience in other disease entities, 4-week intervals can be suggested (Table 9.7).

9.8 Toxic Epidermal Necrolysis

Toxic epidermal necrolysis (TEN), formerly known as Lyell syndrome, is a severe blistering drug reaction that involves the influx of cytotoxic T-cells into the epidermis and a full-blown epidermal necrosis. By definition, patients with TEN present with skin detachment of at least 30% of the body surface. The mucous membranes are usually involved. The mortality of TEN ranges from 25 to 70%, depending on the extent of the disease.

Table 9.7 IVIg in ANCA-associated vasculitis

Indication	Third line, as adjuvant treatment
Dosage	2 g/kg body weight over a period of 2–5 days
Intervals	4 weeks

Table 9.8 IVIg in toxic epidermal necrolysis

Indication	Controversial
Dosage	≥3 g/kg body weight over a period of 2–5 days
Intervals	Single cycle

The mainstay of the treatment of TEN is the cessation of the causative drug and best supportive care. Given the large-scale erosions, patients are usually admitted to a burn intensive care unit. IVIg contains inhibitory antibodies, in particular, anti-FAS antibodies that may, in theory, prevent keratinocyte apoptosis. The available data on the effectiveness of IVIg in TEN is, however, contradictory. Some authorities suggest that IVIg may only be beneficial at high doses in TEN. Indeed, a recent meta-analysis found an inverse relation between the dose of IVIg and mortality (Barron et al. 2015). The recommended dosage is, therefore, a single cycle of at least 3 g/kg body weight IVIg over the course of 2–5 days (Table 9.8). Given the favorable risk profile of IVIg, the harsh prognosis of TEN, and the lack of reliable alternative therapeutics, the current European IVIg guideline states that IVIg treatment is justified in TEN (Enk et al. 2016). If the decision for the application of IVIg is made, however, treatment should commence as early as possible. It is important to stress that, apart from the cessation of the offending drug and best supportive care, no generally accepted treatment guidelines for TEN exist. Alternative treatment options that were very recently labeled promising in a comprehensive meta-analysis by the group of Maja Mockenhaupt (Zimmermann et al. 2017) are systemic steroids and cyclosporine, while insufficient evidence was found to support the use of IVIg in TEN.

References

Ahmed AR, Spigelman Z, Cavacini LA, et al. Treatment of pemphigus vulgaris with rituximab and intravenous immune globulin. N Engl J Med. 2006;355:1772–9.

Amagai M, Ikeda S, Shimizu H, et al. A randomized double-blind trial of intravenous immunoglobulin for pemphigus. J Am Acad Dermatol. 2009;60:595–603.

Amagai M, Ikeda S, Hashimoto T, et al. A randomized double-blind trial of intravenous immunoglobulin for bullous pemphigoid. J Dermatol Sci. 2017;85:77–84.

Barron SJ, Del Vecchio MT, Aronoff SC. Intravenous immunoglobulin in the treatment of Stevens-Johnson syndrome and toxic epidermal necrolysis: a meta-analysis with meta-regression of observational studies. Int J Dermatol. 2015;54:108–15.

Boletis JN, Ioannidis JP, Boki KA, et al. Intravenous immunoglobulin compared with cyclophosphamide for proliferative lupus nephritis. Lancet. 1999;354:569–70.

Dalakas MC, Illa I, Dambrosia JM, et al. A controlled trial of high-dose intravenous immune globulin infusions as treatment for dermatomyositis. N Engl J Med. 1993;329:1993–2000.

Eming R, Sticherling M, Hofmann SC, et al. S2k guidelines for the treatment of pemphigus vulgaris/foliaceus and bullous pemphigoid. J Dtsch Dermatol Ges. 2015;13:833–44.
Enk AH, Hadaschik EN, Eming R, et al. European Guidelines (S1) on the use of high-dose intravenous immunoglobulin in dermatology. J Eur Acad Dermatol Venereol. 2016;30:1657–69.
Feliciani C, Joly P, Jonkman MF, et al. Management of bullous pemphigoid: the European Dermatology Forum consensus in collaboration with the European Academy of Dermatology and Venereology. Br J Dermatol. 2015;172:867–77.
Fortin PM, Tejani AM, Bassett K, et al. Intravenous immunoglobulin as adjuvant therapy for Wegener's granulomatosis. Cochrane Database Syst Rev. 2013; CD007057.
Furusho K, Kamiya T, Nakano H, et al. High-dose intravenous gammaglobulin for Kawasaki disease. Lancet. 1984;2:1055–8.
Group NICRW. Criteria for the clinical use of intravenous immunoglobulin in Australia. 2nd ed. In: 2012.
Hahn BH, Mcmahon MA, Wilkinson A, et al. American College of Rheumatology guidelines for screening, treatment, and management of lupus nephritis. Arthritis Care Res. 2012;64:797–808.
Jayne DR, Chapel H, Adu D, et al. Intravenous immunoglobulin for ANCA-associated systemic vasculitis with persistent disease activity. QJM. 2000;93:433–9.
Mulhearn B, Bruce IN. Indications for IVIG in rheumatic diseases. Rheumatology (Oxford). 2015;54:383–91.
Neudorf U, Lilienthal E. Vaskulitiden – Kawasaki-Syndrom. In: AWMF – Leitlinien. 2013.
Newburger JW, Takahashi M, Burns JC, et al. The treatment of Kawasaki syndrome with intravenous gamma globulin. N Engl J Med. 1986;315:341–7.
Newburger JW, Takahashi M, Gerber MA, et al. Diagnosis, treatment, and long-term management of Kawasaki disease: a statement for health professionals from the Committee on Rheumatic Fever, Endocarditis and Kawasaki Disease, Council on Cardiovascular Disease in the Young, American Heart Association. Circulation. 2004;110:2747–71.
Perricone R, De Carolis C, Kroegler B, et al. Intravenous immunoglobulin therapy in pregnant patients affected with systemic lupus erythematosus and recurrent spontaneous abortion. Rheumatology (Oxford). 2008;47:646–51.
Provan D, Chapel HM, Sewell WA, et al. Prescribing intravenous immunoglobulin: summary of Department of Health guidelines. BMJ. 2008;337:a1831.
Sunderkotter C, Nast A, Worm M, et al. Guidelines on dermatomyositis—excerpt from the interdisciplinary S2k guidelines on myositis syndromes by the German Society of Neurology. J Dtsch Dermatol Ges. 2016;14:321–38.
Tunnicliffe DJ, Singh-Grewal D, Kim S, et al. Diagnosis, monitoring, and treatment of systemic lupus erythematosus: a systematic review of clinical practice guidelines. Arthritis Care Res. 2015;67:1440–52.
Venning VA, Taghipour K, Mohd Mustapa MF, et al. British Association of Dermatologists' guidelines for the management of bullous pemphigoid 2012. Br J Dermatol. 2012;167:1200–14.
Zimmermann S, Sekula P, Venhoff M, et al. Systemic Immunomodulating therapies for Stevens-Johnson syndrome and toxic epidermal necrolysis: a systematic review and meta-analysis. JAMA Dermatol. 2017;153(6):514–22. https://doi.org/10.1001/jamadermatol.2016.5668.

Part II

Basics of IgG Concentrates

Historical Aspects of Polyclonal IgG Preparations

10

Volker Wahn and Peter Späth

10.1 Introduction

Today we can choose between several polyclonal IgG products for both replacement and immunomodulation. However, it was a long way to go to reach this stage. In this chapter, we try to illustrate the major stages of IgG product development which began more than 70 years ago.

10.2 Development of Standard IgG

The development of plasma fractionation was a WW II effort with a primary aim to provide human albumin for battlefield injuries. The technique was developed in Boston under the lead of Edwin Joseph Cohn (1892–1953) and was made possible through the strong support of the US Department of Navy, the Office of Scientific Research and Development, and the wartime blood donor program of the American Red Cross (Cohn et al. 1944). Gamma globulin was enriched at high purity in fraction II of the Cohn-Oncley cold ethanol fractionation method (Oncley et al. 1949). This "standard IgG" at increasing amounts became available from 1943 onward, a time point when the fractionation of albumin has been transferred to industry (Armour Pharma at Kankakee, IL, USA). Indeed, between 1944 and 1948, approximately 1 mio doses of "standard IgG" were applied in the USA.

V. Wahn (✉)
Department of Pediatric Pneumology and Immunology, Charité University Hospital, Augustenburger Platz 1, 13353 Berlin, Germany
e-mail: Volker.Wahn@charite.de

P. Späth
Institute of Pharmacology, University of Bern, Bern, Switzerland
e-mail: peter.spaeth@pki.unibe.ch

P. Imbach (ed.), *Antibody Therapy*, https://doi.org/10.1007/978-3-319-68038-5_10

10.3 The Early Days of Clinical Development of IgG Therapies

From 1941 onward, therapies with protein concentrates from fractioned plasma were developed under contract between the Office of Scientific Research and Development and Boston Harvard University. Charles A. Janeway (1909–1981) was put in charge. At that time, he was running the infectious and immunology laboratory at the Peter Bent Brigham Hospital and was member of the Harvard Medical School Department of Bacteriology and Immunology, and in 1940 he furthermore joined the laboratory of Edwin J. Cohn in the Harvard Medical School Department of Physical Chemistry (Geha 2005; Rosen and Janeway 1994). After initial studies in 1941 in humans with bovine (fatal outcomes) and human serum albumin (successful), in 1943 he turned to study Cohn fraction II (+III), the plasma fraction(s) enriched in IgG. The initial studies largely remained restricted to the prevention or attenuation of viral infections, particularly of measles infections (Ordman et al. 1944). The initial restriction to viral diseases probably was because from the late 1930s onward, the dawn of antibiotic treatment, Janeway built up an outstanding expertise in the treatment of bacterial infections with these emerging new drugs (Smith 1977).

The first human ever receiving an IgG concentrate was Janeway himself—with almost fatal consequences as the lot was contaminated with bacterial toxin (Rosen and Janeway 1994). Aiming for rapid increase of antibodies in the circulation and pursuing the "tradition" set, the "lot-release" for intravenous application of toxin free preparations was a self-infusion to one or the other collaborators of Janeway. Repeated severe and one almost fatal adverse event let Janeway note: "One mystery about normal serum gamma globulin which has defied explanation is its toxicity on intravenous injection. Although reactions have been practically nonexistent on intramuscular injection for measles prophylaxis, intravenous injection of the most highly purified preparations into normals in moderate doses and into patients ill with acute infections in much smaller doses has led to acute vasomotor reactions followed by severe chills and hyperpyrexia. This has occurred so regularly that one wonders whether it has genuine physiologic significance" (cited from Janeway 1948). Therefore, intravenous application of "standard IgG" was given up in favor of the intramuscular route.

10.4 From Intramuscular "Standard IgG" to Intravenous Preparations

Until the early 1950s, two slightly different cold ethanol fractionation methods were established. In the USA the Cohn-Oncley method provided a highly pure "standard IgG." The method was a lavish one with high volumes during fractionation and a low recovery of IgG (Cohn et al. 1944; Oncley et al. 1949). The other was the Kistler-Nitschmann method established as the "European" method for plasma fractionation (Nitschmann et al. 1954). With this method, volumes to handle during fractionation were considerable lower and the recovery higher at cost of some impurities, mainly IgA. Both methods provided a "standard IgG" concentrate.

Most likely gamma globulin therapy would have stayed in the shadow of antibiotic treatment, if not agammaglobulinemia would have been described in 1952 by OC Bruton. Applying plasma electrophoresis to the serum of an 8-year-old boy, he realized an association between recurrent severe infections (starting at an age of four and a half years of age) and a very low gamma globulin in serum. In an attempt to reduce susceptibility to infections, he administered "standard IgG" subcutaneously and demonstrated an increase of gamma globulin in blood, clinically a decrease of infections. Some remarkable facts of Bruton's work have to be highlighted: (a) despite the overwhelming position of the Boston group, he selected the less painful subcutaneous route of administration for his young patient; (b) he detected a new disease; and (c) he provided the therapy. Although less painful, at that time, only low doses of "standard IgG" could be administered via this route, and the need for i.v. preparations allowing administration of larger doses became evident (again).

10.5 Initial Problems with IVIG Administration

The first human immunoglobulin preparations were Cohn fraction II at 16% strength without any dedicated polishing step, i.e., a "crude" IgG concentrate. The effort of Barandun and colleagues shed light on Janeways "mystery about normal serum gamma globulin": "standard IgG" contained IgG aggregates capable of activating the complement system. This activation process generated anaphylatoxins like C3a and C5a and caused acute intolerance reactions if "standard IgG" was given intravenously. Thus, from the beginning of the 1960s onward, research focused on the reduction of aggregates as the cause of anticomplementary activity (ACA) in order to create preparations that were tolerated upon intravenous use. Even today, ACA assessment is a release criterion for IVIG lots.

10.6 Chemical Procedures to Improve Tolerance

Within this chapter, it is impossible to discuss all details of industrial procedures developed in order to make human immunoglobulins applicable by i.v. the route. Thus, only some principles of polishing "standard IgG" are summarized (historical examples mostly with modification of the molecules):

- Harsh pepsin digestion leading to 5S $F(ab')_2$ fragments devoid of Fc-effector functions and shortened half-life in vivo (Schultze and Schwick 1962)
- Plasmin digestion (Sgouris 1967)
- Limited sulfitolysis (Masuho et al. 1976)
- Reduction and alkylation (Wright 1978)
- Anion exchange chromatography and PEG precipitation
- Treatment with ß-propiolactone (Stephan 1969), an IgM/IgA enriched product remained on the market in some countries

Only a very few of these products are still available in some regions of the world, mainly because the above measures to achieve i.v. tolerability provided markedly impaired structures and functions of IgG. Some procedures destroyed IgG3. Currently, the plasma fractionating companies use combinations of procedures to achieve high recovery as well as high purity and leave their product as native as possible, nevertheless well-tolerated by the i.v. route (see Chaps. 12 and 13).

10.7 The First Conference on IVIG Quality

In pivotal trials, rarely placebo controlled, the biological activity of most of the older products was assessed measuring protection from infections of antibody-deficient patients. Head-to-head comparisons of different products in vivo or placebo-controlled trials were rarely performed. A few clinical trials in patients with primary Immunodeficiencies illustrating developmental steps should be mentioned: Ammann et al. 1982; Steele et al. 1987; Garbett et al. 1989; Schiff et al. 1997; Lamari et al. 2000; Roifman et al. 2003; Kallenberg 2007).

In order to define some quality characteristics for IgG preparations a WHO/IUIS expert committee met in 1983 and defined minimal requirements for IVIG products (IUIS 1983):

- Obtained from plasma pools from at least 1000 donors
- Prekallikrein activator (PKA) activity below a predefined threshold level
- Kinins below a predefined threshold level
- Anticomplementary activity (ACA) below a predefined threshold level (a general lot release criterion)
- Plasmin content below a predefined threshold level
- No accumulative preservatives (i.e., Merthiolate)
- IgG content at least 90% (monomers + dimers, low aggregate content)
- IgG as native as possible, i.e., chemically unmodified, retained biological functions such as antigen recognition and Fc functions
- Physiological IgG subclass distribution
- Titer of some selected specific antibodies guaranteed, a lot release criterion varying from brand to brand
- Low IgA, absence or minute amounts of IgE
- Isohemagglutinins below a predefined threshold level
- Alloantibodies (i.e., anti-D and others) below a predefined threshold level

At that time, not all products fulfilled these requirements. However, keeping these goals in mind the different companies intensified their research heading for products that came as close to these requirements as possible. After a one and half decade of development, the first "native" 7S IgG concentrate came to the market in Switzerland: Ig-SRC (SRC = Swiss Red Cross). The clue to reach intravenous tolerability was the polishing of "standard IgG" at low pH and traces of pepsin. This step rendered remaining aggregates ineffective. Other manufacturers applied other techniques to get rid of IgG aggregates or to render them non-complement activating. Much progress in polishing steps was made leading to different products with lyophilized or liquid formulation needing different stabilizers (Cherin et al. 2016).

10.8 Adverse Events

Severe adverse events (sAEs) from the very beginning of transfusion science and its clinical application have been a threat to the recipients. sAEs encompass incompatible transfusion reactions, TRALI, anaphylactic reactions, organ damage, and transmission of pathogens. Plasma products mediate some of these sAEs as well. Back in the early 1940s, an elevated risk for "homologous serum jaundice" was associated with the use of pooled serum (for stabilizing yellow fever vaccine). The same was true for the first product prepared from pooled plasma, albumin (Spurling et al. 1946). Great efforts made already in 1945 available a virus inactivation method for albumin concentrates, pasteurization at 60 °C for 10 h (Gelli et al. 1948). Unfortunately, this method was not applicable to "standard IgG" and sporadic transmission of hepatitis occurred (see below).

The recommendations by the WHO/IUIS expert committee in 1983 were based on causes of adverse events known at that time. A major problem at that time were immediate anaphylactoid reactions caused by anti-IgA antibodies (IgG or IgE isotype) in the patients and "phlogistic" reactions delayed by about 2–3 h after start of the infusion (= patient-related) or anticomplementary, PKA or kinin activity in the products (= product-related).

10.8.1 Pathogen Transmission

The worst of the adverse events with IgG concentrates which occurred after the WHO/IUIS recommendation was the transmission of hepatitis C virus (HCV; "hepatitis non-A, non-B" termed at that time) by some polyvalent IgG preparations (Lane 1983; Lever et al. 1984; Stephan and Dichtelmüller 1983; Weiland et al. 1986; Welch et al. 1983; Williams et al. 1989) as well as with an anti-D immunoglobulin prepared in the former German Democratic Republic. It became apparent that Cohn fractionation II of human plasma alone was limited in its capacity to inactivate transmissible viruses while products remained free from the threat of virus transmission, particularly those prepared by the Kistler-Nitschmann fractionation technique, most likely due to the low pH applied at polishing. Several patients infected by HCV experienced a severe course of infection and a few died (Björkander et al. 1988; Razvi et al. 2001) making viral safety a crucial issue for IgG products (Cuthbertson et al. 1987). Driven by the virus transmission risks of blood transfusion and the obvious elevated risk of virus transmission by coagulation factor concentrates, authorities always orient themselves to the highest risk level and require accordingly measures to guarantee product safety. IgG therapy on one hand comprises a particular set of risks, while on the other hand the fractionation technique and the polishing steps offer particular opportunities for virus inactivation/removal. The particular risks with IgG therapy are:

- Economic reasons force manufacturers to manipulate at once large volumes of pooled plasma.
- One contaminated plasma unit can contaminate thus a large pool.
- One lot of IgG concentrate has many vials for clinical use.
- The many vials are applied to a certain (high) number of patients and in case of contamination infections are usually clustered in a patient population.
- Recipients might be individuals with genetically impaired antibody production. Such patients are particularly vulnerable to infections. Such patients receive IgG concentrates for replacement therapy possibly lifelong, and patients are prolonged and repeatedly exposed to (a theoretical) risk of pathogen transmission.
- Patients with inherited immunodeficiency might need lifelong replacement therapy which exposes them to repeated risk of virus transmission.
- Patients with chronic autoimmune and/or inflammatory diseases are treated with "immunomodulatory" doses of IgG. The doses are high and usually are applied repeatedly, and this again exposes patients to an elevated level of risk for pathogen transmission (Table 10.1).

Table 10.1 Transfusion medicine from the very early days onward was struggling with transmission of pathogens, particularly viruses

Genus	Viruses
Herpesviruses	Epstein-Barr virus (EBV), cytomegalovirus (CMV), human herpesviruses (HHV)-6, -7, -8
Papovaviruses	John Cunningham (JC) and BK (initials patients) viruses
Parvoviruses	**Parvovirus B19V**, adeno-associated virus (AAV)
Hepadnaviruses	**Homologous serum jaundice (HBV)**
Circoviruses	Transfusion transmitted virus (TTV), TTV-like mini virus or torque teno mini virus (TLMV)
Retroviruses	**Human immunodeficiency virus (HIV)-1,-2**, human T-cell lymphotropic virus (HTLV III, LAV)
Flaviviruses	**Hepatitis C virus (HCV)**, **West Nile virus (WNV)**, **Zika virus (ZIKV)**, yellow fever virus (YFV), other arboviruses
Alphaviruses	Chikungunya virus (CHIKV), (W,E,V) equine encephalosis viruses (EEVs)
Coronaviruses	**SARS-associated virus**
Bornaviruses	Borna disease virus
Picornaviruses	**Hepatitis A virus (HAV)**, human enteroviruses
Bunyaviruses	La Crosse, Sin Nombre, Hantaan
Arenaviruses	Lassa fever, Junin, Machupo
Hepaviridae	**Hepatitis E virus (HEV)**

Listed are some viruses found in blood donations. Pooling of plasma elevates the risk of infecting clusters of recipients by a single lot of a plasma product. Those viruses, which might represent a potential threat for transmission by plasma products, are depicted in bold

In order to lower the risk of pathogen transmission, validated processes for elimination/inactivation of pathogens became mandatory for plasma products (see Chap. 12).

It needs to be mentioned that up to date not a single case of HIV infection acquired through IgG preparations even before dedicated virus inactivation and removal steps have been introduced to the fractionation and polishing processes. Furthermore, no case of variant CJD transmission by plasma products has been reported worldwide (Helbert et al. 2016). The problem with hepatitis C seems to be solved because since more than 25 years no new cases of HCV transmission have been reported. Nevertheless all companies producing IgG concentrates are extremely alert with respect to pathogens possibly emerging/re-emerging in the future.

10.8.2 Noninfectious Adverse Events

A coevolution of noninfectious adverse event profiles with "improved" products, routes of application, doses applied, increased infusion rate, and the more broad therapeutic use of IgG concentrates has occurred (Feldmeyer et al. 2010; Berger 2013; Dantal 2013). Reasons for the adverse effects are multiple (Späth et al. 2015).

Parameters controllable by, e.g., polishing steps or the use of appropriate stabilizers:

- Harming of the IgG molecules inherent to any fractionation process.
- Chemicals to stabilize the concentrates during their shelf life.
- Inappropriate handling of the concentrates during their shelf life.
- Alteration of the IgG molecules due to inappropriate handling before infusion (foam).
- Presence of too high amounts of preformed dimers in the preparation.
- Skin reactions at site of infusion/injection.
- Too rapid increase of exogenous IgG in the circulation, a combination of infusion rate and strength of the solution infused.
- Increase in recovery might lead to an altered population of IgG molecules resulting in an altered adverse event profile.

Parameters not controllable:

- The immune status of the diseased patient at the time point of the infusion, i.e., the subtle and extreme wide array of recognition by infused IgG of the patients' immune structures and vice versa, the recognition by patients' immune system, the exogenous IgG (for details see P. Späth et al. 2015).

Delayed adverse reactions might all be associated with risk factors the diseased patient brings along. These factors are discussed to render patients particularly sensitive to effects of the interrelation of applied IgG and patient's immune status. Such "risk factors" may exist subclinically. Some of the more common adverse events seen primarily with IVIG are (modified from Cherin et al. 2016):

- Migraine headaches
- Aseptic meningitis (patient dehydrated? Local meningeal inflammation induced by IgG on the basis of infused IgG recognizing "risk factors?") (Sekul et al. 1994; Scribner et al. 1994; Hopkins and Jolles 2005; Berg and Fuellenhals 2016)
- Osmotic nephrosis caused by sugars like saccharose in the products, associated with "risk factors" of the kidney
- Other renal impairments due to diuretics and renin–angiotensin system inhibitors
- Thrombosis/embolic events and myocardial infarction (probably caused by activated faxtor XI, high sodium content, and high osmolality) (Hefer and Jaloudi 2004; Elkayam et al. 2000; Ammann et al. 2016)
- Hemolysis (probably caused by isohemagglutinins and alloantibodies)
- Neutropenia (cause unknown)
- Transfusion-related acute lung injury (TRALI; speculation on pathogenetic role of anti-neutrophil antibodies)
- Hyponatremia, pseudohyponatremia (rare, defect in urinary free water excretion?)
- Hyperviscosity syndrome (possibly caused by preexisting very high levels of IgG in patients) (Hague et al. 1990; Oh et al. 1997)
- Necrotizing enterocolitis in newborn babies (cause unknown, immaturity?) (Figueras-Aloy et al. 2010; Kara et al. 2013; Navarro et al. 2009; Yang et al. 2016)

These observations have stimulated further improvements of the products: Saccharose was replaced by other stabilizers, by validation studies elimination of potential procoagulant activity (demonstrating activated factor XI) during the manufacturing process has had to be shown by each company; some of these studies have been published (José et al. 2013; Williams et al. 2013). The rate of hemolytic adverse events has increased with chromatographically produced IgG concentrates. Attempts to reduce these rates include screening of individual plasma donations and withholding from pooling very high isohemagglutinin titer donations and/or polishing by affinity column chromatography steps to lower these titers (Dhainaut et al. 2013; Siani et al. 2014; Gerber et al. 2016). With the expanding use of IgG concentrates for subcutaneous application, any adverse events have declined considerably.

10.9 Summary

Manufacturing and safe clinical use of IgG concentrates has gone a long stony but finally successful way. Compared to "old" products currently available, IgG concentrates combine better recovery and higher purity, are more convenient in their use due to liquid formulation and storage at room temperature during their shelf life, and have a higher pathogen safety, tolerability, purity, and efficacy than the products 40 years ago (Gelfand 2006; Cherin et al. 2016).

The development of products for s.c. administration expanded the spectrum of treatment options. The option of self-administration by patients increased their quality of life because this treatment can be given at home. S.c. products also help to treat patients who have repeated intolerance reactions to IVIG. S.c. products are increasingly studied in chronic autoimmune/inflammatory conditions, e.g., chronic inflammatory demyelinating polyradiculoneuropathy (CIDP), multifocal motor neuropathy (MMN), and various dermatological and collagen-vascular diseases. Results from clinical trials will be available soon. Whether or not ITP can be treated by s.c. route remains to be clarified. One boy with ataxia telangiectasia developed ITP while being on s.c. replacement for his immunodeficiency (Heath and Goldman 2010).

The availability of human IgG has enabled clinicians all over the world to treat several diseases with relatively low toxicity. Nevertheless, the obstacles illustrated in this chapter should be kept in mind to motivate authorities and the plasma industry to enforce efforts to further optimize their products.

References

Ammann AJ, Ashman RF, Buckley RH, Hardie WR, Krantmann HJ. Use of intravenous gammaglobulin in antibody immunodeficiency: results of a multicenter controlled trial. Clin Immunol Immunopathol. 1982;22(1):60–7.

Ammann EM, Haskins CB, Fillman KM, Ritter RL, Gu X, Winiecki SK, Carnahan RM, Torner JC, Fireman BH, Jones MP, Chrischilles EA. Intravenous immune globulin and thromboembolic adverse events: a systematic review and meta-analysis of RCTs. 2016. Am J Hematol. 2016;91(6):594–605.

Berg R, Fuellenhals E. Aseptic meningitis following therapy with immune globulins: a combination of product features and patient characteristics? Transfusion (Paris). 2016; 56(12):3021–8.

Berger M. Adverse effects of IgG therapy. J Allergy Clin Immunol Pract. 2013;1(6):558–66.

Björkander J, Cunningham-Rundles C, Lundin P, Olsson R, Söderström R, Hanson LA. Intravenous immunoglobulin prophylaxis causing liver damage in 16 of 77 patients with hypogammaglobulinemia or IgG subclass deficiency. Am J Med. 1988;84(1):107–11.

Bruton OC. Agammaglobulinemia. Pediatrics. 1952;9(6):722–8.

Cherin P, Marie I, Michallet M, Pelus E, Dantal J, Crave JC, Delain JC, Viallard JF. Management of adverse events in the treatment of patients with immunoglobulin therapy: a review of evidence. Autoimmun Rev. 2016;15(1):71–81.

Cohn EJ, Oncley JL, Strong LE, Hughes WL, Armstrong SH. Chemical, clinical and immunological studies on the product of human plasma fractionation. I. The characterization of the protein fractions of human plasma. J Clin Invest. 1944;23:417–32.

Cuthbertson B, Perry RJ, Foster PR, Reid KG, Crawford RJ, Yap PL. The viral safety of intravenous immunoglobulin. J Infect. 1987;15(2):125–33.

Dantal J. Intravenous immunoglobulins: in-depth review of excipients and acute kidney injury risk. Am J Nephrol. 2013;38(4):275–84.

Dhainaut F, Guillaumat PO, Dib H, Perret G, Sauger A, De Coupade C, et al. In vitro and in vivo properties differ among liquid intravenous immunoglobulin preparations. Vox Sang. 2013;104(2):115–26.

Elkayam O, Paran D, Milo R, Davidovitz Y, Almoznino-Sarafian D, Zeltser D, Yaron M, Caspi D. Acute myocardial infarction associated with high dose intravenous immunoglobulin infusion for autoimmune disorders. A study of four cases. Ann Rheum Dis. 2000;59(1):77–80.

Feldmeyer L, Benden C, Haile SR, Boehler A, Speich R, French LE, et al. Not all intravenous immunoglobulin preparations are equally well tolerated. Acta Derm Venereol. 2010;90(5):494–7.

Figueras-Aloy J, Rodríguez-Miguélez JM, Iriondo-Sanz M, Salvia-Roiges MD, Botet-Mussons F, Carbonell-Estrany X. Intravenous immunoglobulin and necrotizing enterocolitis in newborns with hemolytic disease. Pediatrics. 2010;125:139–44.

Garbett ND, Currie DC, Cole PJ. Comparison of the clinical efficacy and safety of an intramuscular and an intravenous immunoglobulin preparation for replacement therapy in idiopathic adult onset panhypogammaglobulinaemia. Clin Exp Immunol. 1989;76(1):1–7.

Geha RS. Charles A. Janeway and Fred S. Rosen: the discovery of gamma globulin therapy and primary immunodeficiency diseases at Boston Children's Hospital. J Allergy Clin Immunol. 2005;116(4):937–40.

Gelfand EW. Differences between IGIV products: impact on clinical outcome. Int Immunopharmacol. 2006;6(4):592–9.

Gelli SS, Neefe JR, Stokes J, Janeway CA, Scatchard G. Chemical, clinical, and immunological studies on the products of human plasma fractionation. XXXVI. Inactivation of the virus of homologous serum hepatitis in solutions of normal human serum albumin by means of heat. J Clin Invest. 1948;27(2):239.

Gerber S, Gaida A, Spiegl N, Wymann S, Antunes AM, Menyawi IE, et al. Reduction of isoagglutinin in intravenous immunoglobulin (IVIG) using blood group A- and B-specific immunoaffinity chromatography: industry-scale assessment. BioDrugs. 2016;30(5):441–51.

Hague RA, Eden OB, Yap PL, Mok JY, Rae P. Hyperviscosity in HIV infected children--a potential hazard during intravenous immunoglobulin therapy. Blut. 1990;61(2–3):66–7.

Heath J, Goldman FD. Idiopathic thrombocytopenic purpura in a boy with ataxia telangiectasia on immunoglobulin replacement therapy. J Pediatr Hematol Oncol. 2010;32(1):e25–7.

Hefer D, Jaloudi M. Thromboembolic events as an emerging adverse effect during high-dose intravenous immunoglobulin therapy in elderly patients: a case report and discussion of the relevant literature. Ann Hematol. 2004;83(10):661–5.

Helbert MR, Bangs C, Bishop M, Molesworth A, Ironside J. No evidence of asymptomatic variant CJD infection in immunodeficiency patients treated with UK-sourced immunoglobulin. Vox Sang. 2016;110(3):282–4.

Hopkins S, Jolles S. Drug-induced aseptic meningitis. Expert Opin Drug Saf. 2005;4:285–97.

IUIS/WHO NOTICE. Appropriate uses of human immunoglobulin in clinical practice. Clin Exp Immunol. 1983;52:417–22.

Janeway CA. The plasma proteins; their functions and clinical uses. Pediatrics. 1948;2(4):489–97.

José M, Marzo N, Pons B, Herrerias A, López L, Faro M, López M, Jorquera JI. Pasteurization inactivates clotting enzymes during Flebogamma® and Flebogamma® DIF production. Biologicals. 2013;41(6):393.

Kallenberg CGM. A 10% ready-to-use intravenous human immunoglobulin offers potential economic advantages over a lyophilized product in the treatment of primary immunodeficiency. Clin Exp Immunol. 2007;150(3):437–41.

Kara S, Ulu-ozkan H, Yilmaz Y, Arikan FI, Dilmen U, Bilge YD. Necrotizing enterocolitis in a newborn following intravenous immunoglobulin treatment for haemolytic disease. J Coll Physicians Surg Pak. 2013;23(8):598–600.

Lamari F, Karamanos NK, Papadopoulou-Alataki E, Kanakoudi-Tsakalidou F, Dimitracopoulos G, Anastassiou ED. Monitoring of two intravenous immunoglobulin preparations for immunoglobulin G subclasses and specific antibodies to bacterial surface antigens and relation with their levels in treated immunodeficient patients. J Pharm Biomed Anal. 2000;22(6):1029–36.

Lane RS. Non-A, non-B hepatitis from intravenous immunoglobulin. Lancet. 1983; 2(8356):974–5.

Lever AM, Webster AD, Brown D, Thomas HC. Non-A, non-B hepatitis occurring in agammaglobulinaemic patients after intravenous immunoglobulin. Lancet. 1984;2(8411):1062–4.

Masuho Y, Tomibe K, Matsuzawa K, Watanabe T, Ishimoto S. Reconstruction of intact gamma-globulin from S-sulfonated gamma-globulin in vivo. J Biochem. 1976;79(6):1377–9.

Navarro M, Negre S, Matoses ML, Golombek SG, Vento M. Necrotizing enterocolitis following the use of intravenous immunoglobulin for haemolytic disease of the newborn. Acta Paediatr. 2009;98:1214–7.

Nitschmann H, Kistler P, Lergier W. Vereinfachtes Verfahren zur Gewinnung von humanem Albumin und g-Globulin aus Blutplasma mittels Alkoholfällung – [Simplified method for isolation of human albimin and g-globulin from plasma using the ethnol precipitation method]. Helv Chim Acta. 1954;37:866–73.

Oh KT, Boldt HC, Danis RP. Iatrogenic central retinal vein occlusion and hyperviscosity associated with high-dose intravenous immunoglobulin administration. Am J Ophthalmol. 1997;124(3):416–8.

Oncley JL, Melin M, Richert DA, Cameron JW, Gross PM. The separation of the antibodies, isoagglutinins, prothrombin, plasminogen and b1-lipoprotein into subfractions of human plasma. J Am Chem Soc. 1949;71:541–50.

Ordman CW, Tenning CG, Janeway CA. Chemical, clinical and immunological studies on the products of human plasma fractions. XII. The use of concentrated normal human serum gamma globulin (human immune serum globulin) in the prevention and attenuation of measles. J Clin Immunol. 1944;23(4):541–9.

Razvi S, Schneider L, Jonas MM, Cunningham-Rundles C. Outcome of intravenous immunoglobulin-transmitted hepatitis C virus infection in primary immunodeficiency. Clin Immunol. 2001;101(3):284–8.

Roifman CM, Schroeder H, Berger M, Sorensen R, Ballow M, Buckley RH, et al. Comparison of the efficacy of IGIV-C, 10% (caprylate/chromatography) and IGIV-SD, 10% as replacement therapy in primary immune deficiency. A randomized double-blind trial. Int Immunopharmacol. 2003;3(9):1325–33.

Rosen FS, Janeway CA. J Pediatr. 1994;125(1):167–8.

Schiff RI, Williams LW, Nelson RP, Buckley RH, Burks W, Good RA. Multicenter crossover comparison of the safety and efficacy of Intraglobin-F with Gamimune-N, Sandoglobulin and Gammagard in patients with primary immunodeficiency diseases. J Clin Immunol. 1997;17(1):21–8.

Schultze HE, Schwick G. Über neue Möglichkeiten intravenöser Gammaglobulin-Applikation – [on new possibilities of intravenous gamma globulin administration]. Dt Med Wochenschr. 1962;87(34):1643–50.

Scribner CL, Kapit RM, Phillips ET, Rickles NM. Aseptic meningitis and intravenous immunoglobulin therapy. Ann Intern Med. 1994;121:305–6.

Sekul EA, Cupler EJ, Dalakas MC. Aseptic meningitis associated with high-dose intravenous immunoglobulin therapy: frequency and risk factors. Ann Intern Med. 1994;121:259–62.

Sgouris JT. The preparation of plasmin-treated immune serum globulin for intravenous use. XXIst Scientific Meeting of the Protein Foundation, Cambridge, 1966 Nov 21-1966 Nov 22;1967:p. 71–84.

Siani B, Willimann K, Wymann S, Marques AA, Widmer E. Isoagglutinin reduction in human immunoglobulin products by donor screening. Biol Ther. 2014;4(1–2):15–26.

Smith CA. Dr. Janeway and American pediatrics. Pediatrics. 1977;59(2):149–50.

Späth PJ, Granata G, La Marra F, Kuijpers TW, Quinti I. On the dark side of therapies with immunoglobulin concentrates: the adverse events. Front Immunol. 2015;6:11.

Spurling N, Shone J, Vaughan J. The incidence, incubation period, and symptomatology of homologous serum jaundice. Br Med J. 1946;2(4472):409.

Steele RW, Augustine RA, Tannenbaum AS, Charlton RK. A comparison of native and modified intravenous immunoglobulin for the management of hypogammaglobulinemia. Am J Med. 1987;293(2):69–74.

Stephan W. Beseitigung der Komplementfixierung von g-globulin durch chemische Modifizierung mit b-Propiolacton – [Elimination of complement fixation of g-globulin by chemical modification with b-propiolactone]. Z Klin Chem Klin Biochem. 1969;7(3):282–6.

Stephan W, Dichtelmüller H. Non-A, non-B hepatitis from intravenous immunoglobulins. Lancet. 1983;2(8365–66):1488.
Weiland O, Mattsson L, Glaumann H. Non-A, non-B hepatitis after intravenous gammaglobulin. Lancet. 1986;1(8487):976–7.
Welch AG, Cuthbertson B, McIntosh RV, Foster PR. Non-A, non-B hepatitis from intravenous immunoglobulin. Lancet. 1983;2(8360):1198–9.
Williams M, Willey J, Tull K, Stevenson G, Parks M, McElrath LT, Golovko L, Russ C, Griffin J, Vandeberg P. Removal of coagulation factors by the Gamunex®-C purification process. J Allergy Clin Immunol. 2013;131(2, Suppl.) AB10 [Congress abstract].
Williams PE, Yap PL, Gillon J, Crawford RJ, Urbaniak SJ, Galea G. Transmission of non-A, non-B hepatitis by pH4-treated intravenous immunoglobulin. Vox Sang. 1989;57(1):15–8.
Wright JK. Reduced immunoglobulin G activates complement system with decreased cooperativity. Biochem Biophys Res Commun. 1978;83(4):1284–90.
Yang Y, Pan JJ, Zhou XG, Zhou XY, Cheng R, YH H. The effect of immunoglobulin treatment for hemolysis on the incidence of necrotizing enterocolitis – a meta-analysis. Eur Rev Med Pharmacol Sci. 2016;20(18):3902–10.

11 Basics of Immunoglobulins as Effector Molecules and Drugs

Tchavdar L. Vassilev, Victor Kostov, Stephan von Gunten, and Anastas D. Pashov

11.1 Introduction

Immunoglobulins (antibodies) are glycoprotein molecules that play a key role in adaptive immunity. They protect us in the hostile environment of bacteria, viruses, and parasites. There are five classes of human immunoglobulins—IgM, IgG, IgA, IgE, and IgD. Most IgM antibodies (1.5 mg/mL plasma) are "natural"—i.e., they are produced even without an antigenic stimulus. Their antigen-binding polyspecificity ensures them a role as a first line of defense mechanism against invading pathogens. The therapeutic potential of pooled IgM has not been utilized in clinical practice yet. IgG is the most abundant immunoglobulin isotype in human plasma (12 mg/mL), and this chapter is devoted mostly to it. The ability of IgG antibodies to bind with a high affinity and specificity to a remarkably large variety of antigens is their main feature. Serum IgA (3 mg/mL, 90% as monomers, 10% dimeric) has effects similar to these of IgG, while secretory IgA antibodies are resistant to proteases and protect all mucosal surfaces. IgE is the class with the lowest plasma concentration (0.05 mcg/mL). The contact of mast cell-bound IgE with the specific antigen results in an acute inflammatory reaction that might help to expel parasites from the gut. IgE antibodies are also believed to have a role in the host defense against noxious environmental substances, including venoms, environmental xenobiotics, and irritants (Palm et al. 2012). The plasma concentration of IgD is highly variable (mean value 25 mg/mL), and the biological role of antibodies of this isotype is poorly understood.

T.L. Vassilev (✉)
UniMed Medical Center, Sevlievo, Bulgaria
e-mail: tchavdar@gmail.com

V. Kostov • A.D. Pashov
Stephan Angelov Institute of Microbiology, Sofia, Bulgaria

S. von Gunten
Institute of Pharmacology, University of Bern, Bern, Switzerland

P. Imbach (ed.), *Antibody Therapy*, https://doi.org/10.1007/978-3-319-68038-5_11

The future of the use of antibodies as drugs for the prevention and treatment of infectious, autoimmune diseases and cancer is bright. The global normal pooled intravenous immunoglobulin (IVIg) market grows by 6.8% each year and is expected to reach $11.6 billion (230 tons) by 2021 (see http://www.prnewswire.com/news-releases).

11.2 Structure and Functions of IgG Molecules

11.2.1 The $F(ab)_2$ Fragment

IgG is composed of two heavy and two light polypeptide chains linked to each other by disulfide bonds. Each of the two antigen-binding (Fab) fragments is composed of a light chain and a portion of a heavy chain. The light chain has two immunoglobulin domains—regions of compactly folded structure—while the heavy chain has four (see Fig. 11.1). The amino-terminal domains of both chains are highly variable (V domains), while the others are referred to as "constant." The variable (V) domains of both form the antigen-binding site (paratope). They are not encoded in full in the genome, but by a combination of multiple variants of different gene segments. Two or three gene segments (for the V regions of light and heavy chains, respectively) are assembled by a process known as gene rearrangement forming a complete V-region sequence. There are 34–38 V-kappa and 5 J-kappa; 29–33 V-lambda and 4–5 J-lambda light chain V segments, as well as

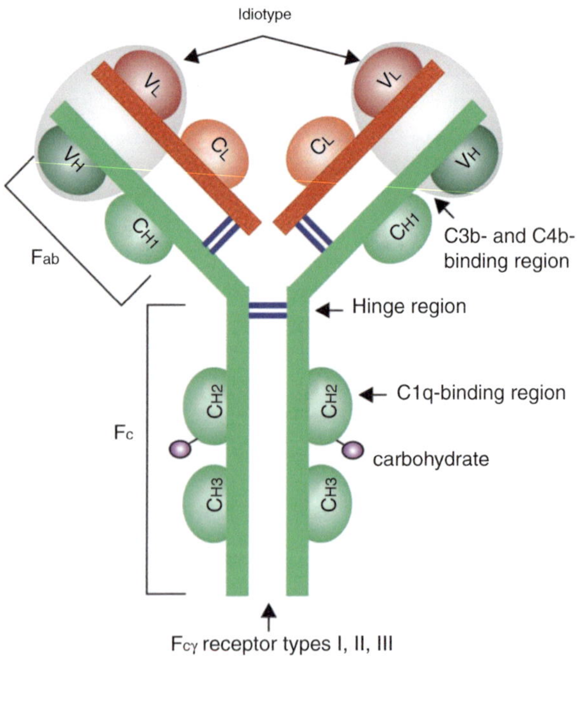

Fig. 11.1 The structure of an IgG molecule. The heavy immunoglobulin chain and its four domains are shown in *green* and the light in *red*. The inter-chain disulfide bonds are in *blue*. The variable (*V*) regions of both chains of the Fab fragments shape the two antigen-binding sites (paratopes) of the antibody. Its idiotypic determinants (idiotopes) are in the same area. The biding sites of complement components and Fc receptors are also shown

36–46 V-, 23 D-, and 6 J functional heavy chain V-gene segments. The combination of any V-light chain variant with any V-heavy chain should result in approx. 2.10^6 antigen-binding site specificities. Further diversity is generated by the subtraction (by endonucleases) and by the addition (by the enzyme terminal deoxynucleotidyl transferase (TdT) and by the incorrect DNA chain repair) of nucleotides during the process of gene fragment recombination. The somatic hypermutation of the already rearranged V-region genes of the activated B cells in the secondary lymphoid organs increases the diversity still further. These processes result in the ability to generate about 10^{12} different specificities of immunoglobulin B cell receptors and of circulating immunoglobulins. B cells with strong anti-self reactivities are eliminated, become anergic, or change their receptors by receptor editing in the bone marrow. The repertoire of immunoglobulin B cell receptors and circulating immunoglobulins is regarded as being quasi-complete—i.e., although purged of strong self-reactivities, they can still interact with practically any xenoantigen. The same is true for the antibody diversity in pooled therapeutic immunoglobulins produced from healthy donor plasma pools. The antibody repertoire is discussed in more detail below.

Between 15 and 25% of all Fab variable regions have additional complex branched glycans linked to N-glycosylation sites that emerge during somatic hypermutation. These glycans affect antigen binding by both BCR and circulating immunoglobulins (van de Bovenkamp et al. 2016).

11.2.2 The Fc Fragment

The Fc fragments are built of a pair of the CH2 and CH3 heavy chain domains (Fig. 11.1). The two CH3 domains are paired, while the two CH2 are not. Fc fragments are much less variable than the Fab antibody fragments. In addition to isotypic and allotypic differences, there are also hundreds of variants of the glycans coupled to it. The "hinge" region is located in between the $F(ab)_2$ and Fc fragments. Its length and flexibility determine the ability of both Fab arms to assume different arm angles—from 0^0 to 180^0. IgG1 and IgG3 antibodies have longer and flexible hinge regions, and this relates to their strong ability to activate complement and antibody-dependent cell cytotoxicity. IgG2 and IgG4 have short hinge regions and are weak complement activators.

The IgG binding to a toxin or to a virus particle can prevent the interaction with their surface receptors on target cells, thus neutralizing them. For other pathogens, however binding is not sufficient to disarm them. To fight them the Fc-fragment-dependent activation of complement and/or Fc receptors on immune cells is needed. This has as a result the launching of effector molecules—reactive oxygen species, cytokines, as well as antibody-mediated killing by complement-dependent cytotoxicity (CDC), by antibody-dependent cell cytotoxicity (ADCC), and by the antibody-dependent cellular phagocytosis (ADCP).

While monomeric IgG does not bind the C1q complement component, IgG that is part of immune complexes does so efficiently. Activating the complement system through its classical pathway results in the complement-mediated killing of the pathogen. Other component cascade components—C3b and C4b—attach to a site between the CH1 and VH domains of the heavy immunoglobulin chain and might interact with the corresponding receptors.

The IgG Fc fragments also allow for an active transport of these molecules to parts of the body which would have been otherwise unreachable—e.g., the human fetus.

The glycans attached to asparagine 297 of both heavy chain CH2 domains represent 3% (by weight) of IgG molecules. Their backbone structure is biantenary and carries N-acetylglucosamine, mannose, fucose, galactose, and sialic acid and other residues. The glycans of both heavy chains of an IgG molecule could have identical or different structures. These structures depend also on the diet and are modified in patients with autoimmune diseases.

The removal of the Fc-linked glycan suppresses the effector functions of the IgG molecule. Removal of the N-glycan impairs binding to activating FcR's and complement activation. The infusion of the bacterial IgG glycan-hydrolyzing enzyme EndoS has been shown to have the potential to suppress anti-self antibody-mediated autoimmunity (Hirose et al. 2012). Even minor changes in the glycan structure result in strong modification of these functions. These modifications could be clinically relevant, e.g., the engineered anti-CD20 antibody obinutuzumab with reduced fucosylation is used for the treatment of patients with chronic lymphocytic leukemia and follicular lymphoma who have not responded to a fucosylated anti-CD20 antibody (rituximab) (Quast et al. 2017).

11.2.3 Fc-Gamma Receptors

While the antigen-binding specificity of IgG molecules is only $F(ab)_2$ dependent, most biological effects depend on the ability of the Fc portion to engage various receptors on immune cells.

The neonatal Fc receptor for IgG (FcRn) stays apart from the other human Fcγ receptors because of its peculiar structure and functions. Unlike the others its structure resembles that of a MHC class I molecule. It binds to all IgG subclasses, and this interaction is not dependent on the glycosylation state of the immunoglobulin molecules. The FcRn receptor is responsible for the transplacental transport of IgG to the fetus. This receptor binds IgG in acidic vesicles at a $pH < 6.5$ and releases IgG at a $pH > 7.4$ in the blood. The long half-life of these maternal antibodies in the newborn child ensures a sufficient degree of protection until the start of the production of its own antibodies. Another important function of FcRn is its role in continuous IgG recycling which contributes toward the long half-life of immunoglobulins of this class in the circulation—21 days. In addition FcRn also binds and recirculates albumin.

The classical type I Fc receptors (FcγRI, FcγRIIa, FcγRIIb, FcγRIIc, FcγRIIIa, and FcγRIIIb), being members of the big immunoglobulin superfamily, are present in unequal combinations on many cells of the immune system (see Table 11.1). In addition, their expression levels vary on different cell types. FcγRIIb is the only known inhibitory receptor of this group. This activity is due to the ITIM (immunoreceptor tyrosine inhibitory motif) on its cytoplasmatic tail. It suppresses signaling through other stimulatory FcγRs, immunoglobulin receptors on B cells, etc. FcγRIIb binds weakly monomeric IgG, but interacts with IgG-containing immune complexes. The co-ligation of FcγRIIb and the BCR receptors of B cells results in the recruitment of SHIP (SH2-containg inositol phosphatase) to the BCR receptor complex, resulting in blocking the PI3-kinase. Blocking the PI3-kinase in turn reduces the availability of 3-phosphorylated phosphoinositide second messengers, critical for a variety of signaling pathways including phospholipase C activation and cell survival.

FcγRI is the only receptor with high affinity to IgG that allows it to bind monomeric IgG molecules. The FcγRII and FcγRIII are binding with low-affinity and high-avidity immune complexes and aggregated IgG, but not monomeric IgG. IgG complexes are generated during an ongoing immune response to invading pathogens and induce various inflammatory reactions by signaling through the abovementioned receptors. In a healthy individual, such FcγRII and FcγRIII activation does not occur, and thus, highly undesirable excessive signaling and inflammatory reactions are avoided.

CD23 and DC-SIGN belong to the group of nonclassical type II C-lectin receptors. They bind a site between the CH2 and CH3 regions of the Fc fragments. CD23 has been known as a receptor for IgE, but has recently been show to bind also to sialylated IgG. The functional consequences of these interactions remain poorly understood. DC-SIGN binds glycosylated proteins. The group of F. Nimmerjahn has claimed over the last years that the binding of Fc-sialylated IgG to DC-SIGN leads to the upregulation of the inhibitory FcγRIIB on macrophages and dendritic cells. The authors consider this upregulation as the main mechanism responsible for the beneficial immunomodulatory effects of immunoglobulin therapy in autoimmune diseases (Schwab and Nimmerjahn 2013). We and others have argued that the mechanisms of action of IVIg—a very complex and pluripotent drug—could hardly be explained by such a simplistic approach (von Gunten et al. 2014).

Table 11.1 Overview of the cell expression and Fc-binding affinity of human type 1 FcγRs

Type 1 FcγRs						
	FcγRI	FcγRIIa	FcγIIb	FcγRIIc	FcγRIIIa	FcγRIIIb
Expression	Monocytes, macrophages, granulocytes	Myeloid and dendritic cells, platelets	B, myeloid, and dendritic cells	NK cells	NK cells, macrophages, monocytes	Granulocytes
Fc-binding affinity	High	Low	Low	Low	Low	Low

11.2.4 IgG Subclasses

There are four subclasses of human IgG—IgG1 (approximately 7 mg/mL plasma), IgG2 (3 mg/mL), IgG3 (1 mg/mL), and IgG4 (0.5 mg/mL). While their amino acid sequences are 90% identical, they all have different heavy chains, hinge regions, and differing functional properties: placental transport, antigen binding, immune complex formation, ability to activate complement, ability to interact with activating and inhibitory Fc-gamma receptors on cell surfaces, and different half-lives in the plasma. The production of different IgG subclasses after immunization depends on the nature of the antigen and the cytokine milieu during the ongoing immune response. Cases of selective deficiency of each IgG subclass are rare but are informative about their roles in vivo.

Most protein-binding antibodies belong to the IgG1 subclass. Its decreased levels in primary and secondary immune deficiencies result in frequent infections. Most of the antibodies to carbohydrate antigens are of the IgG2 isotype. Their placental transfer and binding to Fc receptors is weak. The consequences of IgG2 deficiency are repeated infections caused by encapsulated bacteria—*Streptococci*, *Meningococci*, etc. The polysaccharide capsule protects these microorganisms from being engulfed by phagocytes. The efficiency of phagocytosis and killing depends on the presence of IgG2 anti-capsule antibodies.

Antibodies of the IgG3 subclass are strong activators of the complement system and bind to all activating Fc-gamma receptors. This makes them strongly pro-inflammatory. The production of specific IgG3 is generally in parallel with that of specific IgG1. IgG4 molecules have an unusual feature—they can exchange their Fab arms in vivo. As a result, they might become bi-specific and their two antigen-binding sites can bind different epitopes. Such antibodies lose the ability to cross-link antigens and the avidity of their antigen binding decreases considerably. The biological role of this phenomenon remains poorly understood. IgG4 antibodies are often produced in parasitic diseases as well as after the repeated administration of the same antigen. This is the case during immunotherapy of allergy by the continuous injection of increasing doses of an allergen. These specific IgG4 antibodies are often referred to as "blocking" as they compete with IgE with the same specificity for binding to the allergen, and as a result the immediate hypersensitivity reactions to it are suppressed or even prevented.

Pharmacopoeia rules oblige immunoglobulin producers to ensure that the ratio of IgG subclasses in the pooled IgG preparations corresponds to that in healthy plasma donors. The fractionation technologies used allow this requirement to be easily met.

11.2.5 IgG Monomers, Dimers, and Aggregates in Therapeutic Immunoglobulins

Some IgG molecules tend to aggregate in concentrated solutions. While IgG monomers and dimers are normal components of therapeutic immunoglobulin concentrates for intravenous administration, the percentage of aggregates is strictly controlled. The "art" of plasma fractionation is to apply technologies that result in as little aggregation as possible in the final product and which ensure the prevention of further aggregation during the shelf-life of a preparation.

The immunoglobulin plasma fraction obtained by cold ethanol fractionation in the early 1940s of the last century has been infused to volunteers. All developed a severe anaphylactic type of reaction (see Chap. 12). It took 20 more years to define the responsible mechanism. The drop of blood pressure has been shown to be linked to the presence of complement-activating IgG aggregates in the intravenously injected preparation. The activation of the complement system results in the generation of anaphylatoxins (C3a and C5a, released from the parent molecules). Both anaphylatoxins trigger the release of pre-formed mediators from basophils and mast cells. The mediators released (mainly histamine) cause dilatation of postcapillary venules, increased permeability of blood vessels, and hypotension.

IgG dimers are a regular component of all therapeutic immunoglobulins. They form spontaneously when two (or more) IgG molecules engage in, e.g., idiotype/anti-idiotype binding (Roux and Tankersley 1990). The affinity of these interactions is low and dimers take time to form. The percentage of dimers increases with the number of individual donors the plasma pool for fractionation comes from, as well as after storage of the IgG solution at 4 °C. The optimal pH for their formation is around 7.

The intravenous infusion of a preparation with a dimeric fraction above 8–10% has been shown to cause a cytokine storm in healthy volunteers (Späth et al. 2015). Control of dimer formation was achieved through L-proline at moderately lowered pH of the liquid IVIg (Bolli et al. 2010).

11.2.6 Non-immunoglobulin Molecules in Therapeutic IgG Preparations

Immunoglobulin preparations from different manufacturers may contain sugars (sucrose, maltose, etc.) or amino acids (glycine, L-proline, L-isoleucine, etc.), added to improve IgG long-term stability and diminish the formation of IgG aggregates and dimers.

In addition to pooled IgG, therapeutic immunoglobulins contain some amounts of human serum albumin, IgM and IgA, traces of IgE as well as fragments from immunoglobulins, and other plasma proteins. Their contribution to the overall antibody repertoire of the preparation is negligible. Anti-IgA antibodies are found in about 25% of individuals with selected IgA or IgA plus IgG deficiency. Non-IgE-mediated anaphylactic reactions may develop in them after IVIg infusions. R. Rachid et al. report that out of 22 IgA-deficient patients, three had anti-IgA antibodies and only one of them has had an anaphylactic reaction in the past. All of the studied patients tolerated subcutaneous administration of immunoglobulin (Rachid et al. 2011).

Numerous research groups have used sensitive analytical methods to look for the presence of non-immunoglobulin human molecules in therapeutic IVIg—cytokines, HLA and CD molecules, etc. (Blasczyk et al. 1993; Lam et al. 1993; Sherer et al.

2001). The existence of traces of these molecules comes as no surprise as most of them are members of the big immunoglobulin superfamily. Authors of these publications generally speculate that the non-immunoglobulin molecules may contribute to some of the immunomodulating effects of the therapeutic immunoglobulins. The concentration of these impurities is, however, low, and they can hardly be expected to have a biological effect.

11.2.7 Specific High-Titer Immunoglobulin Preparations

While most immunoglobulin preparations used today contain pooled human IgG isolated from plasma of healthy donors, there is still a small niche for specific high-titer immunoglobulins of animal (mostly equine) origin, as well as increasing niches for high-titer preparations of polyclonal human IgG as well as of human monoclonal immunoglobulins for passive prophylactic immunization and immunotherapy of infectious diseases.

Normal pooled IgG preparations contain antibodies neutralizing various bacterial toxins, viruses, etc. The levels of the respective protective antibodies in individual production lots are only known when being parameters of lot release. High-titer preparations are from reconvalescent plasma, from plasma of immunized volunteers, or from pre-screened individual donors. The levels of respective antibodies are standardized and the optimal doses to be administered are well known.

A hundred and twenty five years after the first use of hyperimmune horse serum in children with diphtheria, animal immunoglobulins are still used for the treatment of patients with diphtheria, tetanus, food-borne botulism, venomous snakebites, etc. The side effects and dangers of injecting animal antibodies to humans are serious and very well known. Their half-lives are short (approx. 5 days) and the lifelong sensitization to the administered animal proteins is inevitable. These preparations have an additional disadvantage—they could not be injected intravenously, but only intramuscularly. Passive immunization is an emergency procedure which works well when the antibodies are injected intravenously and reach the tissues quickly (Bayry et al. 2004). The reason for the continuous production and use of animal immunoglobulins is that they are cheaper and more easy to produce, while their human analogs are expensive, are not available worldwide, or are even nonexistent.

Several specific high-titer human immunoglobulins are available for intravenous administration: anti-D, anti-tetanus, anti-cytomegalovirus, anti-botulism, etc. (Lazarus et al. 1998); Arnon et al. 2006; Alexander et al. 2010). A human specific intravenous immunoglobulin for the treatment of Crimean/Congo hemorrhagic fever has been shown to be effective in a small clinical trial (Vassilenko et al. 1990), but its orphan drug status prevented its further production. The therapeutic potential of reconvalescent serum and monoclonal anti-Ebola virus monoclonal antibodies for Ebola virus disease has been proved in recent epidemic in sub-Saharan Africa (Moekotte et al. 2016).

A good recent example for the successful use of a human monoclonal antibody in a bacterial-caused disease is that of bezlotoxumab in severe *Clostridium difficile* infection. The administration of this antibody, specific for the A toxin of the pathogen, has resulted in a significantly lower rate of recurrent infections (Wilcox et al. 2017).

11.3 Antibody Repertoires in Therapeutic Immunoglobulins

11.3.1 Anti-protein Antibodies in Therapeutic Immunoglobulins

The extremely diverse repertoire of antibody specificities in each production batch of immunoglobulins keeps track of all previous immune activities during the lifetime of the plasma donors (Lacroix-Desmazes et al. 1995; Fesel and Coutinho 1999). The techniques for the indirect antibody repertoire profiling have evolved from immunoblot through phage libraries to microarrays.

In healthy people the total IgG reactivity with bacterial antigens was shown to be highly diversified both between individuals and as a function of age (Lacroix-Desmazes et al. 1995). Furthermore the repertoire can be probed through immunoglobulin variable region gene sequencing. It can also be explored by the combined profiles of binding to known antigens or to the proteome. Studying therapeutic immunoglobulin antibody repertoires in detail can detect unexpected antigen-binding specificities which might have therapeutic relevance. The patterns of binding to large arrays of mimotopes observed in the sera of patients have been referred to as immunosignatures. They have been shown to carry information beyond that provided by defined sets of well-known antigens (Merbl et al. 2009).

Thus, probing the entire Ig repertoire is more than just exploring a bunch of humoral immune responses. Natural antibodies (of IgG, IgM, and IgA isotypes) bind a variety of xeno- and autoantigens in a polyspecific manner (Fig. 11.2). Even without an antigenic stimulation, they are an essential, nonredundant factor of the defense against viral infections (Baumgarth et al. 2000). On the other hand, induced or adaptive anti-protein antibodies are not only elicited by specific antigens, but they are also T cell-dependent and, thus, of high affinity and high specificity. In most repertoire binding assays, it is hard to distinguish natural from induced antibodies.

11.3.2 The Repertoire of Carbohydrate-Specific Antibodies in IVIg

The surface of all living cells is covered by a layer of complex carbohydrates (glycans) also referred to as glycocalyx. Exposed to the cellular environment, these carbohydrates, often attached to glycoproteins or glycolipids, harbor multiple functions including charge repulsion effects, ligand-receptor interactions, adhesion, immunological identification (e.g., blood group antigens), and protection. Microbes often carry characteristic glycan structures, such as contained in bacterial cell walls or capsules, which are exploited for diagnostic purposes or as targets of antimicrobial therapy. In multicellular organisms there are species-dependent and interindividual differences of glycosylation, with carbohydrate xenoantigens and blood group

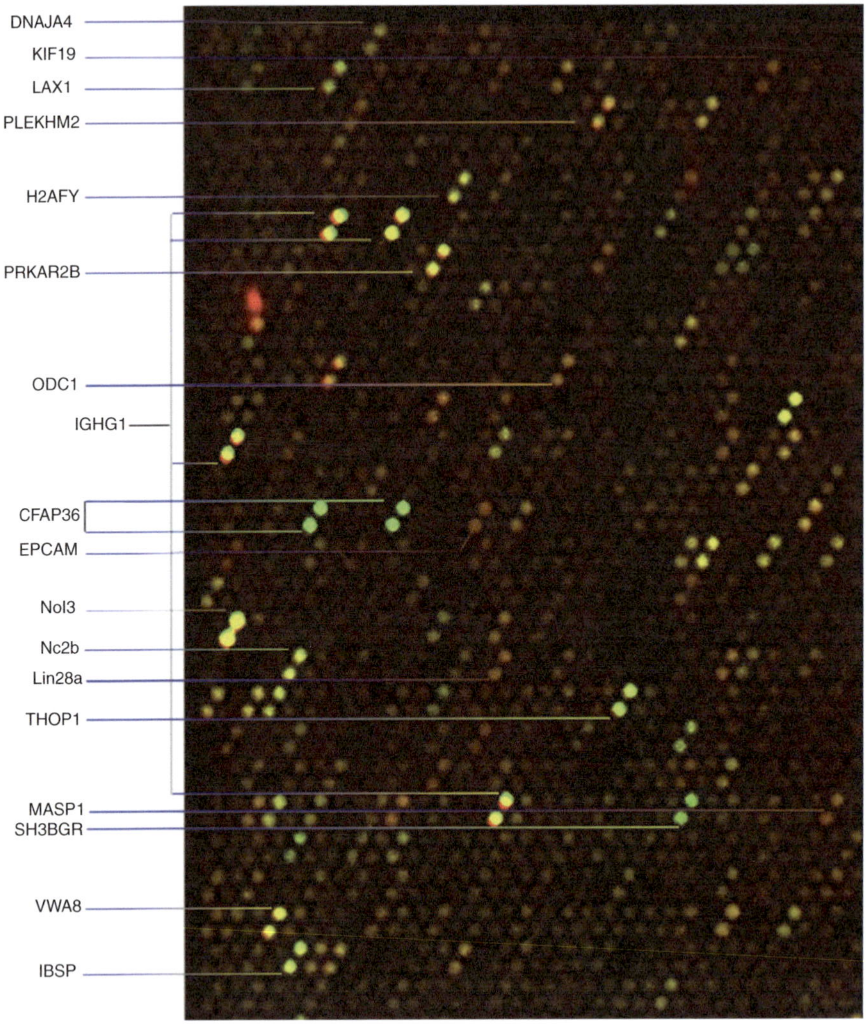

Fig. 11.2 Typical IVIg reactivity with a human protein array. Multiple natural anti-self reactivities are observable. Human proteome arrays (HuProt™, Cambridge Protein Arrays) were treated with 0.7 μM IgG from native or Fe^{2+}-exposed IVIg. Only block #19 (out of 24 blocks) is shown as an example. The labeled proteins indicate that the natural reactivities include not only sequestered intracellular proteins but also some receptors and secreted proteins (see Table 11.2)

determinants providing challenges to the fields of transfusion and transplantation medicine. Furthermore, intraindividual differences in cell surface glycosylation patterns exist, which explains the organotropism of certain microbes. Aberrant surface glycosylation is observed in essentially all human malignancies, and so-called tumor-associated carbohydrate antigens (TACA) have not only diagnostic significance but

Table 11.2 Identity and function of the self-proteins bound by IVIg (see Fig. 11.2)

Gene	Protein name	Notes
DNAJA4	DnaJ heat shock protein family (Hsp40) member A4	Heat shock protein
LAX1	Lymphocyte transmembrane adaptor 1	Membrane, regulator or TCR and BCR signaling
KIF19	Kinesin family member 19	Role in platelet development, motor protein in cilia
PLEKHM2_frag	Pleckstrin homology and RUN domain containing M2	Golgi, membrane movements, salmonella-induced filaments
H2AFY	H2A histone family member Y	Medulloblastoma antigen MU-MB-50.205
PRKAR2B	Protein kinase CAMP-dependent type II regulatory subunit beta	
ODC1	Ornithine decarboxylase 1	
CFAP36	Cilia- and flagella-associated protein 36	
EPCAM	Epithelial cell adhesion molecule, CD326	Tumor-associated GI tract, interaction between intestinal epithelial cells and intraepithelial lymphocytes
Nol3	Nucleolar protein 3	Antiapoptotic
Nc2b	Downregulator of transcription 1	Chromatin organization
Lin28a	Zinc finger CCHC domain-containing protein 1	Posttranscriptional regulator of genes involved in developmental timing and self-renewal in embryonic stem cells, tumor antigen
THOP1	Thimet oligopeptidase 1	Cleaves cytosolic peptides, making them unavailable for display on antigen-presenting cells
SH3BGR	SH3 domain-binding glutamate-rich protein	Skeletal muscles, myocytes, proline rich, glutamate rich
MASP1	Mannan-binding lectin serine peptidase 1	Lectin pathway of C′
VWA8	von Willebrand factor A domain containing 8	
IBSP	Integrin-binding sialoprotein	Rich in bone. Acidic amino acid clusters

also influence tumor progression (Boligan et al. 2015). IVIg contains reactivity to an extensive range of complex carbohydrates (Schneider et al. 2015). Recognized glycans included certain blood group antigens, tumor and microbial antigens, including bacterial cell wall, and capsular or exopolysaccharides. IVIg reactivity is not restricted to microbes, but include bacterial and viral glycan receptors (attachment sites), as well as carbohydrate tissue attachment sites of the exotoxins Shiga toxin from *Shigella dysenteriae* type 1 and the verotoxins SLT-I and SLT-II from

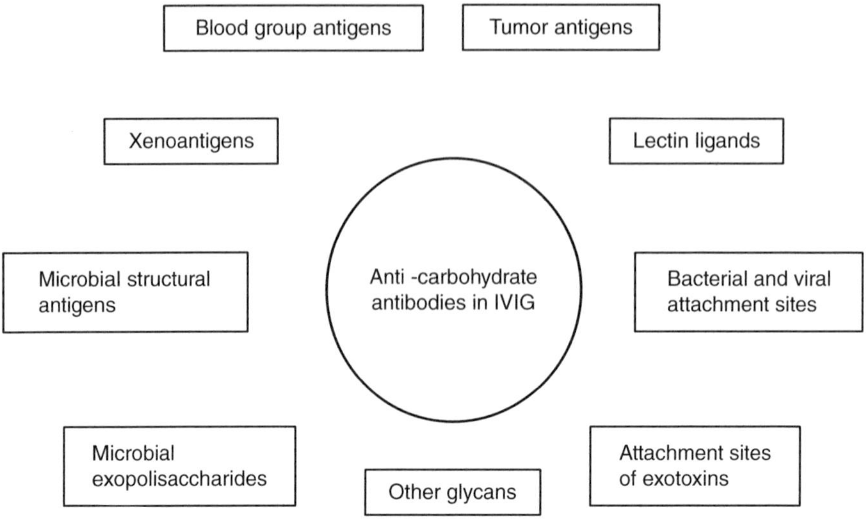

Fig. 11.3 Overview on proposed carbohydrate antigens (*rectangles*) recognized by glycan-specific antibodies in intravenous immunoglobulin (IVIg)

Escherichia coli, suggesting a potential role of glycan-specific antibodies by preventing adhesion processes and sequelae of infection (Schneider et al. 2015).

The comparison of different intravenous and subcutaneous immunoglobulin preparations using glycan array technology revealed a universal architecture of the human IgG anti-carbohydrate repertoire. A striking association between IVIg-binding capacity and terminal carbohydrate moieties was found, showing an association between structural features and glycan immunogenicity or tolerance (Schneider et al. 2015). Textbooks often refer to glycans as only poorly immunogenic and T cell-independent antigens. However, studies of the anti-carbohydrate repertoire indicate that class-switched IgG antibodies in IVIg, including non-IgG1 IgG antibodies, recognize a broad variety of glycans, thus indicating T cell involvement (Fig. 11.3). In line with IVIg-derived data, in a recent system biology study, the meningococcal polysaccharide vaccine MPSV4 was shown to induce higher IgG titers than a conjugate vaccine, and the analysis of blood transcription modules (BTM) revealed evidence for T cell signaling (Li et al. 2014). Furthermore, there is evidence for carbohydrate-specific T cells, also referred to as "Tcarbs," that specifically recognize presented carbohydrate epitopes from glycoconjugate vaccines (Avci et al. 2011). Research on the repertoire of carbohydrate-specific antibodies in IVIg revealed more insights into the composition and mechanisms of IgG concentrates as pluripotent drugs (Pashova et al. 2017).

11.3.3 Anti-idiotype Antibodies

Immunoglobulins are big, variable, and complex molecules and—therefore—immunogenic. Their antigenic determinants (epitopes) are divided into three groups—isotypic, allotypic, and idiotypic. The isotypic ones are present in all members of a given immunoglobulin class or subclass. The allotypic ones are inherited as alleles and each person inherits particular allotypes.

The idiotypic determinants (idiotopes) are unique antigen determinants of an antibody variable region. The idiotype of an individual antibody molecule is the combination of all its idiotopes. All antigen-binding molecules, free circulating immunoglobulins, membrane-bound immunoglobulin receptors of B cells, as well as T cell antigen receptors, have idiotopes. The latter can be "public"—when they are shared between several antibody clones— or "private" when they are unique for the antigen receptor of a cell and the antibodies produced by its progeny. Immunoglobulin preparations contain a vast diversity of IgG molecules that can network by idiotype-anti-idiotype interactions. This results in the formation of dimers during the shelf-life of a liquid preparation (see above).

Niels Jerne (Nobel prize for 1984) has hypothesized in 1974 that the self-recognition of antigen-binding cell receptors and circulating immunoglobulins based on idiotype/anti-idiotype interactions ensures their connectivity and is the main control mechanism in the immune system. According to this "network" theory, the immune system is self-controlled by using signals generated within itself. The immune response to an antigen is considered as a temporary imbalance between the antigen-specific clone and the anti-idiotypic clones (Jerne 1974). Autoimmune diseases are believed to be the result of defective self-control of the immune network. The network hypothesis might in part explain the beneficial effects of infusions of large doses of normal pooled IgG to patients with autoimmunity. Beneficial effects are provided by the introduction of components of a healthy immune network that helps repair their dysfunctional ones. The philosophical beauty of these ideas is evident. However, quarter of century ago, the interest in them faded after the discovery of the main mechanisms of immune tolerance and memory. The new knowledge rendered the immune function explanation by network emergent properties largely dispensable.

Nevertheless, discarding idiotype interactions as biologically irrelevant may be premature. Their role in the beneficial effects of pooled immunoglobulins cannot be ruled out. A single IVIg infusion to patients with autoimmune hemophilia has resulted in the rapid disappearance of 95% of the disease-associated anti-factor VIII antibodies. The effect was proven to be due to the binding of anti-idiotype IgG antibodies from the administered preparation to the idiotypes of pathological IgG with anti-factor VIII reactivity in the patients (Rossi et al. 1989).

11.3.4 Antibodies with Natural (Innate) and with Induced Polyspecificity

The father of immunochemistry Karl Landsteiner has proven 90 years ago that antibodies can bind an antigen with exclusive specificity, but he has never claimed that all antibodies are monospecific. In the next five decades, however, that was the conventional paradigm. The ability of an individual immunoglobulin molecule to bind to two or more structurally unrelated antigens was formally proven only by studying monoclonal immunoglobulins. Monoclonal antibodies were produced using the progeny of a single malignant B cell or clones of engineered single B cells, constructed using the hybridoma technology. A large percentage of the B cell clones produced IgG antibodies able to bind more than one antigen. While all IgM were polyspecific, only part of those belonging to the IgG, IgA, and IgE isotypes displayed such antigen-binding promiscuity. Interestingly, there is still no universally accepted definition of a polyspecific antibody. The proof of binding to two or more foreign or self-antigens that are structurally unrelated is regarded so far as sufficient to classify an antibody as being polyspecific. Yet, may be any antibody could be shown to interact with two or more antigens were the testing panels large enough (Van Regenmortel 2014).

Polyspecific antibodies are often neglected as "background," "silent," "sticky," etc. Recent studies have proven, however, their important role in the first line of innate defense against the dissemination of pathogens in the pre-immune host. The knowledge on the biophysical mechanisms of polyspecific antigen binding by IgG antibodies and their biological properties have been recently summarized (Dimitrov et al. 2013).

Apart from "innate," the polyspecificity of IgG molecules can be also "induced." Such antibodies are referred to as "masked," "hidden," "cryptic" or "latent." The IgG exposure to acid pH buffers is known to result in enhanced polyspecificity (Bouvet et al. 2001). This phenomenon may not be directly related to in vivo events. However, some of the licensed therapeutic intravenous immunoglobulin preparations are produced utilizing a protein fractionation stage at acid pH used as a supplemental virus-neutralizing and IgG aggregation-preventing step. They have enhanced antigen-binding polyspecificity (see Fig. 11.4)

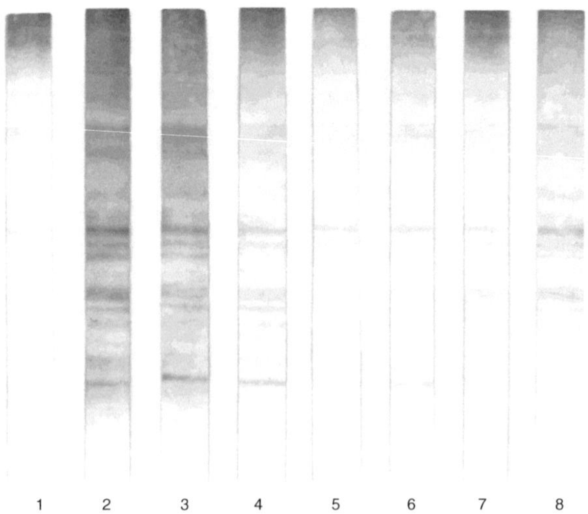

Fig. 11.4 Immunoblot analysis of the reactivity of seven different licensed IVIg preparations to human liver antigens (the first two are produced using a fraction stage at acid pH). *1* human serum, *2* Octagam, *3* Sandoglobulin, *4* Gammagard S/D, *5* Endobulin S/D, *6* Intraglobin F, *7* Immunovenin Intact, *8* Venimmun N (from Scand. J. Immunol. (2005), 61, 357)

that includes the newly acquired binding to at least one pro-inflammatory cytokine—interferon gamma. The comparative study of the effects of passive immunotherapy in mice with bacterial lipopolysaccharide-induced systemic inflammation (endotoxemia) has shown that while the administration of intact IVIg had no effect on survival, a single dose of the same preparation, exposed to a pH 4.0 buffer, significantly decreased the mortality (Djoumerska et al. 2005; Djoumerska-Alexieva et al. 2010). This is an important observation, as it points to the fact that commercially available immunoglobulin preparations may have different antigen binding as well as different therapeutic properties. To the best of our knowledge, no clinical trials have been conducted so far to compare the therapeutic effects of "unmodified" IVIg and preparations exposed to acidic conditions during its production.

Reactive oxygen species (ROS), ferrous ions, and free heme are aggressive protein-modifying molecules that are released in vivo at sites of inflammation, severe trauma, hemolysis, etc. This led us to formulate the hypothesis that the circulation of IgG molecules through a local inflammation site might modify their antigen-binding behavior. The experimental testing fully confirmed this prediction—both in vitro (Dimitrov et al. 2006, 2007) and in vivo (Mihaylova et al. 2008).

Sepsis and other aseptic severe inflammatory response syndromes (SIRS) are medical disasters that respond poorly to available treatments. The unfavorable prognosis of these patients is now believed to be due to the quick and dramatic change in gene expression affecting more than 80% of all cellular functions and pathways referred to as "genomic storm" (Xiao et al. 2011). This "storm" could well explain the failure of treatment approaches targeting single inflammation-related molecules. Passive immunotherapy with pooled IgG is a logical therapeutic approach because of its broad specificity that encompasses many pathogens—as well as self-antigens. The results from clinical trials on patients with SIRS are, however, inconclusive. If the anti-inflammatory effects of IVIg are partially attributable to its polyspecific natural antibody reactivity, could it be that by additionally enhancing the polyspecificity would improve its effectiveness? IVIg, preexposed in vitro to pro-oxidative ferrous ions, was used for the passive immunotherapy of mice with experimental sepsis or aseptic SIRS induced by the injection of bacterial lipopolysaccharide (LPS), of live *E. coli*, of zymosan or by the colon puncture and ligation technique. The low single dose of only 50 mg/kg of the modified preparation but not of the native, commercially available IVIg significantly increased survival in all models of severe generalized inflammation (Fig. 11.5). IVIg exposed to pro-oxidative ferrous ions was more efficient than the acid pH-exposed IVIg (Djoumerska-Alexieva et al. 2015).

The intravenous injection of pooled human IgG antibodies to the treated patient ensures the administration of the quasi-complete IgG antibody repertoire of a big healthy donor population. There are many questions regarding this treatment that are still waiting to be answered and mysteries to be solved. One is sure—the better understanding of the mechanisms of action of normal human immunoglobulins will result in the optimization of presently used therapeutic approaches and in increasing the range of potential new ones.

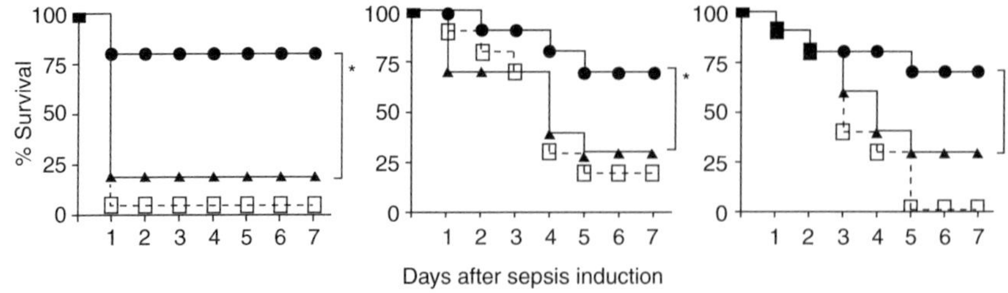

Fig. 11.5 The administration of a single dose of IVIg with additionally enhanced polyspecificity improves survival in experimental sepsis and aseptic severe inflammatory syndromes. Survival curves in endotoxemia (*left panel*), zymosan-induced systemic inflammation (*middle panel*), and polymicrobial sepsis (*right panel*). Animals were injected intravenously with a single dose of the native IVIg (*black triangles*), of the Fe(II)-exposed IVIg (*black circles*), or with PBS pH 7.4 (*open squares*), $*p < 0.05$, Mantel-Haenszel log-rank test (from Molec. Med. (2014), 21, 1002)

References

Alexander BT, Hladnik LM, et al. Use of cytomegalovirus intravenous immune globulin for the adjunctive treatment of cytomegalovirus in hematopoietic stem cell transplant recipients. Pharmacotherapy. 2010;30(6):554–61.

Arnon SS, Schechter R, et al. Human botulism immune globulin for the treatment of infant botulism. N Engl J Med. 2006;354(5):462–71.

Avci FY, Li X, et al. A mechanism for glycoconjugate vaccine activation of the adaptive immune system and its implications for vaccine design. Nat Med. 2011;17(12):1602–9.

Baumgarth N, Herman OC, et al. B-1 and B-2 cell-derived immunoglobulin M antibodies are nonredundant components of the protective response to influenza virus infection. J Exp Med. 2000;192(2):271–80.

Bayry J, Lacroix-Desmazes S, et al. Intravenous immunoglobulin for infectious diseases: back to the pre-antibiotic and passive prophylaxis era? Trends Pharmacol Sci. 2004; 25(6):306–10.

Blasczyk R, Westhoff U, et al. Soluble CD4, CD8, and HLA molecules in commercial immunoglobulin preparations. Lancet. 1993;341(8848):789–90.

Boligan KF, Mesa C, et al. Cancer intelligence acquired (CIA): tumor glycosylation and sialylation codes dismantling antitumor defense. Cell Mol Life Sci. 2015;72(7):1231–48.

Bolli R, Woodtli K, et al. L-Proline reduces IgG dimer content and enhances the stability of intravenous immunoglobulin (IVIG) solutions. Biologicals. 2010;38(1):150–7.

Bouvet J, Stahl D, et al. Induction of natural autoantibody activity following treatment of human immunoglobulin with dissociating agents. J Autoimmun. 2001;16:163–72.

Dimitrov JD, Ivanovska ND, et al. Ferrous ions and reactive oxygen species increase antigen-binding and anti-inflammatory activities of immunoglobulin G. J Biol Chem. 2006;281(1):439–46.

Dimitrov JD, Planchais C, et al. Antibody polyreactivity in health and disease: statu variabilis. J Immunol. 2013;191(3):993–9.

Dimitrov JD, Roumenina LT, et al. Antibodies use heme as a cofactor to extend their pathogen elimination activity and to acquire new effector functions. J Biol Chem. 2007;282(37):26696–706.

Djoumerska I, Tchorbanov A, et al. The autoreactivity of therapeutic intravenous immunoglobulin (IVIG) preparations depends on the fractionation methods used. Scand J Immunol. 2005;61(4):357–63.

Djoumerska-Alexieva IK, Dimitrov JD, et al. Exposure of IgG to an acidic environment results in molecular modifications and in enhanced protective activity in sepsis. FEBS J. 2010;277(14):3039–50.

Djoumerska-Alexieva I, Roumenina L, et al. Intravenous immunoglobulin with enhanced polyspecificity improves survival in experimental sepsis and aseptic systemic inflammatory response syndromes. Mol Med. 2015. https://doi.org/10.2119/molmed.2014.00224.

Fesel C, Coutinho A. Structured reactions of serum IgM repertoires to immunization are dependent on major histocompatibility complex genes. Scand J Immunol. 1999;49(3):251–7.

Hirose M, Vafia K, et al. Enzymatic autoantibody glycan hydrolysis alleviates autoimmunity against type VII collagen. J Autoimmun. 2012;39(4):304–14.

Jerne NK. Towards a network theory of the immune system. Ann Inst Pasteur Immunol. 1974;125C:373–89.

Lacroix-Desmazes S, Mouthon L, et al. Analysis of the natural human IgG antibody repertoire: life-long stability of reactivities towards self antigens contrasts with age-dependent diversification of reactivities against bacterial antigens. Eur J Immunol. 1995;25(9):2598–604.

Lam L, Whitsett CF, et al. Immunologically active proteins in intravenous immunoglobulin. Lancet. 1993;342(8872):678.

Lazarus AH, Freedman J, et al. Intravenous immunoglobulin and anti-D in idiopathic thrombocytopenic purpura (ITP): mechanisms of action. Transfus Sci. 1998;19(3):289–94.

Li S, Rouphael N, et al. Molecular signatures of antibody responses derived from a systems biology study of five human vaccines. Nat Immunol. 2014;15(2):195–204.

Merbl Y, Itzchak R, et al. A systems immunology approach to the host-tumor interaction: large-scale patterns of natural autoantibodies distinguish healthy and tumor-bearing mice. PLoS One. 2009;4(6):e6053.

Mihaylova NM, Dimitrov JD, et al. Inflammation-induced enhancement of IgG immunoreactivity. Inflamm Res. 2008;57(1):1–3.

Moekotte AL, Huson MA, et al. Monoclonal antibodies for the treatment of Ebola virus disease. Expert Opin Investig Drugs. 2016;25(11):1325–35.

Palm NW, Rosenstein RK, et al. Allergic host defences. Nature. 2012;484(7395):465–72.

Pashova S, Schneider C, et al. Antibody repertoire profiling with mimotope arrays. Hum Vaccin Immunother. 2017;13(2):314–22.

Quast I, Peschke B, et al. Regulation of antibody effector functions through IgG Fc N-glycosylation. Cell Mol Life Sci. 2017;74(5):837–47.

Rachid R, Castells M, et al. Association of anti-IgA antibodies with adverse reactions to gammaglobulin infusion. J Allergy Clin Immunol. 2011;128(1):228–230 e221.

Rossi F, Dietrich G, et al. Anti-idiotypes against autoantibodies in normal immunoglobulins: evidence for network regulation of human autoimmune responses. Immunol Rev. 1989;110:135–49.

Roux KH, Tankersley DL. A view of the human idiotypic repertoire. Electron microscopic and immunologic analyses of spontaneous idiotype-anti-idiotype dimers in pooled human IgG. J Immunol. 1990;144(4):1387–95.

Schneider C, Smith DF, et al. The human IgG anti-carbohydrate repertoire exhibits a universal architecture and contains specificity for microbial attachment sites. Sci Transl Med. 2015;7(269):269–1.

Schwab I, Nimmerjahn F. Intravenous immunoglobulin therapy: how does IgG modulate the immune system? Nat Rev Immunol. 2013;13(3):176–89.

Sherer Y, Wu R, et al. Cytokine levels in various intravenous immunoglobulin (IVIg) preparations. Hum Antibodies. 2001;10(2):51–3.

Späth PJ, Granata G, La Marra F, Kuijpers TW, Quinti I. On the dark side of therapies with immunoglobulin concentrates. The adverse events. Front Immunol. 2015;6:11.

van de Bovenkamp FS, Hafkenscheid L, et al. The emerging importance of IgG Fab glycosylation in immunity. J Immunol. 2016;196(4):1435–41.

Van Regenmortel MH. Specificity, polyspecificity, and heterospecificity of antibody-antigen recognition. J Mol Recognit. 2014;27(11):627–39.

Vassilenko SM, Vassilev TL, et al. Specific intravenous immunoglobulin for Crimean-Congo haemorrhagic fever. Lancet. 1990;335(8692):791–2.

von Gunten S, Shoenfeld Y, et al. IVIG pluripotency and the concept of Fc-sialylation: challenges to the scientist. Nat Rev Immunol. 2014;14(5):349.

Wilcox MH, Gerding DN, et al. Bezlotoxumab for prevention of recurrent clostridium Difficile infection. N Engl J Med. 2017;376(4):305–17.
Xiao W, Mindrinos MN, et al. A genomic storm in critically injured humans. J Exp Med. 2011;208(13):2581–90.

Essentials of the Production of Safe and Efficacious State-of-the-Art Polyclonal IgG Concentrates

12

Peter J. Späth

12.1 Introduction

From the very beginning of the clinical use of plasma-derived protin concentrates severe noninfectious adverse events (AEs) and transmission of pathogens by plasma-derived protein concentrates were threats to recipients (see Chap. 10 for additional information). First anti-infectious plasma potein concentrates were the "standard IgG" preparations. They were produced by the cold-ethanol fractionation methods and did not make an exception to the above: noninfectious severe AEs occurred while infectious AEs were rarely reported. Indeed, prior to the introduction of mass screening for infection markers of plasma donations, inadvertent transmission of HIV to recipients of factor VIII and factor IX concentrates did occur, while IgG concentrates obtained from the same plasma pool did rarely transmit HIV (Morgenthaler 2001). Rare transmissions were restricted to products not exposed to low pH. The very few incidences of HIV and some incidences of HCV transmission by IgG concentrates in the early 1990s, together with many cases of coagulation factor concentrates transmitted viral disease, clearly demonstrated the need to establish standardized measures to render plasma products pathogen safe. In the second half of the 1990s, authorities shifted regulatory emphasis from a scientific review of the processes to a focus on compliance to current good manufacturing practice (cGMP). The focus on cGMP compliance was applied to all aspects of plasma fractionation and the clinical use of plasma products. Court injunctions and warning letters were the consequences of this paradigm shift by authorities. This in turn resulted in a paradigm shift how the modern plasma industry operates (Steinhardt 1998).

The strict implementation of the recommendations by authorities resulted in today's immunoglobulin concentrates in general being well tolerated and safe regarding the transmission of known blood-borne viruses, the agent of the

P.J. Späth
Institute of Pharmacology, University of Bern, Bern, Switzerland
e-mail: peter.spaeth@pki.unibe.ch

P. Imbach (ed.), *Antibody Therapy*, https://doi.org/10.1007/978-3-319-68038-5_12

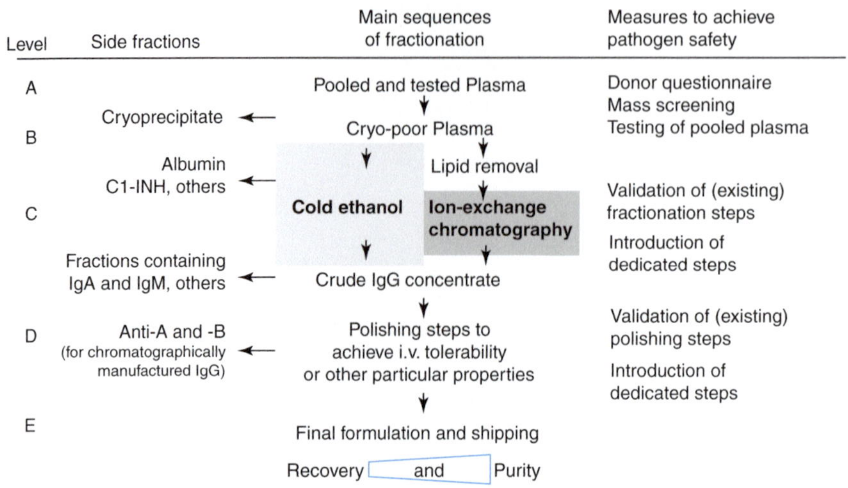

Fig. 12.1 Strongly simplified outline of fractionation of pooled plasma to pathogen free, well-tolerated IgG concentrates. Side fractions of the process are starting material for plasma products other than IgG. Level A of manufacturing: generating a large volume of plasma with optimal safety. Level B: plasma deprived of cryoprecipitate that contains relevant blood-clotting factors. Level C: a series of steps resulting in a crude IgG concentrate that is not tolerated intravenously. Level D: a sequence of steps rendering an IgG concentrate clinically well tolerated. Level E: lyophilized products are adjusted to the appropriate concentration, the excipient is added, the solution is filled into the vials, and the product is lyophilized. Liquid formulations are finalized similarly while leaving the freeze-drying process. Bottles with lyophilizate or IgG solutions are labeled and are ready for shipping

transmissible spongiform encephalitis (TSE) or even emerging and reemerging zoonotic viruses. Furthermore, moden IgG concentrates have an excellent noninfectious adverse event record, particularly when used in chronic conditions.

Manufacturing of IgG concentrates is a flow of processes as outlined in Fig. 12.1. Along this flowchart, particular measures can serve to obtain clinical tolerability and to achieve reduction in pathogens potentially contaminating the starting material. Below the efforts undertaken to provide for patients IgG concentrates safe in all aspects are outlined.

12.2 Plasma Fractionation: Regulatory Agencies' Requests

Plasma protein concentrates, typically prepared from plasma of thousands of donors, inevitably are associated with the risk of transmitting blood-borne pathogens (see Chap. 10). Therefore, modern fractionation of human plasma for clinical use is embedded in a tight network of quality assurance (QA) put in place by recommendation of authorities. Good manufacturing practice (GMP) is part of a QA program (Slopecki et al. 2007). GMP is a guidance for industry. GMP ensures consistency in production. It describes the minimal requirement a product must fulfill for obtaining a marketing authorization and covers procedures for receipt of materials, production, packaging, labeling, quality control, release, storage, and distribution. The procedures and laws of GMP are defined by each country. GMP is a "moving target" and current GMP (cGMP) includes the most recent developments and knowledge of the field; as technology and information capabilities change, so do the requirements for maintaining good manufacturing practices. On a solid fundament of GMP, the elements for a state-of-the-art plasm product are:

- Good clinical practice (GCP).
- Good laboratory practice (GLP).
- Standard operation procedures (SOPs).
- Training of staff.
- Donor selection, deferral and inventory hold.
- Mass screening of donation for infection markers by serology and nucleic acid amplification technology (NAT) testing. Recently one company added isoagglutinin titer screening in plasma donations in order to obtain plasma pools for chromatographic fractionation low in isoagglutinins anti-A and anti-B (Siani et al. 2014).
- In-process controls (production parameters and infection markers).
- Validation studies (manufacturing steps and dedicated pathogen reduction).
- Polishing steps (clinical tolerability and pathogen reduction).
- Labeling and shipment.
- Cleaning and segregation.
- Look back.
- Pharmacovigilance.
- Audits by internal and external inspectors.

A plasma fractionation, which is compliant with GMP, has undergone process validation for each manufacturing step. Process validation helps to ensure that systems are performing in the intended manner. Process validation ensures that the product has the required potency, purity, and safety. The parameters of a single process step are defined on a laboratory scale. The parameters obtained during the validation process help to define the elements of process control and provide a mechanism for ongoing quality assurance, quality control, training, competency review, and continuous improvement (Preti 1999).

Ensuring pathogen safety of a plasma product needs a tripod of measures: (1) donor selection, (2) mass screening for pathogen markers, and (3) pathogen elimination and inactivation during manufacturing. As an example how to implement pathogen safety of plasma products, the view of the European Medicines Agency is cited: "The safety of a product has to be demonstrated experimentally by validation studies on a laboratory scale. Such studies are based on the principle of deliberate contamination of the intermediate product by model viruses at given stages of the manufacturing process and monitoring the reduction in infectivity produced by the production step under consideration." At the time when GMP was introduced, well-established fractionation procedures were in place. For validation studies, the processes had to be downscaled to a laboratory scale. In a first step, it had to be demonstrated that the scaled-down process mimics the process in production, i.e., ideally has identical process parameters. Furthermore, authorities request at least two "dedicated" virus removal/inactivation steps in sequence during the fractionation. The two methods should represent two different principles of action thereby assuring that virus reduction is complementary.

When fractionating plasma on the fundaments of cGMP and applying the "full package" of complementary recommendations a state-of-the-art immunoglobulin preparation results.

Any activity from plasma collection to delivery at the door of a customer that is not performed and documented according to the standards may have severe consequences to the noncompliant company. Deficiencies in adherence to GMP detected during inspections of companies can lead to consent decrees, and severe deviations can have the consequence of a company forced to cease distribution of its products (http://www.ema.europa.eu/docs/en_GB/document_library/Press_release/2010/09/WC500097037.pdf; https://wayback.archive-it.org/7993/20161023082812/http://www.fda.gov/mw/ucm223968.htm; both accessed April 2017).

The leading regulatory agencies, which are enforcing the adherence to QA fractionation recommendations, are the US Food and Drug Administration (FDA; https://www.fda.gov/) and the European Medicines Agency (EMA; www.ema.europa.eu), while in all countries own agencies govern the enforcement of recommendations. A list of regional offices for Africa, for the Americas, for the Eastern Mediterranean, for Europe, for Southeast Asia, and for the Western Pacific can be found under: http://www.who.int/medicines/areas/quality_safety/regulation_legislation/ListMRAWebsites.pdf (accessed April 2017).

12.3 Plasma Collection: The Starting Point for Quality and Safety of a Plasma-Derived Product

IgG concentrates belong to the stable blood products. Ensuring quality of an IgG concentrate starts with collection of plasma, its correct handling, and cautious pooling.

Donor selection (*level A*, Fig. 12.1): Plasma fractionated to current best practice IgG concentrates all are from donors donating blood or plasma from free will. There are two types of donations: whole blood from which plasma is collected after centrifugation (recovered plasma) or plasma obtained by apheresis device (apheresis or source plasma) (Table 12.1). There is epic, for several decades' ongoing debate which of the two ways of plasma collection is of higher ethical and better biological quality. There is no reason to step into this discussion in this book chapter. However, it has to be acknowledged that apheresis plasma collection of volumes at the upper end of what is allowed might have an influence on protein composition of the donated plasma (Laub et al. 2010). As GMP covers minimal requirements for quality, and because having been accused remunerated

Table 12.1 Some characteristics of collection of plasma for fractionation[a]

	Recovered plasma	Apheresis plasma
Collection method	Whole blood donations; nothing is returned to the donor's circulation; plasma is separated by centrifugation and the cellular components serve therapies by these "labile blood products"	Plasmapheresis; the cellular components are returned to the donor by continuous machine-aided separation of plasma form blood cells
Remuneration	Predominantly none (especially in the European Union)	Most (especially in the USA)
Collection frequency and max. number of donations per year	Max. every 2 months	Intervals differ in various regions of the world
	4–6	USA: up to 104[b]
		EU: 15–50[b]
Collected volumes of plasma in one session and allowed maximal volume per year	Approx. 250 mL	Approx. 600 mL
	1.5 L (including anticoagulants)	USA: 90 L[c]
		EU: 10–35 L[c]
Extent to which worldwide plasma requirements are covered	20–25%	75–80%

[a]Donor suitability is defined by national regulatory authority requirements for whole blood donation *plus* additional special requirements for plasma donation

[b]Donation is allowed when total plasma protein content is >60 g/L (the USA, Germany) and when level is IgG > 6 g/L (Germany)

[c]EU: to be assessed after every fifth donation; USA, serum protein electrophoresis every 4 months; the protein quality of donations from donors donating very high volumes per year having low plasma protein content has been addressed recently (Laub et al. 2010)

donations being of lesser quality and safety, the apheresis plasma collecting and fractionating industry has introduced additional voluntary regulations. These are the International Quality Plasma Program (IQPP) introducing qualified donor standard, implementation of a donor deferral registry, and a drug abuse screening and the Quality Standards of Excellence, Assurance, and Leadership (QSEAL). QSEAL covers control on incoming plasma, inventory hold, NAT testing, intermediates purchased form external suppliers, recovered plasma specification, qualified donor, and viral markers (http://www.pptaglobal.org/safety-quality/standards/qseal; accessed June 2017). With the implementation of these voluntary standards, no relevant differences are found in pathogen marker frequencies of either type of plasma donation (EMEA 2002). In summary, the main goal of donor selection is to ensure that donors with high risk are excluded form donating, or their donation is withheld from further processing (Table 12.2). The donor is informed if HIV positive.

Finally yet importantly, plasma donations require careful handling to prevent formation and accumulation of vasoactive (e.g., prekallikrein activator (PKA)) or coagulation promoting (e.g., coagulation factor FXIa) substances. Due to their physicochemical properties, their removal during the manufacturing process may remain imperfect, and they may induce severe adverse events.

Table 12.2 Outline of the main measures of safe donor selection

• Physical examination
• Donor questionnaire, confidential self-exclusion
Detailed health history questionnaire relative to current known safety risks, designed to obtain information, e.g., about acute infections, (silently progressing), chronic illness, or elevated risk, for having acquired blood-borne pathogens (e.g., social behavior, sexually transmitted diseases, or having had tattoos, acupuncture, or ear/body piercing in the past 12 months) or having received xenotransplants (cornea) of animal origin or having been treated by pituitary (growth) hormones of human origin
• Donor deferral, e.g., donors having traveled or lived in endemic regions; donor deferral is a moving target (Yang et al. 2017)
• Inventory hold, e.g., allow for the retrieval of plasma prior to use if new post-donation information becomes available regarding the donor's health status
The apheresis plasma collecting industry has in addition established the IQPP[a] and QSEAL[b] standards that in addition to the above add
1. Qualified donor standard; donor successfully passing two donor medical history screenings and required viral testing
2. Community-based donors; only donors accepted with proof of a permanent address
3. The use of PPTA Source's National Donor Deferral Registry (NDDR) helps ensure that deferred donors cannot donate their plasma again, e.g., at another center
4. Education of donors at risk for infectious disease; education how to avoid behavior that is believed to lead to an increased risk of (HIV) infection
5. Personnel education and training standards
6. Professional medical facility criteria
7. Quality assurance
8. Viral marker standard

As 2/3 of plasma for fractionation is obtained from remunerated plasmapheresis donations, additional voluntary standards have been introduced by the corresponding plasmapheresis collecting industry to minimize the risk of infections remunerated donations might harbor

Donor deferral can be established, e.g., a donor has lived for a certain time in a given region of the world and has received a xenotransplant, a drug (D'Aignaux et al. 1999) or medical devices with parts of animal origin. Donor deferral is a moving object (Yang et al. 2017)

[a]*IQPP* International Quality Plasma Program

[b]*QSAEL* Quality Standards of Excellence, Assurance, and Leadership; a certification program to which donation centers have to comply

Mass screening of donations (*level A*, Fig. 12.1): Mass screening is the measure to exclude donations potentially contaminated by pathogens such as virus(es). Stable blood products inherit a particular risk for transmission of viruses because the staring material being a pool of thousands of individual donations (Table 12.3). Parameters of mass screening for virus markers are outlined in Table 12.4 and include serological and nucleic acid amplification technology (NAT) testing. NAT testing in addition to serological screening was introduced in order to shorten the time period of "window donations." During a window period, a donor already harbors the infective agent and is infective while seroconversion has not occurred yet, i.e., antibody formation has not set in, or antibodies are at a titer not detectable by validated serological methods. By introducing NAT testing, the estimated risk of an undetected infectious donation entering the blood supply dropped as given in

Table 12.3 Some human pathogens transmissible or theoretically transmissible by blood and plasma products[a]

Ascertained transmission by blood or plasma products with possibly severe clinical consequences	Ascertained transmission by blood or plasma products with no known clinical consequences	No report of transmission by transfusion	Suspected cases of transmission most likely through non-leukocyte-depleted red blood cell concentrates or contaminated plasma-derived factor VIII concentrate
Hepatitis B virus (enveloped, HBV)	Hepatitis D virus (enveloped)	TSE agent of classical/ sporadic CJD (sCJD)[d,g]	TSE agent of the variant form of CJD (vCJD)[d,f]
Hepatitis C virus (enveloped, HCV)	Hepatitis F virus (non-enveloped)	Severe acute respiratory syndrome-associated coronavirus (SARS-CoV, enveloped)	
Human immunodeficiency virus 1/2 (HIV 1/2, enveloped)	GBV-C/hepatitis G virus (enveloped)	Chikungunya virus (CHIKV, enveloped)	
Human T cell leukemia virus HTLV I/II	SEN virus (enveloped)		
West Nile virus (WNV, enveloped)	TT virus (enveloped)		
Hepatitis A virus (non-enveloped, HAV)			
Hepatitis E virus (HEV, non-enveloped)[b]			
Erythrovirus B19 (B19V, non-enveloped)[c]			
Zika virus (ZIKV, enveloped)[e]			

[a]After implementation of virus reduction steps in the fractionation process of plasma-derived medicinal products and thorough the enforcement by authorities of the rigorous implementation of good manufacturing practice (GMP) rules, no further proven transmission of (enveloped) viruses was reported. Criteria invariably present in true virus transmission by stable plasma products are (1) several patients infected with the same virus, (2) cluster of transmission (e.g., a restricted number of hospitals), (3) it is possible to identify one/a few lots that were used in all of the affected hospitals, and (4) the same virus is identified in the relevant product lot(s) and in patients treated with these lots. If these criteria are not fulfilled, transmission by plasma products of pathogen remains uncertain

[b]HEV infection by genotypes 1 and 2 cause large epidemics in in tropical and subtropical regions. The transmission is via the fecal-oral route. Infections by genotypes 3 and 4 are an emerging threat in countries of the northern hemisphere and are a food-borne disease. Pigs are the animal reservoir for this zoonotic virus. These genotypes have been identified in blood donors in Europe. Transfusion associated with HEV infection was reported (Tamura et al. 2007). Significant acute hepatitis can be the result of chronic HEV infection in immune compromised patients (Motte et al. 2012), while in immunocompetent patients, HEV infection has been associated to neurological complications

(continued)

Table 12.3 (continued)

[c]Human parvovirus B19

[d]*CJD* = Creutzfeldt-Jakob disease; aberrantly folded prion proteins (PrP^{Sc}) are considered to be the infectious agent of transmissible spongiform encephalopathy (TSE) diseases, *sCJD* sporadic CJD, *vCJD* variant CJD

[e]Reports on transfusion, solid organ transplantation, or sexually transmitted ZIKV disease are available (Barjas-Castro et al. 2016; Nogueira et al. 2017; Venturi et al. 2016). Prenatal infection is associated with microcephaly, while infection in adults can be fatal or be associated with Guillain-Barré syndrome or severe thrombocytopenia

[f]The transmission by non-leukocyte depleted erythrocyte concentrates might represent a risk for transmission. Four possible transmission events by non-leukocyte-depleted erythrocyte concentrates have been reported. In one case of probable transmission, the most likely route of infection was by contaminated plasma-derived factor VIII concentrate

[g]In May 2017 a report on two patients receiving blood-clotting factor concentrates dying form sCJD was posted electronically (Urwin et al. 2017). A causal link between the treatment with plasma products and the development of sCJD has not been established

Table 12.4 Mass screening on plasma for fractionation[a]

Parameters	All individual donations	Pooled plasma before fractionation
Serological		
Anti-human immunodeficiency virus (HIV)-1/-2 antibodies	Yes	Yes
Anti-hepatitis C virus (HCV) antibodies	Yes	Yes
Hepatitis B virus surface antigen (HBsAg)	Yes	Yes
Nucleic acid testing (NAT) by mini-pool		
HIV-1 RNA	Yes	Yes
HCV RNA	Yes	Yes
HBV DNA	Yes	Yes
HAV RNA	Not mandatory for plasma donations for fractionation	No
B19 Virus DNA	Not mandatory for plasma donations for fractionation	No

[a]Mass screening for the agent of variant Creutzfeldt-Jakob disease has become feasible; however, it is not practiced (Jackson et al. 2014)

Fig. 12.2. In addition to the minimal requirements given by GMP, most manufacturers request human parvovirus B19 and HAV NAT testing of plasma donations.

NAT testing is performed in mini-pools and largely can be automated. Aliquots from bar code labeled pilot tubes are transferred to, e.g., a micro titer plate. In such an X/Y layout, each aliquot is unequivocally associated to an individual donation. Starting NAT testing, aliquots from the aliquots are pooled, undergo validated amplification of part(s) of pathogen's genome, and the resulting genome equivalents are quantified. The size of the mini-pool depends on amplification efficiency and minimal infectious dose of the given pathogen. In case a mini-pool is reactive, pooling is repeated, this time by rows and columns. From the row and the column pool

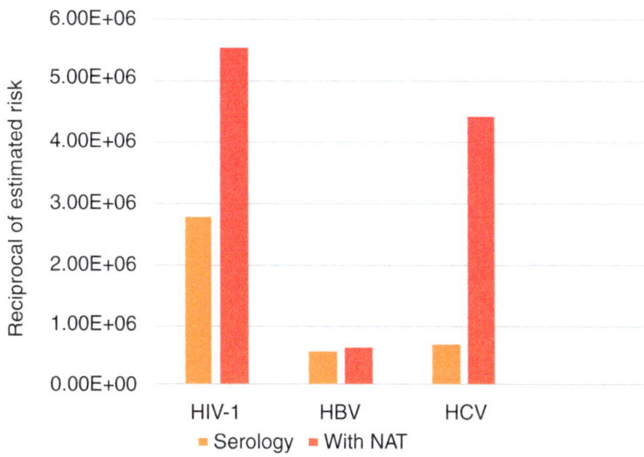

Fig. 12.2 Estimated risk of an undetected donation entering the blood supply when mass screening is by serology only or NAT is performed in addition (Offergeld et al. 2005). The reciprocal of risk rate of undetected infectious donations is given; the higher the bar, the lower the risk rate

being reactive, the X/Y layout allows the identification of the reactive donation. The contaminated donation is withheld from pooling and is destroyed safely.

Plasma fractionation starts with pooling of individual donations to an appropriate volume. Before starting the fractionation process, an in-process control is performed to ascertain absence of potential contaminating viruses (Table 12.4). This reduces the risk of pathogen transmission and reduces the financial risk of losing an entire lot of IgG concentrate.

12.4 Fractionation Methods in Use to Obtain From Plasma Well-Tolerated, Highly Pure IgG Concentrates

Over many decades, the development of IgG fractionation was driven to achieve intravenous tolerability and increase recovery and purity of the concentrates. Today two different main methods are in place how to fractionate plasma: the cold-ethanol fractionation and the ion-exchange chromatography process (Fig. 12.1). Before applying either method, frozen plasma is thawed at 0 °C. The part remaining insoluble at 0 °C is separated and represents the cryoprecipitate that harbors the blood coagulation factors (level A to B in Fig. 12.1). The supernatant is the cryo-poor plasma that contains a wide array of plasma proteins, including immunoglobulins and albumin.

Cold-ethanol fractionation is either according to Cohn/Oncley or to Kistler-Nitschmann (Oncley et al. 1949; Nitschmann et al. 1954) (see Chap. 10 as well). From cryo-poor plasma, a precipitate is obtained which contains the immunoglobulins (level B, Fig. 12.1). The supernatant is the starting material for albumin fractionation. Further suspension/precipitation steps of the precipitate containing the

Table 12.5 Polishing steps to achieve particular properties of clinically applicable IgG, e.g., intravenous tolerability

• Polyethylene glycol precipitation, removes aggregates
• pH 4 and traces of pepsin; alters aggregates; low pH is a virus inactivating step
• pH 4; virus inactivation; reduction of aggregates
• Depth-/ultra-/diafiltration; not to confound with virus filtration
– Depth filtration uses a filter on which the precipitated protein is separated from the supernatant using "filter aids." Filter aids help to maintain high flow rates during the filtering process and at the same time may adsorb pathogens and or pathogen-protein complexes quite efficiently: is predominantly applied during cold-ethanol preparation of crude IgG, and can remove aggregates and adsorb viruses
– Diafitration serves to remove, e.g., salts from an IgG solution with the help of semipermeable membranes
– Ultrafiltration uses pressure or concentration gradients and semipermeable membranes
• Reduction of isoagglutinins anti-A and anti-B by immunoaffinity chromatography step (Dhainaut et al. 2013; Höfferer et al. 2015); elevated isoagglutinin titers are associated with the chromatographic fractionation method; reduction in rate of hemolytic adverse events

immunoglobulins finally end up what is termed "IgG bulk" (level C, Fig. 12.1). This crude IgG concentrate then undergoes various polishing steps (Table 12.5). Polishing steps and the final formulation are those differing the most among various companies (levels D and E, Fig. 12.1).

The early "standard" IgG concentrates underwent only few polishing steps of the "IgG bulk" material. They contained aggregates that rendered them not tolerable when applied intravenously. Typically, these i.m. products were of a solution strength of 16–16.5%. By introducing virus inactivation/removal steps to the original manufacturing process, some of these products survived to our days.

A "first generation" of IgG products for intravenous use (IVIGs) was deprived of unwanted Fc-effector functions by harsh enzyme treatment. The digested IgG molecules were heavily impaired in their biological functions however were well tolerated. One product still available posted on a Japanese website (see Chap. 13). For a "second generation" of IVIGs, intact IgG molecules were chemically modified in order to prevent overt spontaneous complement activation in the recipients' circulation. Only a very few of these chemically modified products are still available in some regional markets. They are mentioned in Chap. 13 of this book. The "third generation" of IVIGs was made intravenously tolerable by gentle polishing steps (level D, Fig. 12.1).

Although in many aspects excellent, the two cold-ethanol fractionation methods reach their limits when pushing for improved recovery without loss of purity. For this reason, the plasma industry is moving toward the *ion-exchange chromatography* fractionation of IgG. This manufacturing method allows relative high recoveries at high purity. Before cryo-poor plasma or the intermediate fraction deprived of albumin can be fed onto ion-exchange columns, they must be free of lipids (level B,

Fig. 12.1). The most widely used technique to get rid of lipids is by octanoic acid (=caprylic acid) precipitation. Caprylic acid precipitation was the first to be used in combination with DEAE cellulose columns for the isolation of IgG from plasma at good yield (Steinbuch and Audran 1969).

During chromatographic fractionation, lipid-free plasma undergoes several anion- and/or cation-exchange chromatography steps (Bertolini 1998; Dhainaut et al. 2013; Cramer et al. 2009; Trejo et al. 2003). The resulting IgG solutions again undergo polishing steps in order to achieve tolerability (Table 12.5).

With some chromatographically obtained preparations, an elevated frequency of hemolytic reactions emerged. These adverse events were supposed being related to the presence of higher titers of isoagglutinins than seen in products obtained with the cold-ethanol fractionation. In order to reduce levels of isoagglutinins anti-A and anti-B, a particular polishing step was introduced by some manufacturers: immunoaffinity chromatography using columns with corresponding trisaccharides coupled to the matrix (Dhainaut et al. 2013; Höfferer et al. 2015; Späth et al. 2015).

12.5 Widening the Pathogen Safety Margins During Fractionation and Polishing

Donor selection, mass screening, and implementation of added voluntary quality measures are important for pathogen safety of a plasma product. However, by far they are not sufficient for an optimal safety bill. "Building in" safety to the fractionation process is what finally can render a product pathogen safe.

Among the stable plasma products, the manufacturing of IgG concentrates offers the most steps effective enough to reduce or inactivate viruses without harming too much the biologic function of the molecules. Indeed, IgG concentrates largely remained free from transmitting viruses. This was remarkable as patients with impaired immune defense may require monthly administration of immunoglobulins lifelong, or patients with autoimmune/inflammatory diseases might require high to very high doses of immunoglobulin therapy sometimes over a prolonged period and nevertheless remained virus free. Beside donor selection and mass screening the third pillar on which pathogen safety is built on is the reduction of potentially present pathogens during manufacturing (levels B and C, Fig. 12.1). Either an existing fractionation step is validated accordingly, or dedicated virus inactivation/removal steps are introduced to the manufacturing process. Aspects of the validation process are outlined in Table 12.6.

There are three, in their principles different, mechanisms that contribute to the elimination or inactivation of viruses potentially present during manufacturing of plasma products (Kempf et al. 2007), namely:

Table 12.6 The essentials of validation of viruses inactivation/removal

A. Downscaling
• Validation studies are performed on a laboratory scale and this implements downscaling the fractionation process
• The lab-scale process has to undergo validation by demonstrating that critical parameters of that step correspond in large-scale and laboratory conditions
B. Virus stocks (Table 12.7)
• Model viruses should be selected for their biologic and physiologic similarities to plasma-borne viruses; they should be well characterized in size, purity, and aggregate level; the term model virus defines that all viruses used for validation studies are grown in cell cultures, event those being human pathogen
• For safety reasons, the use of human pathogen viruses should largely be avoided
• Must cover a wide range of physicochemical properties of viruses in an effort to test the ability of the system to cope with pathogen diversity, e.g., enveloped, non-enveloped, various size, DNA and RNA viruses, and viruses with high resistance to physicochemical treatment
• Animal viruses in their physicochemical properties should closely resemble the human pathogen viruses of interest and should represent a range of physicochemical properties as wide as ever possible
• The virus stock should be of high titer
• When validating IgG manufacturing processes, cross-reacting antibodies to the virus used should be always considered
C. Cell cultures for read out
• The assay system should be convenient, i.e., cell cultivation should be easy, sensitivity to virus should be high, and the read out system should be convenient for (electronic) documentation
• Cell cultures are best prepared in micro titer plates
• Staining of cells not destroyed by virus
D. Validation of a partitioning or filtration step
• The starting material is spiked by a corresponding virus, and the spiked material is assessed for infectivity, i.e., spiked material is diluted by tenfold ($\log_{10}$ dilution steps) and is titrated for the tissue culture infectious dose 50% ($TCID_{50}$)
• The resulting materials (e.g., precipitate and supernatant or filtrate and retained material/solution) are separately tested for residual infectivity as descried above
• The logarithmic reduction factor (LRF) for a virus is calculated as follows: $\log_{10}$ inoculated virus – $\log_{10}$ residual virus in, e.g., supernatant
• The sum of residual virus infectivity found in, e.g., supernatant and precipitate, must equal the titer of inoculation; if this is not the case, either an explanation has to be found and the explanation itself has to be validated or the validation failed
E. Validation of a virus inactivation step
• The inoculated material is incubated while changing an appropriate parameter such as temperature, and aliquots are taken at various incubation times
• Each aliquot is assessed for remaining infectivity, and the kinetics of virus inactivation is calculated
• The appropriateness of results is proven by calculation of inactivation constants, transformation into natural logarithms, and plotting against the reciprocal of absolute temperature (Arrhenius plot). The fitting of calculated values on a regression line is an excellent internal control for quality of data

Table 12.7 Human viruses and their model viruses[a] recently used for validation studies

Human pathogen	Model virus	Size of the viruses (nm)
B19 virus (*Parvoviridae*)	Minute virus of mice (MVM); canine parvovirus (CPV)	18–25
Hepatitis A, poliovirus (*Picornaviridae*)	Encephalomyocarditis virus (EMCV)	30
Hepatitis B virus (enveloped DNA viruses)	Infectious bovine rhinotracheitis virus (IBRV)	200
Hepatitis C, West Nile (*Flaviviridae*)	Bovine viral diarrhea virus (BVDV); WNV[b]; Sindbis virus (SINV)	40–60 70
Human immunodeficiency virus (*Retroviridae*)	HIV[b]	80–100
Herpes 1 and 2, HHV-8 (*Herpesviridae*)	Pseudorabies virus (PRV)	100–180
Vaccinia, cowpox, smallpox (*Poxviridae*)		Approx. 250 and higher
TSE agent (PrP^{Sc})		1 IU is assumed to contain ≥20 aggregated proteins having a calculated size of 16–56 nm

[a]Viruses used in validation studies should be well characterized in size, represent as closely as possible viruses which might be present in plasma, cover a wide range of physicochemical properties of viruses, e.g., enveloped, non-enveloped, various size, DNA and RNA viruses, and viruses with high resistance to physicochemical treatment. In validation studies with immunoglobulins, care has to be taken that results are not misleading due to the presence of cross-reactive and/or neutralizing antibodies

[b]Although human pathogen, viruses grown in cell cultures are all considered "model"

1. Inactivation
   - Solvent/detergent (S/D) treatment: disruption of virus envelope
   - Caprylic (octanoic) acid treatment
   - Treatment a low pH: destructive conformational changes of structural proteins
   - Heat: dry or wet (wet = pasteurization), disruption of envelope *and* destructive conformational change of structural proteins (e.g. capsid proteins)
2. Elimination based on size: virus filtration (formerly termed nanofiltration). Elimination at large scale of possibly contaminating pathogens based on size is the most recent technique to free plasma products form pathogens. Virus filtration at large scale was introduced by the Central Laboratory of the Swiss Red Cross, Blood Transfusion Service in the late 1990s (virus filtration on a modest size (Stucki et al. 1997); virus filtration at large scale: submission dossier for Sandoglobulin NF in 1999). With the progress in manufacturing of filters with smaller and smaller pores, virus filtration has become a universal key process in assuring pathogen safety—size matters only.

3. Partitioning, e.g., virus in the precipitate while the supernatant, is processed further. Filtration with filter aids can take advantage of the filter aids tightly binding and adsorbing viruses in precipitates and despite their small size retaining them (technical term: depth filtration). Partitioning involving filtration techniques are not to confound with virus filtration that is a dedicated virus removal principle.

The highest level of product safety is achieved when all three principles are applied in a stepwise and diligent manner during the fractionation process (Table 12.8). As an example the LRFs obtained by various methods are listed in Table 12.9. LFRs obtained on basis of varying principles are additive in defining the safety margin of an entire manufacturing process.

Table 12.8 Aspects of dedicated virus inactivation/removal processes

	S/D	Low pH	Heat/pasteurization	Virus filtration
Enveloped viruses	+[a]	+	+	+
Non-enveloped viruses	–	±	±/(−)	+
Prions	–	–	–	+

[a]Except on *Poxviridae*

Table 12.9 Examples are depicted of margins of pathogen inactivation and removal during fractionation of IVIG staring from possibly contaminated starting material

Principal mechanism and methods of pathogen reduction	HIV	HAV	HCV	HHV	B19V
Partitioning (separation into different physical phases)					
Depth filtration with filter aids (A)	11.5		4.6–10.2	12.4	
Depth filtration with filter aids (B)	≥5.3	4.2	2.1	≥6.3	2.3
Ion-exchange chromatography (1)					
Ion-exchange chromatography (2)	≥3.0	≥1.4	4.0 ± 0.3	≥3.3	
Inactivation by alteration of structures which are essential for the infectivity of the pathogen					
Pasteurization (wet heat)	≥5.5	≥5.4	≥5.7		
Low pH	≥5.4		4.6	≥5.9	>3
Low pH and traces of pepsin	6.1	<1.0	>4.4 and >6.7	>5.3	n.a.
Solvent/detergent treatment	≥6.0	n.a.	≥7.8	≥8.4	n.a.
Caprylate incubation	≥4.5	n.a.	≥4.5	≥4.6	n.a.
Combination of partitioning and inactivation	4.0	3.4	1.4–3.6	3.6	
Elimination based on size					
Virus filtration A	≥5.3	>5.1	>5.1 and >7.5		
Virus filtration B	≥5.3	≥3.7	≥2.7		≥5.5

Numbers indicate logarithmic reduction factors (LRFs). Examples are taken from literature and package inserts. The human pathogen viruses aimed to eliminate or inactivate are indicated on column heads. The effectively used model viruses are given in Table 12.6

The results published by various manufacturers of the various virus inactivation and removal steps allow to conclude that by applying the various techniques sequentially:

- Inactivation of enveloped viruses is usually achieved well.
- Current inactivation methods show limited efficiency for non-enveloped viruses.
- Virus filtration has the potential to completely remove the smallest and most robust non-enveloped viruses known.
- Partitioning processes additionally contribute to viral safety.

The combination of these pathogens elimination methods also provides confidence that the various fractionation processes can cope with newly emerging viruses.

12.6 Emerging Human Pathogens

So far, no proven transmission by IgG concentrates of (re-)emerging viruses in the last two decades occurred. This might be credited to the tightly implemented QA framework. The (re-)emerging pathogens are predominantly of zoonotic nature. Hence, their reservoirs are animals and their (re-)emergence is associated with hygienic conditions. Transmission of enveloped zoonotic viruses over the species barrier with severe consequences for man have been described for Chikungunya virus, MERS coronavirus, avian influenza virus (bird flu; H5N1), SARS coronavirus, West Nile virus, Ebola virus, Zika virus, others. The presence of these viruses in blood donors were reported for West Nile virus, *SARS coronavirus* and Zika virus which persists in the cellular blood compartment. Validation studies have assured the safety regarding transmission by plasma products of relevant enveloped zoonotic viruses (Table 12.10). In general, enveloped viruses can relatively easily be inactivated, e.g., by solvent/detergent treatment.

For non-enveloped viruses, gene mutations are a prerequisite to cross the species barrier. Hepatitis E virus (HEV) is a non-enveloped zoonotic virus of pigs. Four genotypes are known. Genotypes 3 and 4 are recognized as zoonotic pathogens in industrialized countries. Transmissions are by pork blood (in rare cooked meat). Transmission of HEV by plasma exchange has been reported (Mallet et al. 2016). Prevention of HEV transmission is relevant as infection can have severe neurological consequences, even in immunocompetent individuals (Blasco-Perrin et al. 2015; Higuchi et al. 2015; Pérez Torre et al. 2015; Scanvion et al. 2017). Elimination or inactivation of HEV during the manufacturing of plasma products apparently is sufficient in preventing pathogen transmission (Table 12.10).

In general non-enveloped viruses do mutate slowly, with one known exception, the DNA of *Parvoviridae* which shows a similar mutation frequency to RNA viruses (Boschetti et al. 2005; Shackelton and Holmes 2006). Under distinct immune and

Table 12.10 Emerging zoonotic human pathogen viruses and their model viruses used for validation studies

Human pathogen	Model virus	Size of the viruses (nm)	Validation studies[a]
Chikungunya virus (CHIKV, enveloped; *Flaviviridae*)	Bovine viral diarrhea virus (BVDV)	40–60	Leydold et al. (2012)[c]
	Sindbis virus (SINV)[b]	50–70	
	CHIKV strain "LR2006-OPY1"		
Hepatitis E virus (HEV, non-enveloped; *Herpesviridae*)	Feline calicivirus (FCV)	32–34	Farcet et al. (2016)
Severe acute respiratory syndrome-associated coronavirus (SARS-CoV, enveloped)	Frankfurt-1 strain of SARS-CoV		Yunoki et al. (2004)
	SARS-CoV isolate FFM-1		Rabenau et al. (2005)
West Nile virus (WNV, enveloped; *Flaviviridae*)	Bovine viral diarrhea virus (BVDV)	40–60	Kreil et al. (2003)
Zika virus (ZIKV, enveloped; *Flaviviridae*)	ZIKV strain PF13/251013-18	40–60	Blümel et al. (2017)
	ZIKV isolate H/PF/2013	40–60	Kühnel et al. (2017)

Except for HEV, all are enveloped viruses
[a]The logarithmic reduction factors (LRFs) are given in the publications.
[b]A model virus of the early days of validation studies
[c]This study provides solid reassurance for the safety of plasma products in regard to emerging viruses. Furthermore, the results verify that the use of model viruses is appropriate to predict the inactivation characteristics of newly emerging viruses when their physicochemical properties are well characterized

adaptive pressures, specific amino acid changes in parvoviruses endowed tropism shifts in the animal world (Lopez-Bueno et al. 2006). Hence, new variants/species tropisms have to be expected. Theoretically, small non-enveloped viruses represent the biggest threat for transfusion incidences in the future, and hopefully the technique of virus filtration is sufficient or will be improved to eliminate eventually emerging *Parvoviridae* with human tropism.

12.7 Transmissible Spongiform Encephalopathies (TSEs)

Also of animal origin is the agent of the variant Creutzfeldt-Jakob disease (vCJD), a TSE. vCJD with great certainty was transmitted from cow (mad cow disease or bovine spongiform encephalitis = BSE) to humans (Bruce et al. 1997). BSE emerged due to an "optimized" production process of animal carcass-derived material fed to cows (Wilesmith et al. 1991). Other forms of human spongiform encephalitides exist and can be iatrogenic/sporadic, inherited/genetic, or acquired/infectious (Table 12.11).

Spongiform encephalitides are mediated by the misfolded isoform "scrapie" of a normal cellular prion protein, PrP^{C} which is ubiquitous in cells and is a protein highly conserved over the evolution. The misfolded "scrapie" prion protein (PrP^{Sc})

results in fatal neurodegenerative diseases of mammals. Although a protein-only agent, PrP^{Sc} is “infectious” in a sense that the misfolded protein might induce conformation changes of the normal PrP^{C} resulting in sticky rod-like and fibrillary particles accumulating in the brain.

Serum, plasma, and leukocytes from vCJD patients might harbor infectious PrP^{Sc}. Indeed, transmission of PrP^{Sc} has been reported in three symptomatic and one non-symptomatic cases of non-leukocyte-depleted red blood cell concentrates (Hewitt et al. 2006; Peden et al. 2004). Measures to eliminate possibly contaminating PrP^{Sc} during plasma fractionation became mandatory. It is accepted that inactivation of PrP^{Sc} is not possible without destruction of the biological activity of a plasma product. Hence, elimination by partitioning or exclusion by size remains the two possibilities (Cai et al. 2002). Validation studies were performed at different manufacturers' site with different spikes and different detection systems. The manufacturing steps studied for removal capacity of PrP^{Sc} included precipitation, adsorption, chromatography, and filtration, as well as combined steps. They proved to be highly potent in removal of the TSE agents possibly contaminating plasma (Cai et al. 2013). Reduction by individual steps in sequence was additive (Table 12.12).

Table 12.11 Spongiform encephalopathies (SEs) of mammals

Animals	*Humans*
Sheep → Scrapie	Kuru (cannibalism; acquired/infectious)
Deer & Elk → Chronica wasting disease (CWD)	Gerstmann-Sträussler-Scheinker-Syndrome (GSS; inherited)
	Fatal familial insomnia (FFI; inherted)
Mink → MSE	Creutzfeldt-jakob Disease; classical = idiopathic/sporadic form (CJD or cCJD/sCJD)
Cat → FSE	pathogenic prion protein almost exclusively located in the CNS
Live stock carcass derived material fed to ruminants → Bovine → BSE	→ Creutzfeldt-jakob Disease; new variant form (vCJD; acquired/infectious)
	pathogenic prion protein found in CNS but also in abundance in some lymphatic tissue

Table 12.12 Elimination of PrP^{Sc} during manufacturing of IgG concentrates

Principal mechanism and methods of pathogen reduction	PrP^{Sc}
Partitioning (separation into different physical phases)	
Depth filtration with filter aids	7.3
Ion-exchange chromatography	≥5.4
Elimination based on size	
Virus filtration (A)	4.4
Virus filtration (B)	≥4.3

Logarithmic reduction factors (LRFs) are given. Inactivation was never assessed because not applicable (see text)

Furthermore, the declining incidence of vCJD, the stringent donor selection due to geographic donor deferral policy, and the additive nature of removal steps render the agent of vCJD unlikely to be transmitted by plasma products. Indeed, no proven transmission of vCJD by IgG concentrates was ever reported (Ritchie et al. 2016), even not when the administration of a possibly PrP^{Sc} contaminated IgG concentrate occurred (El-Shanawany et al. 2009). Ascertained transmission by other plasma products has not been described neither.

The sporadic/iatrogenic CJD (sCJD) is not the same as vCJD (Table 12.11). sCJD represents about 85% of all spongiform encephalitides of humans and affects elderly people. There exist several surveillance studies on the transmission of sCJD by blood and blood products. These are conducted by the American Red Cross, in the UK and in France (Crowder et al. 2017; Martin and Trouvin 2013; Urwin et al. 2016). These studies did not report sCJD in patient populations treated with blood and plasma products. This was the basis not to consider sCJD transmissible by blood transfusion or by plasma products. However, the *Emerging Infectious Disease Journal* in May 2017 posted in electronic form a report on two patients receiving coagulation factor concentrates and dying from sCJD. Authors conclude (citation): "A causal link between the treatment with plasma products and the development of sCJD has not been established, and the occurrence of these cases may simply reflect a chance event in the context of systematic surveillance for CJD in large populations." It will be of outmost importance whether and how many new cases will be reported in future.

12.8 Completing the Full Package for a Safe and Efficacious Immunoglobulin Concentrate

Final formulation: To ensure stability/tolerability of a product over its shelf life, the right selection of stabilizers is of particular importance. Products can by lyophilized (=freeze-dried). The basic physicochemical process of freeze-drying is the replacement of the layer of water surrounding the IgG molecules. This layer, which is also termed "hydration shell" or "hydration sphere," keeps the IgG molecules in solution (Makarov et al. 2002). In dehydrated products, e.g., oxidation of the preparation is largely prevented, and aggregation or dimer formation is suppressed. Hence, the excipient only to a part serves stabilization of a freeze-dried product, while its major role is to make sure the lyophilized protein can be reconstituted entirely within reasonable time (no aggregates remaining). The compounds that can be injected intravenously with the best physicochemical properties to simulate water are sugars followed by some amino acids. Although associated with osmotic nephrosis in patients at risk, several lyophilized products containing sucrose are still on some markets (see also Chap. 13).

In response for the request of more convenient handling, the liquid preparations were developed. In liquid preparations, aging and continuous interaction of molecules are inherent. The stabilizer has to preserve the characteristics without hampering their quality by preventing oxidation and IgG-IgG interactions, e.g., limiting

IgG dimer formation. The most widely used stabilizers for liquid preparations are glycine, L-proline, maltose, and sorbitol.

Cleaning and sanitation of a production line: Prevention of cross-contamination through surface-adsorbed infectious agent is a measure to be taken under cGMP. Cleaning validations involving infectious agents are problematic, e.g., because the cleaning process has to be scaled down. This in most cases is impossible, e.g., because the rheological properties are different on a small scale. Typically NaOH or sodium hypochlorite (NaClO) are used for plant sanitation after a run and at appropriate concentrations are sufficient to destroy virus infectivity. However, how about the TSE agent of vCJD? It needed a particular effort to show that there are sanitation measures that can destroy the TSE agent PrP^{Sc}. PrP^{res} served this purpose (Table 12.13). The validation strategy was to show that PrP^{res} after NaOH/NaClO exposure becomes on one hand noninfectious and on the other hand sensitive to proteinase K digestion. NaOH and NaClO treatment both destroy PrP^{res} even at low NaOH and NaClO concentrations. Regulatory agencies consider current cleaning regimes adequate to assure batch-to-batch segregation.

Traceability: GMP requirements for blood and plasma derivatives include the traceability of batches from donor to recipient. The industry is responsible for interlinking a given batch of plasma product with information such as responses of the donor has given on the medical questionnaire, results of mass screening and pooling information. Traceability also has to interconnect batches and the hospital where the product was delivered. It is the responsibility of the hospital to complete traceability by documenting which IVIG batch has been given to which individual patient(s).

Table 12.13 Some physicochemical properties of prion proteins of mammals in health and disease[a]

Origin	Condition/prion protein (agent)	Some properties
Mammals	Health/PrP^C	An ubiquitous, normal, native, noninfectious protein of cells encoded on the short arm of chromosome 20
		No tendency to aggregate
		Complete degradation by proteinase K
Mammals	Spongiform encephalitides/ PrP^{Sc}	Aberrantly folded prion protein
		Tendency to convert PrP^C into the misfolded form thereby aggregating and forming filaments and plaques that destroy CNS cells
		Only partially digested by proteinase K
		Detection by Western-blotting indicates infection of the tissue examined
		Various strains known
Artificial	No biological function/PrP^{res}	Fragment of PrP^{Sc} resistant to digestion upon prolonged incubation with proteinase K; $PrP^{Sc} \neq PrP^{res}$

[a]General term of disease = transmissible spongiform encephalopathy (TSE) mediated by PrP^{Sc}; PrP^{Sc} is a generic term for aberrantly folded, "infectious" prion proteins and does not refer exclusively to the suspected agent of scrapie of sheep

This enables "look backs" in case any problem should be identified at the donor or recipient end. The basis of the traceability is a bar code identification system. A proper traceability system ensures that each lot can be recalled, should this be necessary. It further allows the handling of post-donation information and pharmacovigilance in an efficient and safe manner.

Obtaining the final proof of clinical efficacy and pathogen safety of an IgG concentrate: Quality assurance through surveillance programs extends product quality after its distribution. Pharmacovigilance, post-marketing studies and surveillance programs are the pillars on which the final proof for the quality of an IgG concentrate stands. Pharmacovigilance ensures the continued safety of medicinal products in use by collecting, monitoring, and assessing any type of adverse drug reactions related to the product (Ball et al. 2016), http://ec.europa.eu/health/human-use/pharmacovigilance_en. For some infections, incubation time might be long. Surveillance programs are currently the only means to conclusively obtain long-ranging safety information. Clinicians are encouraged to report adverse events, especially those that are unexpected or unusual.

Acknowledgments The help of Christoph Kempf, University of Berne, is greatly appreciated, as well as information kindly provided by Roland Hubner, The Federal Public Service (FPS) Health, Food Chain and Environment, Belgium.

Some web sites for additional information:
http://www.cjd.ed.ac.uk
http://www.eurocjd.ed.ac.uk
http://www.who.int/home-page/
http://www.ukhcdo.org/patient-information
http://case.edu/med/pathology/centers/npdpsc
http://www.who.int/medicines/areas/quality_safety/regulation_legislation/ListMRAWebsites.pdf

References

Ball R, Robb M, Anderson SA, Dal PG. The FDA's sentinel initiative—a comprehensive approach to medical product surveillance. Clin Pharmacol Ther. 2016;99:265–8.

Barjas-Castro ML, Angerami RN, Cunha MS, Suzuki A, Nogueira JS, Rocco IM, Maeda AY, Vasami FG, Katz G, Boin IF, Stucchi RS, Resende MR, Esposito DL, de Souza RP, da Fonseca BA, Addas-Carvalho M. Probable transfusion-transmitted Zika virus in Brazil. Transfusion. 2016;56:1684–8.

Bertolini J. Chromatographic purification of immunoglobulins. Downstream. 1998;31:21–2.

Blasco-Perrin H, Cintas P, Abravanel F, Gérolami R, D'Alteroche L, Raynal J-N, Alric L, Dupuis E, Prudhomme L, Vaucher E, Couzigou P, Liversain J-M, Buscail L, Bureau C, Vinel J-P, Kamar N, Izopet J, Péron JM. Neurologic disorders in immunocompetent patients with autochthonous acute hepatitis E. Emerg Infect Dis. 2015;21:1928–34.

Blümel J, Musso D, Teitz S, Miyabayashi T, Boller K, Schnierle BS, Baylis SA. Inactivation and removal of Zika virus during manufacture of plasma-derived medicinal products. Transfusion. 2017;57:790–6.

Boschetti N, Stucki M, Späth PJ, Kempf C. Virus safety of intravenous immunoglobulin: future challenges. Clin Rev Allergy Immunol. 2005;29:333–44.

Bruce ME, Will RG, Ironside JW, McConnell I, Drummond D, Suttie A, McCardle L, Chree A, Hope J, Birkett C, Cousens S, Fraser H, Bostock CJ. Transmissions to mice indicate that 'new variant' CJD is caused by the BSE agent. Nature. 1997;389:498–501.

Cai K, Gröner A, Dichtelmüller HO, Fabbrizzi F, Flechsig E, Gajardo R, von Hoegen I, Jorquera JI, Kempf C, Kreil TR, Lee DC, Moscardini M, Polsler G, Roth NJ. Prion removal capacity of plasma protein manufacturing processes: a data collection from PPTA member companies. Transfusion. 2013;53:1894–905.

Cai K, Miller JL, Stenland CJ, Gilligan KJ, Hartwell RC, Terry JC, Evans-Storms RB, Rubenstein R, Petteway SR, Lee DC. Solvent-dependent precipitation of prion protein. Biochim Biophys Acta. 2002;1597:28–35.

Cramer M, Frei R, Sebald A, Mazzoletti P, Maeder W. Stability over 36 months of a new liquid 10% polyclonal immunoglobulin product (IgPro10, Privigen©) stabilized with L-proline. Vox Sang. 2009;96:219–25.

Crowder LA, Schonberger LB, Dodd RY, Steele WR. Creutzfeldt-Jakob disease lookback study: 21 years of surveillance for transfusion transmission risk. Transfusion. 2017;57(8):1875–8. [Epub ahead of print].

D'Aignaux JH, Costagliola D, Maccario J, De Villemeur TB, Brandel JP, Deslys JP, Hauw JJ, Chaussain JL, Agid Y, Dormont D, Alpérovitch A. Incubation period of Creutzfeldt-Jakob disease in human growth hormone recipients in France. Neurology. 1999;53:1197–201.

Dhainaut F, Guillaumat PO, Dib H, Perret G, Sauger A, De Coupade C, Beaudet M, Elzaabi M, Mouthon L. *In vitro* and *in vivo* properties differ among liquid intravenous immunoglobulin preparations. Vox Sang. 2013;104:115–26.

El-Shanawany T, Jolles S, Unsworth DJ, Williams P. A recipient of immunoglobulin from a donor who developed vCJD. Vox Sang. 2009;96:270.

EMEA. CPMP Position Statement: Non-remunerated and remunerated donors: Safety and supply of plasma-derived medicinal products. European Agency for the Evaluation of Medical Products EMEA/CPMP/BWP/1818/02; 2002. p. 1–2.

Farcet MR, Lackner C, Antoine G, Rabel PO, Wieser A, Flicker A, Unger U, Modrof J, Kreil TR. Hepatitis E virus and the safety of plasma products: investigations into the reduction capacity of manufacturing processes. Transfusion. 2016;56:383–91.

Hewitt PE, Llewelyn CA, Mackenzie J, Will RG. Three reported cases of variant Creutzfeldt-Jakob disease transmission following transfusion of labile blood components. Vox Sang. 2006;91:348.

Higuchi M-A, Fukae J, Tsugawa J, Ouma S, Takahashi K, Mishiro S, Tsuboi Y. Dysgeusia in a patient with Guillain-Barre syndrome associated with acute hepatitis E: a case report and literature review. Intern Med. 2015;54:1543–6.

Höfferer L, Glauser I, Gaida A, Willimann K, Marques Anuntes A, Siani B, Wymann S, Widmer E, El Menyawi I, Bolli R, Spycher M, Imboden M. Isoagglutinin reduction by a dedicated immunoaffinity chromatography step in the manufacturing process of human immunoglobulin products. Transfusion. 2015;55(Suppl 2):S117–21.

Jackson GS, Burk-Rafel J, Edgeworth JA, Sicilia A, Abdilahi S, Korteweg J, Mackey J, Thomas C, Wang G, Schott JM, Mummery C, Chinnery PF, Mead S, Collinge J. Population screening for variant Creutzfeldt-Jakob disease using a novel blood test: diagnostic accuracy and feasibility study. JAMA Neurol. 2014;71:421–8.

Kempf C, Stucki M, Boschetti N. Pathogen inactivation and removal procedures used in the production of intravenous immunoglobulins. Biologicals. 2007;35:35–42.

Kreil TR, Berting A, Kistner O, Kindermann J. West Nile virus and the safety of plasma derivatives: verification of high safety margins, and the validity of predictions based on model virus data. Transfusion. 2003;43:1023–8.

Kühnel D, Müller S, Pichotta A, Radomski KU, Volk A, Schmidt T. Inactivation of Zika virus by solvent/detergent treatment of human plasma and other plasma-derived products and pasteurization of human serum albumin. Transfusion. 2017;57:802–10.

Laub R, Baurin S, Timmerman D, Branckaert T, Strengers P. Specific protein content of pools of plasma for fractionation from different sources: impact of frequency of donations. Vox Sang. 2010;99:220–31.

Leydold SM, Farcet MR, Kindermann J, Modrof J, Polsler G, Berting A, Howard MK, Barrett PN, Kreil TR. Chikungunya virus and the safety of plasma products. Transfusion. 2012;52:2122–30.

Lopez-Bueno A, Villarreal LP, Almendral JM. Parvovirus variation for disease: a difference with RNA viruses? Curr Top Microbiol Immunol. 2006;299:349–70.

Makarov V, Pettitt BM, Feig M. Solvation and hydration of proteins and nucleic acids: a theoretical view of simulation and experiment. Acc Chem Res. 2002;35:376–84.

Mallet V, Sberro-Soussan R, Vallet-Pichard A, Roque-Afonso AM, Pol S. Transmission of hepatitis E virus by plasma exchange: a case report. Ann Intern Med. 2016;164:851–2.

Martin M, Trouvin JH. Risk of transmission of Creutzfeldt-Jakob disease via blood and blood products. The French risk-analysis over the last 15 years. Transfus Clin Biol. 2013;20:398–404.

Morgenthaler JJ. Securing viral safety for plasma derivatives. Transfus Med Rev. 2001;15:224–33.

Motte A, Roquelaure B, Galambrun C, Bernard F, Zandotti C, Colson P. Hepatitis E in three immunocompromized children in southeastern France. J Clin Virol. 2012;53:162–6.

Nitschmann H, Kistler P, Lergier W. Vereinfachtes Verfahren zur Gewinnung von humanem Albumin und γ-Globulin aus Blutplasma mittels Alkoholfällung - [Simplified method for isolation of human albimin and γ-globulin from plasma using the ethnol precipitation method]. Helv Chim Acta. 1954;37:866–73.

Nogueira ML, Estofolete CF, Terzian ACB, Mascarin do Vale EPB, da Silva RCMA, da Silva RF, Ramalho HJ, Fernandes Charpiot IMM, Vasilakis N, Abbud-Filho M. Zika virus infection and solid organ transplantation: a new challenge. Am J Transplant. 2017;17:791–5.

Offergeld R, Faensen D, Ritter S, Hamouda O. Human immunodeficiency virus, hepatitis C and hepatitis B infections among blood donors in Germany 2000–2002: risk of virus transmission and the impact of nucleic acid amplification testing. Euro Surveill. 2005;10:8–11.

Oncley JL, Melin M, Richert DA, Cameron JW, Gross PM. The separation of the antibodies, isoagglutinins, prothrombin, plasminogen and β1-lipoprotein into subfractions of human plasma. J Am Chem Soc. 1949;71:541–50.

Peden AH, Head MW, Ritchie DL, Bell JE, Ironside JW. Preclinical vCJD after blood transfusion in a PRNP codon 129 heterozygous patient. Lancet. 2004;364:527–9.

Pérez Torre P, Acebrón F, Monreal E, Viedma GE, Martinez UP, FC E+®v, Alonso CA, Avil+®s O, I, Buis+ín CJ. Guillain-Barré syndrome following acute hepatitis E in a Western European man. Eur J Neurol. 2015;22:291.

Preti RA. Process validation. Cytotherapy. 1999;1:481–3.

Rabenau HF, Biesert L, Schmidt T, Bauer G, Cinatl J, Doerr HW. SARS-coronavirus (SARS-CoV) and the safety of a solvent/detergent (S/D) treated immunoglobulin preparation. Biologicals. 2005;33:95–9.

Ritchie DL, Gibson SV, Abee CR, Kreil TR, Ironside JW, Brown P. Blood transmission studies of prion infectivity in the squirrel monkey (Saimiri sciureus): the Baxter study. Transfusion. 2016;56:712–21.

Scanvion Q, Perez T, Cassim F, Outteryck O, Lanteri A, Hatron PY, Lambert M, Morell-Dubois S. Neuralgic amyotrophy triggered by hepatitis E virus: a particular phenotype. J Neurol. 2017;264:770–80.

Shackelton LA, Holmes EC. Phylogenetic evidence for the rapid evolution of human B19 erythrovirus. J Virol. 2006;80:3666–9.

Siani B, Willimann K, Wymann S, Marques AA, Widmer E. Isoagglutinin reduction in human immunoglobulin products by donor screening. Biol Ther. 2014;4:15–26.

Slopecki A, Smith K, Moore S. The value of good manufacturing practice to a blood service in managing the delivery of quality. Vox Sang. 2007;92:187–96.

Späth PJ, Granata G, La Marra F, Kuijpers TW, Quinti I. On the dark side of therapies with immunoglobulin concentrates. The adverse events. Front Immunol. 2015;6:11.

Steinbuch M, Audran R. The isolation of IgG from mammalian sera with the aid of caprylic acid. Arch Biochem Biophys. 1969;134:279–84.

Steinhardt B. Blood plasma safety. Plasma product risks are low if good manufacturing practices are followed. B-278739. Washington: GAO/HEHS; 1998. p. 1–47. Ref Type: Report.

Stucki M, Moudry R, Kempf C, Omar A, Schlegel A, Lerch PG. Characterisation of a chromatographically produced anti-D immunoglobulin product. J Chromatogr B Biomed Sci Appl. 1997;700:241–8.

Tamura A, Shimizu YK, Tanaka T, Kuroda K, Arakawa Y, Takahashi K, Mishiro S, Shimizu K, Moriyama M. Persistent infection of hepatitis E virus transmitted by blood transfusion in a patient with T-cell lymphoma. Hepatol Res. 2007;37:113–20.

Trejo SR, Hotta JA, Lebing W, Stenland C, Storms RE, Lee DC, Li H, Petteway S, Remington KM. Evaluation of virus and prion reduction in a new intravenous immunoglobulin manufacturing process. Vox Sang. 2003;84:176–87.
Urwin P, Thanigaikumar K, Ironside JW, Molesworth A, Knight RS, Hewitt PE, Llewelyn C, Mackenzie J, Will RG. Sporadic Creutzfeldt-Jakob disease in 2 plasma product recipients, United Kingdom. Emerg Infect Dis. 2017;23:893.
Urwin PJ, Mackenzie JM, Llewelyn CA, Will RG, Hewitt PE. Creutzfeldt-Jakob disease and blood transfusion: updated results of the UK Transfusion Medicine Epidemiology Review Study. Vox Sang. 2016;110:310–6.
Venturi G, Zammarchi L, Fortuna C, Remoli ME, Benedetti E, Fiorentini C, Trotta M, Rizzo C, Mantella A, Rezza G, Bartoloni A. An autochthonous case of zika due to possible sexual transmission, Florence, Italy, 2014. Eurosurveillance. 2016;21:1–4.
Wilesmith JW, Ryan JB, Atkinson MJ. Bovine spongiform encephalopathy: epidemiological studies on the origin. Vet Rec. 1991;128:199–203.
Yang H, Huang Y, Gregori L, Asher DM, Bui T, Forshee RA, Anderson SA. Geographic exposure risk of variant Creutzfeldt-Jakob disease in US blood donors: a risk-ranking model to evaluate alternative donor-deferral policies. Transfusion. 2017;57:924–32.
Yunoki M, Urayama T, Yamamoto I, Abe S, Ikuta K. Heat sensitivity of a SARS-associated coronavirus introduced into plasma products. Vox Sang. 2004;87:302–3.

13 Current IgG Products and Future Perspectives

Peter J. Späth

13.1 Introduction

Most international IG products are FDA and/or EMA approved. For some countries, some IG products might have formulation characteristics that allow their safe use although the supply chain might be less well standardized as in others. In case a country might not be willing to build up the complex organization necessary for plasma fractionation, an established fractionation company might be willing to offer a fractionation technique they formerly have used. In such a case, the country designs a dedicated organization that is responsible for plasma collection under supervision of authorities, and the collected plasma is shipped to a fractionating company for fractionation. The final product is shipped back to the country and is distributed to hospitals. The entire process is termed "toll manufacturing."

Progress in IG manufacturing and formulations always are driven by enhancing recovery without losing in purity. Liquid formulation and storage at room temperature are important for hospital pharmacies and bedside activities. Tolerability at high infusion rates/high strength of the IG solutions is a hospital and medical preference. Subcutaneous application first reported in 1952 (Bruton 1952) and not practiced for the next 30 years (Berger et al. 1980) has meanwhile enhanced convenience and partly shifted the IG administration from hospital to home.

The tables intend giving an overview and serve as an orientation. The tables were generated from summaries of product characteristics, prescribing information, form package inserts, websites of regulatory agencies, and the literature. It has to be stressed that the tables do not replace a package insert and that they should not serve a basis for therapies.

Excluded from the tables are the maximal infusion rates of the different products, which are the main source for adverse events (Späth et al. 2015).

P.J. Späth
Institute of Pharmacology, University of Bern, Bern, Switzerland
e-mail: peter.spaeth@pki.unibe.ch

P. Imbach (ed.), *Antibody Therapy*, https://doi.org/10.1007/978-3-319-68038-5_13

Availability of IG products: It is the great merit of the International Patient Organization for Primary Immunodeficiencies (IPOPI) updating accurately and continuously the availability of immunoglobulin concentrates around the world. It is possible to look up which products companies provide or which products are available in a given country (http://www.ipopi.org/index.php?page=immunoglobulin-countries; accessed July 2017). For particular countries/markets or IgG concentrates, it is further recommended to search on the website of the WHO mentioning all local registration agencies around the world http://www.who.int/medicines/areas/quality_safety/regulation_legislation/ListMRAWebsites.pdf (accessed July 2017).

13.2 Update on Available IgG Concentrates

Tables below provide the update on available IgG concentrates. The tables focus on the characteristics and contents of the IG preparations.

The first Table 13.1 lists the products obtained by processes mainly using ion-exchange chromatography. The roots of isolation of IgG from human plasma by ion-exchange chromatography go back to the late 1950s (Fahey and Horbett 1959). The first industrial applications were small-scale isolations using DEAE-sepharose (Baumstark et al. 1964; Bowman et al. 1980; Hoppe et al. 1973). The chromatographic method allowed obtaining products for intravenous use at relative high recovery (Friesen et al. 1985).

Table 13.2 lists products fractionated with the "cold ethanol" techniques to which the most recent improvements have been added.

Table 13.3 depicts products with which many important clinical breakthroughs were achieved and which represent the fundament for the products in Table 13.2.

Table 13.4 summarizes the subcutaneously applicable IG products for replacement therapy and for immunomodulation in chronic diseases.

Table 13.5 lists hyp erimmune globulins fractionated from plasma of selected (convalescent) donors or donations having high titers in a given antibody specificity.

Table 13.6 lists some "domestic" IgG concentrates.

Additional information regarding some of the products mentioned

Several plasma fractionators have a strong commitment for toll manufacturing. A contract for toll manufacturing includes delivery of plasma collected by, e.g., national services, the processing of the plasma, and shipping back the final product. As an example, plasma collected in Australia, New Zealand, Hong Kong, Singapore, Malaysia, and Taiwan are processed according the Intragam P method and are distributed in their countries of plasma origin under the brand name Intragam P or other. LFB has similar contracts for some North African countries.

Intragam P was the first very large-scale produced IgG concentrate applying the chromatographic technique.

Sandoglobulin: was the first product on the market composed of "native" IgG molecules. Originally, the product was termed "IgG-SRK" (SRK = Swiss Red Cross) (Schnoz et al. 1979). IgG-SRK was the product with which the

Table 13.1 Immunoglobulin concentrates manufactured using the ion-exchange chromatography technique as main fractionation method[$#]

IgG concentrate (manufacturer, financial background)	Polishing and validated pathogen reduction	Formulation	IgG cont. (%)	Strength of the solution ready to use (%)	Storage conditions	Osmolality	Carbohydrate stabilizers	Sodium cont.	pH	IgA cont. (mg/mL)
ClairYg® (LFB Biomedicaments, LFB SA, France)	Initial cold ethanol step, S/D treatment, virus filtration	Mannitol, glycine, polysorbate 80	NR	5	2–8 °C for 2 years (RT[a] for 1 year)	270–330 mOsmol/kg	None	None	4.8 ± 0.1	≤0.022
Gammaked™ (Grifols USA, Kedrion Biopharma, S.p.A, Italy)	Gammaked™ is identical to Gamunex									
Gamunex® (Grifols USA Llc, Grifols SA, Spain)	Initial cold ethanol step; caprylate precipitation and filtration; anion-exchange chromatography; ultrafiltration; low pH	Glycine 0.16–0.24 M	≥98	10	+2 °C to +8 °C (refrigerator) for 3 years; ≤6 months at RT with shelf life ending at this 6-month period	258 mOsmol/kg solvent	None	None added	4.0–4.5	≤0.046
Hizentra® (CSL Behring, CSL Ltd., Australia)	Hizentra® is registered for subcutaneous application (see there); beside the strength of the solution (20%), manufacturing corresponds to Privigen®									

(continued)

Table 13.1 (continued)

IgG concentrate (manufacturer, financial background)	Polishing and validated pathogen reduction	Formulation	IgG cont. (%)	Strength of the solution ready to use (%)	Storage conditions	Osmolality	Carbohydrate stabilizers	Sodium cont.	pH	IgA cont. (mg/mL)
Intragam P®[b] (CSL Behring, CSL Ltd., Australia)	Initial cold ethanol step, delipidation pasteurization, low pH	Liquid maltose, 0.1 g/mL (10% w/v)	≥98	6	2 °C–8 °C (refrigerator); or store below 25 °C and use within 3 months	Isotone	Maltose	NR	4.25	≤0.025
Iqyumune® (LFB Biomedicaments, LFB SA, France)	Initial cold ethanol step; caprylic acid precipitation; immunoadsorption chromatography, S/D treatment; virus filtration, ultrafiltration	Liquid, glycine, polysorbate 80	≥95	10	24 months, RT	281 mOsmol/kg	None	None added	4.6–5.0	≤0.028
Privigen® (CSL Behring, CSL Ltd., Australia)	Initial cold ethanol step; octanoic acid precipitation; pH 4; virus filtration; depth filtration; immunoaffinity chromatography	*L*-proline 210–290 mmol/L	≥98	10	4.8 mL/kg/h (EU) 0.04 mL/kg/min in chronic ITP and 0.08 mL/kg/min in PID (US)	320 mOsmol / kg	None	Traces	4.6–5.0	≤ 0.025

IgG concentrate (manufacturer, financial background)	Polishing and validated pathogen reduction	Formulation	IgG cont. (%)	Strength of the solution ready to use (%)	Storage conditions	Osmolality	Carbohydrate stabilizers	Sodium cont.	pH	IgA cont. (mg/mL)
Rhophylac® (CSL Behring, CSL Ltd., Australia)	Rhophylac is a polyclonal hyperimmune anti-blood group Rh(D) IgG concentrate; for details see Table 13.5									
Tegeline New® (LFB Biomedicaments, LFB SA, France)	Tegeline New is identical to ClairYg and is distributed e.g. in Brazil (http://www.lfb.com.br/atualidades/nova-imunoglobulina-intravenosa-liquida-do-grupo-lfb-tegeline-newy/									

[$]All preparations listed are liquid formulations

[#]Main fractionation by ion-exchange chromatography for most products include pre-purification by cryo-precipitation and one cold ethanol step to separate from the starting material for albumin fractionation (see Chap. 12). This forefront technique allows high recoveries at high purities[c]

cont = content, *max* = maximum, *NR* = not reported, *w/w* = weight/weight, *CSL* Commonwealth Serum Laboratories, *LFB* Laboratoire Français du Fractionnement et des Biotechnologies

[a]*RT* = room temperature, i.e., not over 25 °C

[b]Intragam P was the first large-scale chromatographically purified IgG concentrate. The author knows about earlier attempts for chromatographic purification in Humgary (Human, Gödöllő) using a Pharmacia chromatographic system

[c]The first mainly chromatographically obtained products were WinRho® SDF and Varizig® (Aptevo BioTherapeutics, Emergent BioSolutions, USA). Manifacturing used DEAE-Sephadex a method no more the most forefront chromatographic technique. WinRho SDF and Varizig are polyclonal hyperimmune anti-blood group Rh(D) and anti-varizella IgG concentrates, respectively- For details, please consult Table 13.5

Table 13.2 Newer IgG concentrates obtained by the cold ethanol fractionation techniques according to Cohn and Onlcey (C&O) or Kistler and Nitschmann (K-N)

IgG concentrate (manufacturer, organization, country)	Type of cold ethanol fractionation	Polishing and validated pathogen reduction	Excipient	IgG cont. (%)	Strength of the protein solution ready for infusion (%)	Osmolality	Sugars	Sodium cont.	pH	IgA cont. (mg/mL)
Line extensions of well introduced liquid IVIGs as indicated in Table 13.3										
Flebogammadif® 10% DIF (Grifols, Grifols SA, Spain) 10%	C&O	PEG precipitation; ion-exchange chromatography; low pH; pasteurization; solvent/detergent; virus filtration	*D*-sorbitol 5%	≥97	10	240–370 mOsmol/L	None	<3.2 mmol/L	5.0–6.0	≤0.006
Gammagard® liquid (Baxalta, Shire plc, Jersey)	C&O	Cation- and anion-exchange chromatography; low pH; S/D; virus filtration	Glycine 250 mmol/L	≥98	10	240–300 mOsmol/kg	None	No added sodium	4.6–5.1	≤0.037
Gammaplex® 10% (BPL, Creat Group Corp., China)[a]	C&O	Ion-exchange chromatography, S/D treatment, virus filtration, low pH	Glycine200–300 mM, polysorbate 80 1–6 mg	≥98	10	Typically 280 mOsmol/kg	None	≤30 mM	4.9–5.2	≤0.02

IgG concentrate (manufacturer, organization, country)	Type of cold ethanol fractionation	Polishing and validated pathogen reduction	Excipient	IgG cont. (%)	Strength of the protein solution ready for infusion (%)	Osmolality	Sugars	Sodium cont.	pH	IgA cont. (mg/mL)
Intragam P 10% (CSL Behring, CSL Ltd., Australia)	C&O	Low pH, pasteurization	Glycine 2.25 g/100 mL	NR	10	350 mOsmol/kg	None	NR	4.25	Typically <0.025
Intratect® 10% (Biotest pharma, Biotest AG, Germany)[a]	C&O	Octanoic acid/ calcium acetate; cation-exchange chromatography; solvent/detergent; ultra and diafiltration	Glycine 300 mMol/L	≥96	10	300 mOsmol/kg	None	<10 mmol/L	NR	≤1.8
Kiovig® (Baxalta, Shire plc, Jersey)	Kiovig® corresponds in its composition to Gammagard liquid, except for the IgA content which is ≤0.14 mg/mL; Kiovig® is the trade name for the EU market; see further details at Gammagard liquid									
Octagam® 10%[a] (Octapharama, Octapharma AG Switzerland)	C&O	Chromatography; pH 4; solvent/ detergent; ultrafiltration	Maltose 90 mg/mL	≥95	10	≥240 mOsmol/ kg	Maltoe	≤30 mmol/L	4.5–5.0	≤0.400
Panzyga® (Octapharma, Octapharama, AG, Switzerland)	K-N	Ion-exchange chromatography S/D treatment 20 nm virus filtration	Glycine 17.0 ± 0.29 mg/mL	≥95	10	≥240 mOsmol/ kg	None	<0.03 mmol (or 0.69 mg)/ mL	4.5–5.0	<0.3

(continued)

Table 13.2 (continued)

IgG concentrate (manufacturer, organization, country)	Type of cold ethanol fractionation	Polishing and validated pathogen reduction	Excipient	IgG cont. (%)	Strength of the protein solution ready for infusion (%)	Osmolality	Sugars	Sodium cont.	pH	IgA cont. (mg/mL)
Recent IVIGs with new formulations										
Bivigam™ (Biotest pharma, Biotest AG, Germany)[b]	C&O	Partitioning, S/D treatment, 35 nm virus filtration	0.20–0.29 M glycine, 0.15–0.25% polysorbate 80	≥96	10	NR	None	0.100–0.140 M	4.0–4.6	≤0.2
Vigam® (BPL, Creat Group Corp., China)	C&O	Cation-exchange chromatography; low pH; S/D	Human albumin 20% Glycine Sucrose	≥95	5	NR	Sucrose added	Sodium added	4.8–5.1	<0.014

In most cases, 5% preparations were developed further to obtain a stable, safe and clinically well-tolerated solution of 10% IgG. Products intended for intravenous use are listed

C&O: (Cohn et al. 1944; Oncley et al. 1949); K-N: (Nitschmann et al. 1954)

BPL Bio Products Laboratory, *CSL* Commonwealth Serum Laboratories

[a]In some countries several distributors for the product might exist

[b]Distribution in the USA of Bivigam™ by Kedrion US terminated as of January 2017: https://www.kedrion.us/bivigam%C2%AE-will-no-longer-be-available-sale-or-distribution-2017

Table 13.3 IgG preparations for i.v. use available for decades

IgG concentrate (manufacturer, organization, country)	Type of cold ethanol fractio-nation	Polishing and validated pathogen reduction	Excipients stabilizer	IgG cont. (%)	Strength of the protein solution ready for infusion (%)	Osmolality	Sugars as excipients	Sodium cont.	pH	IgA cont. (mg/mL)
Liquid polyclonal IgG concentrates registered for intravenous application										
Flebogamma® 5% DIF (Grifols, Grifols SA, Spain)	C&O	PEG precipitation; ion-exchange chromatography; pasteurization	*D*-sorbitol 5%	≥97	5	240–350 mOsmol/L	None	<3.2 mEq/L	5.0–6.0	≤0.05
Gammaplex® 5% (BPL, Creat Group Corp., China)	C&O	Ion-exchange chromatography, S/D treatment, virus filtration, low pH 2–25 °C for 24 months	*D*-sorbitol Glycine Polysorbat 80	≥95	5	NR	None	<0.85%	4.9	≤0.01
IG Vena N (Kedrion, Kedrion Biopharma S.p.A. Italy)	C&O	Low pH; S/D	Maltose 10%	≥95	5	NR	Maltose	3 mmol/L	NR	<0.05
Gammaplex® 5% (BPL, Creat Group Corp., China)	C&O	Ion-exchange chromatography, S/D treatment, virus filtration, low pH	*D*-sorbitol (max 55 mg/mL), glycine, polysorbate 80 Sodium acetate 0.52 mmol/L	≥98	5	NR	Sorbitol	Yes, NR	4.8–5.1	≤0.01

(continued)

Table 13.3 (continued)

IgG concentrate (manufacturer, organization, country)	Type of cold ethanol fractio-nation	Polishing and validated pathogen reduction	Excipients stabilizer	IgG cont. (%)	Strength of the protein solution ready for infusion (%)	Osmolality	Sugars as excipients	Sodium cont.	pH	IgA cont. (mg/mL)
Intragam P (CSL Bioplasma, CSL Ltd., Australia)	K-N	Low pH, pasteurization	Maltose 10 g/100 mL	≥98	6	NR	Maltose	NR	4.25	Nominally ≤0.025
Intratect 5% (Biotest Pharma; Biotest AG, Germany)[a]	C&O		Glycine	≥96	5		None	NR		≤0.9
Octagam® 5% (Octapharma,Octapharma, AG, Switzerland)[a]	C&O	Chromatography; pH 4; solvent/ detergent; ultrafiltration	Maltose 10 mg/mL	≥95	5	310–380 mOsmol/ kg	Maltose	≤0.015 mmol/L	5.1–6.0	≤0.2
Nanogam® (Sanquin, Sanquin Plasma Products B.V., Netherlands)	K-N	pH 4.4/trace pepsin; solvent/ detergent; nanofiltration 3 years at 2 °C–8 °C (in a refrigerator)	Glucose 50 mg/mL	≥95	5	NR	Glucose	NR	NR	≤0.006
Lyophilized polyclonal IgG concentrates for intravenous use after reconstitution										
Carimune/Carimune® NF (CSL Behring, CSL Ltd., Australia)	K-N	Partitioning; pH 4/trace pepsin; nanofiltration	Lyophilized powder	≥96	3, 6, 9, 12	192–1074 mOsmol/ kg (depending on the IgG concentration of the reconstituted preparation)	Sucrose	<20 mg/g of protein	6.6	720

IgG concentrate (manufacturer, organization, country)	Type of cold ethanol fractio-nation	Polishing and validated pathogen reduction	Excipients stabilizer	IgG cont. (%)	Strength of the protein solution ready for infusion (%)	Osmolality	Sugars as excipients	Sodium cont.	pH	IgA cont. (mg/mL)
Gammagard S/D 5% (Baxalta, Shire plc, Jersey)	C&O	DEAE chromatography S/D	Glucose 20%, glycine 0.3 M human albumin 3%	≥90	5	636 mOsmol/L	Glucose	<8.5 mg/mL	6.8 ± 0.4	<0.001
Sandoglobulin®/ Sandoglobulin® NF (CSL Behring, CSL Ltd., Australia)	Sandoglobulin® NF identical to Carimune® NF; see above Carimune®/Sandoglobulin® are virus filtered as well									
Tegéline® LFB, LFB SA, France)	K-N	pH 4/trace pepsin; filtration; virus filtration	Sucrose 2 g/g protein	>97	5	NR	Sucrose	8 mg/10 mL	NR	17 mg/g protein
A chemically treated liquid IgG concentrate (5%) distributed in several markets (see also Table 13.6)										
Pentaglobin a preparation enriched in IgM and IgA (12% each) (Biotest Pharma, Biotest AG, Germany)	C&O	*β*-propiolacton/ UV treated	Glucose 25 g/L		5	NR	Glucose	78 mmol/L	NR	Enriched in IgA (and IgM)

Some of these preparations were instrumental in progress of clinical use of IVIGs. Those of the early native, well-tolerated preparations which still are on the market, all got a brush up in order to comply with viral safety requirements[b]. For checking the availability of the concentrate in a given market, the reader is advised to visit the following website: http://www.who.int/medicines/areas/quality_safety/regulation_legislation/ListMRAWebsites.pdf (accessed April 2017)
BPL Bio Products Laboratory, *CSL* Commonwealth Serum Laboratories, *LFB* Laboratoire Français du Fractionnement et des Biotechnologies, *cont.* = content, *DEAE* = diethylaminoethyl, *max* = maximum, *NR* = not reported, *PEG* = polyethylene glycol, *w/w* = weight/weight
[a]In some countries several distributors for the product might exist
[b]Upon request, reports on more recent clinical studies with some of these older products are available from the author

Table 13.4 IgG concentrates intended for s.c. applications

Brand name/manufacturer	Main fractionation method	Polishing[a]	Formulation and stabilizer	IgG content	Strength (%)	Sugar content	pH	IgA content (mg/mL)
Polyclonal IgG concentrates registered for s.c. use only								
Beriglobin® P(CSL Behring, CSL Ltd., Australia)	Cold ethanol	The measures taken are considered effective for enveloped and non-enveloped viruses	Liquid glycine (contains 100 IU/vial antibodies to hepatitis B virus)	≥98	16	NR	NR	0.8–1.6
Cuvitru®—IGSC 20 (Baxalta, Shire plc, Jersey)	Cold ethanol	S/D virus filtration low pH	Liquid glycine 0.25 M	≥98	20	None	4.6–5.1	≤0.08
Evogam® (CSL Behring, CSL Ltd., Australia)	Cold ethanol	Pasteurization Virus filtration	Liquid Glycine 2.25 g/100 mL	≥98	16	None	5.5	NR
Hizentra®/IgPro20 (CSL Behring, CSL Ltd., Australia)	Ion-exchange chromatography	S/D Low pH Virus filtration	Liquid *L*-proline 250 mmol/L Polysorbate 80 10–30 mg/mL	≥98	20	None	4.6–5.2	≤0.05
Gammanorm® (Octapharma Sweden, Octapharma AG, Switzerland)	Cold ethanol	S/D	Liquid; glycine, polysorbate 80, Refrigerator	≥95	16.5	None		≤0.0825
Octanorm® (Octapharma Sweden, Octapharma AG, Switzerland)	Identical to Gammanorm							

Brand name/manufacturer	Main fractionation method	Polishing[a]	Formulation and stabilizer	IgG content	Strength (%)	Sugar content	pH	IgA content (mg/mL)
Subgam® (BPL, Creat Group Corp., China)	Cold ethanol	The measures taken are considered effective for enveloped viruses and for non-enveloped viruses	Liquid	≥95	16	NR	NR	<0.04% w/w
Subcuvia® (Baxalta, Shire plc, Jersey)[b]	Cold ethanol	S/D	Liquid Glycine	≥90	16	NR	NR	≤4.8
Polyclonal IgG concentrate for large volume application at a single site								
HyQvia® (IGHy) (Baxalta, Shire plc, Jersey)	Cold ethanol HyQvia is a two-component preparation with IgG concentrate (10%) and recombinant human hyaluronidase (rHUPH20), 160 U/mL	Liquid The IgG component of HyQvia corresponds to Gammagard liquid (for details see Table 13.2) HyQvia is applied sequentially, i.e., first the hyaluronidase than the IgG concentrate						
Polyclonal IgG concentrates registered for i.m. and s.c. use								
Gammaplex® 5% and 10%	For details regarding Gammaplex see Tables 13.2 and 13.3							
Polyclonal IgG concentrates intended for i.v. use applied s.c.[c]								
Carimune® NF	For details on Carimune NF, see Table 13.3							
Gammagard® liquid without hyaluronidase	For details regarding Gammagard liquid, see Table 13.2							
Gamunex®	For details regarding Gamunex, see Table 13.1							
Polyclonal IgG concentrates intended for i.m. use applied s.c.								
BayGam®	BayGam is also marketed as GammaSTAN; see below							

(continued)

Table 13.4 (continued)

Brand name/manufacturer	Main fractionation method	Polishing[a]	Formulation and stabilizer	IgG content	Strength (%)	Sugar content	pH	IgA content (mg/mL)
GammaQuin®	Cold ethanol	NR	Liquid for i.m. or s.c. Glycine	≥90	16	None	NR	≤6
GamaSTAN® S/D (Grifols, Grifols SA, Spain))	Cold ethanol	Precipitation, filtration ultrafiltration Diafiltration	Liquid Glycine0.21–0.32 M	NR	15–18	None	6.4–7.2	NR

SCIG is well suited individualizing immunoglobulin dose to enhance outcomes (Shapiro et al. 2017)

BPL Bio Products Laboratory, *CSL* Commonwealth Serum Laboratories, *S/D* solvent/detergent treatment in order to inactivate enveloped viruses

[a]For details about polishing steps, please refer to Chap. 12

[b]Shire in German recommends to replace Subcuvia® in favor of Cuvitru® or HyQvia®. It is foreseeable that in the future Subcuvia® will be taken from the market, as it happened with Vivaglobin® in favor of Hizentra®

[c]In the 1990s IVIGs were applied in order to prevent the use of those days mercury containing 16% i.m. preparations

Table 13.5 Some human hyperimmune globulin preparations

Specificity	Brand name/manufacturer	Strength of the IgG in the solution (mg/mL)	Administration form	IgG content	Ascertained specific antibody content	Virus inactivation and removal steps part of the manufacturing process	Stabilizer sugar content	Sodium content	pH	IgA content
Anti-toxin/toxoid polyclonal hyperimmune globulins										
Tetanus toxin	Tetanus immunoglobulin-VF (CSL Behring, CSL Ltd., Australia) http://www.cslbehring.com.au/docs/436/447/Tetanus%20IVIG-VF%20AU%20PI%2014.00.pdf	55–65	Liquid for i.v.	≥98	4000 IU/vial	Low pH Virus filtration	Maltose 292 mmol/L	NR	4.25	<0.5 mg/mL
Anti-viral polyclonal hyperimmune globulins										
Human CMV	Cytotect® CP (Biotest, Biotest Pharma GmbH, Germany) http://www.biotest.de/en/data/pdf/therapie/produkte/spc-cytotect_cp_en-nov2012.pdf	50	Liquid for i.v.	≥96	100 PEI U./mL	Yes May be of limited value against non-enveloped viruses	Glycine None	NR	NR	≤2 mg/mL
	Cytogam® (CSL Behring, CSL Ltd., Australia) https://www.fda.gov/downloads/BiologicsBloodVaccines/BloodBloodProducts/ApprovedProducts/LicensedProductsBLAs/FractionatedPlasmaProducts/UCM197962.pdf http://labeling.cslbehring.com/PI/US/Cytogam/EN/Cytogam-Prescribing-Information.pdf	5	Liquid for i.v.	NR	NR	S/D	Sucrose 5% Human albumin 1%	20–30 mEq/L		Trace amount
	CMV immunoglobulin-VF (CSL Behring, CSL Ltd., Australia) http://www.cslbehring.com.au/docs/359/8/CMV%20Immunoglobulin%20AU%20PI%2016.00.pdf	55–65	Liquid, for i.v.		1.5 million units per vial	Yes	292 mmol/L maltose		4.25	<0.5 mg/mL

(continued)

Table 13.5 (continued)

Specificity	Brand name/manufacturer	Strength of the IgG in the solution (mg/mL)	Administration form	IgG content	Ascertained specific antibody content	Virus inactivation and removal steps part of the manufacturing process	Stabilizer sugar content	Sodium content	pH	IgA content
Hepatitis B surface antigen (HBsAg)	Hepatect® CP (Biotest, Biotest Pharma GmbH, Germany) https://www.medicines.org.uk/emc/medicine/23171	50	Liquid for i.v.	≥96	50 I.U./mL	Yes May be of limited value against non-enveloped viruses	Glycine None	NR	NR	2 mg/mL
	Zutectra® (Biotest, Bitest Pharma GmbH, Germany) http://www.ema.europa.eu/docs/en_GB/document_library/EPAR_-_Product_Information/human/001089/WC500073708.pdf	150	Prefilled 5 mL syringes for s.c.	≥96	500 I.U./mL	Yes May be of limited value against non-enveloped viruses	Glycine None	NR	NR	6 mg/mL
	Hepatitis immunoglobulin-VF (CSL Behring, CSL Ltd., Australia) http://www.cslbehring.com.au/docs/413/735/Hepatitis%20B%20IMIG-VF%20AU%20PI%208.00.pdf	160	Liquid for i.m.	≥98	≥100 IU/mL	Yes	22.5 mg/mL glycine		6.6	NR
Human varicella zoster	Varitect® CP (Biotest, Biotest Pharma GmbH, Germany) http://www.choroby-zakazne.pl/uploads/Varitect%20CP%20ang.pdf	50	Liquid for i.v.	≥96	25 IU/mL	Yes May be of limited value against non-enveloped viruses	Glycine			2 mg/mL
	Zoster immunoglobulin-VF(CSL Behring, CSL Ltd., Australia) http://www.cslbehring.com.au/docs/118/175/Zoster%20IMIG-VF%20AU%20PI%209.00.pdf	160	Liquid, i.m. s.c.	≥98	200 IU/vial	Pasteurisation Virus filtration	Glycine 22.5 mg/mL		6.6	NR
	Varzig® (Aptevo BioTherapeutics, Emergent BioSolutions Inc., USA) http://varizig.com/VARIZIG%20LQ%20USPI-Aptevo.pdf	NR	Liquid for i.m. use, prepared by anion-exchange chromatography	NR	125 IU/vial	S/D Virus filtration	Maltose 10% Polysorbate 80 0.03%		5.0–6.5	<0.04 mg/mL

Anti-blood group polyclonal hyperimmune globulins										
Rhesus D antigen of red blood cells	Rhophylac® (CSL Behring CSL Ltd., Australia) http://labeling.cslbehring.com/PI/US/Rhophylac/EN/Rhophylac-Prescribing-Information.pdf	20	Liquid for i.v. or i.m. Pre-filled syringes A chromatographically isolated product	≥95%	1500 IU per vial	S/D Chromatography Virus filtration	Human albumin 10 mg/mL Glycine 20 mg/mL	≤0.25 M	NR	<0.005 mg/mL
	Rh(D) immunoglobulin-VF (CSL Behring, CSL Ltd., Australia) http://www.cslbehring.com.au/docs/713/52/Rh(D)%20Immunoglobulin-VF%20AU%20PI%2012.00.pdf	10 or 30	Liquid for i.m.	≥98	250 or 625 IU per vial	Pasteurization Virus filtration	Glycine 22.5 mg/mL		6.6	NR
	WinRho® SDF (Aptevo BioTherapeutics, Emergent BioSolutions Inc., USA) http://www.winrho.com/pdfs/WinRho_SDF_PI_Aptevo.pdf	NR	Lyophilized powder for i.v. after reconstitution A product primarily manufactured by chromatographic method	NR	600, 1500 or 5000 IU/vial	S/D Virus filtration	Glycine 0.1 M Maltose 10% Polysorbate 80 0.03%	0.04 M	NR	0.005 mg/mL

The list is far from being complete

i.m. intramuscular, *i.v.* intravenous, *S/D* solvent/detergent treatment

Table 13.6 "Domestic" IgG concentrates. Toll-manufactured products might be widely used in some of the countries listed

	IgG concentrate (manufacturer, financial background)	Main fractionation method/reference
Australia and New Zealand All "local" products toll manufactured	Normal immunoglobulin-VF (CSL Behring, CSL ltd., Australia)	Formulation: Liquid for i.m. IgG content: ≥98 Strength of the solution for infusion: 160 mg/mL Stabilizer: Glycine 22.5 mg/mL pH: 6.6
	Various "Australian & New Zealand Immunoglobulins" (CSL Behring (Australia) Pty ltd)	(Young et al. 2017)
China	Human immunoglobulin (IM) (Shanghai Raas, blood products Co. Ltd., China)	
	Gammaraas (Shanghai Raas, Blood Products Co. Ltd., China)	Formulation: Liquid for i.v. at pH of 4 with sorbitol Strength of the solution for infusion: 50 mg/mL IgG content: ≥95 Pathogen safety: Low pH and virus filtration Shelf life: 36 mo at 2–8 °C This product has a market penetration in some countries beside China
	Human hepatitis B immunoglobulin (IM) (Shanghai Raas, Blood Products Co. Ltd., China)	Ascertained specific IgG content: 100, 200, 400 IU per flask
	Human tetanus immunoglobulin (IM) (Shanghai Raas, Blood Products Co. Ltd., China)	Ascertained specific IgG content: 250 IU/vial
	Human rabies immunoglobulin (IM) (Shanghai Raas, Blood Products Co. Ltd., China)	Ascertained specific IgG content: 100 IU/mL
	Normal human immunoglobulins	Application: i.v. A comparative study on concentrations of antibodies against β-amyloid 40/42 monomer and oligomers in 11 Chinese IVIGs (Ye et al. 2017)
Cuba	Intacglobin	(Macías-Abraham et al. 2016)

Table 13.6 (continued)

	IgG concentrate (manufacturer, financial background)	Main fractionation method/ reference
India	Immunorel (Reliance Life Science, India)	
	Globucel (INTAS Pharma, Ahmedabad, India)	Formulation: Liquid Strength of the solution for infusion: 50 mg/mL
	Seroglob (Virchow/Gsk Healthcare Pvt. Ltd.)	Strength of the solution for infusion: 50 mg/mL
	Immuglo (Hemarus Therapeutics Limited, Hyderabad, India)	Strength of the solution for infusion: 50 mg/mL
	V-immune (Virchow Healthcare Pvt. Ltd. Mumbai, India)	Formulation: Liquid Strength of the solution for infusion: 50 mg/mL
Japan	Kenketsu Globulin "KAKETSUKEN" (Nihon Pharmaceutical Co., Takeda Pharmaceutical Company Ltd.)	Formulation: Freeze-dried, enzymatically degraded to the $F(ab)_2$ part by harsh pepsin digestion
	Kenketsu Venilon-I (Nihon Pharmaceutical Co., Takeda Pharmaceutical company Ltd.)	Formulation: Freeze-dried, chemically modified by S-sulfonation
	Glovenin-I (Nihon Pharmaceutical Co., Takeda pharmaceutical company Ltd.)	Formulation: Freeze-dried, polyethylene glycol-treated human normal immunoglobulin
	DRIED HB GLOBULIN for I.M. Injection 200 units INICHIYAKU	Formulation: Freeze-dried Strength of the solution for infusion: 200 mg/mL Ascertained specific IgG content: 250 U/vial
	TETANUS GLOBULIN for I.M. Injection 250 units INICHIYAKUJ	Ascertained specific IgG content: 250 U/vial
	ANTI-D GLOBULIN for I.M. Injection 1000 INICHIYAKUJ	Ascertained specific IgG content: 1000 U/vial
South Africa	Intragam[a] (National Bioproducts, South Africa)	(Peter et al. 2014)
	Polygam[b] (National Bioproducts, South Africa)	(Peter et al. 2014)

(continued)

Table 13.6 (continued)

	IgG concentrate (manufacturer, financial background)	Main fractionation method/ reference
South Korea	IV-globulin SN™, (Green Cross Corporation, Yongin, Korea)	Fractionation: Cold ethanol and DEAE-sepharose chromatography Formulation: Liquid, maltose at 100 mg/mL Pathogen safety: S/D treatment and virus filtration Strength of the solution for infusion: 50 mg/mL Marketed in Korea, Brazil, India, and Iran (Yoon et al. 2017; Stein et al. 2015)
	Gamma globulin an i.m. concentrate	(Tejada-Strop et al. 2017)
	GC5101B (Green Cross Corporation, Yongin, Korea, and the Sungkyunkwan University, Suwon, Korea)	A Green Cross product purified further (Park et al. 2017)

Furthermore, in several of the countries "nondomestic" products listed in the above tables are available. The table is not a complete listing of all domestic products
BPL Bio Products Laboratory, *CSL* Commonwealth Serum Laboratories, *LFB* Laboratoire de Fractionnement Bilogique, http://www.cslbehring.com.au/products/product-finder.htm
[a]In Australia and New Zealand, the predecessor preparation of Intragam P was Intragam
[b]Under the trade name Polygam the American Red Cross sold Gammagard in the USA; after the transmission of HCV, the product is no more on the market

immunomodulatory potential of IVIGs was first reported (Imbach et al. 1981). Following a distribution agreement with Sandoz, the product was renamed Sandoglobulin. Sandoglobulin was the first IVIG which came onto the US market after having been tested in the first IVIG registration study ever performed (Cunningham-Rundles et al. 1984). Sandoglobulin was also the first product that underwent large-scale virus filtration during manufacturing (Kempf and Morgenthaler 1999). Sandoglobulin®/Sandoglobulin® NF is identical to Carimune®/Carimune® NF and is also identical to Panglobulin®/Panglobulin® NF. Panglobulin®/Panglobulin® NF was toll manufactured for the American Red Cross (ARC). Panglobulin® /Panglobulin® NF is no more available. In contrast, Sandoglobulin® NF/Carimune® NF is, at least in some markets, still available.

13.3 Future Perspectives

13.3.1 Polyclonal Immunoglobulin Preparations Different from Presently Available Products

Fractionation of plasma to stable blood products generates a series of side fractions some of which contain IgA and IgM. An investigational preparation for topical use enriched in IgA (IgABulin) was clinically tested in a few patients; however, following a company merger and the outcome of a Cochrane systematic review of the project was not further pursued (Foster and Cole 2004). Polyclonal IgA isolated from plasma contains a few percentage of a polymeric (dimeric) form of IgA (pIgA). The combining of pIgA or of plasma-derived polyclonal IgM with recombinant secretory component to form secretory-like IgA or IgM was reported recently (Longet et al. 2013; Longet et al. 2014). To the best of my knowledge not trials in man followed. A recent review regarding the clinical effects in man of human-derived IgM came to the conclusion that the hard facts in knowledge are marginal despite a bunch of clinical data obtained with a chemically modified concentrate enriched in IgM and IgA (Späth et al. 2017). Nevertheless, some progress is made. Biotest AG (Germany) developed a follow-up product to the existing chemically modified IgM/A-enriched product, termed "BT086." Clinical studies addressing community-acquired pneumonia with BT086 have been completed (EudraCT Number: 2010-022380-35 (https://www.clinicaltrialsregister.eu/ctr-search/search?query=BT086) and Clinical Trail Identifier NCT01420744 (https://clinicaltrials.gov/ct2/show/NCT01420744?term=CIGMA&rank=1; both accessed June 2017). The results of this study are eagerly awaited. As BT086 has an isotype distribution of approximately 54% IgG, 23% IgA, and 23% IgG (mean values), enrichment in products of IgM above 25% is an unmet interest. A more recent patent addresses a possible way how to obtain such highly enriched IgM (Rentsch 2000); however no follow-up publications were found.

13.3.2 Resistance to Antibiotics and Polyclonal IgG Therapy

Outside the field of primary immune deficiencies, the clinical use of IgG concentrates in bacterial infection is almost inexistent. Table 13.5 does not list a single antibacterial hyperimmune globulin. However, this might change. There are astonishingly few reports which preemptively address a possible last resort role of IgG therapy in fighting antibiotic-resistant/multiresistant infections (Diep et al. 2016; Farag et al. 2013). Interest in IgG suddenly might awake, i.e., as soon as the spreading of the *mrc-1* gene located on plasmids of Gram-negative bacteria accelerates. The *mrc-1* gene has broken away the very last line of defense against antibiotic-resistant Gram-negative bacteria (Liu et al. 2016).

13.3.3 Polyclonal Immunoglobulin Preparations for Infectious Complications in Emerging Therapies

The past decade has seen a rapid appearance of innovative new immunosuppressive and immunomodulatory drugs in clinics with currently three broad classes of biologic therapies, i.e., tumor necrosis factor-alpha inhibitors, lymphocyte modulators, and interleukin inhibitors. Therapeutic monoclonal antibodies, peptides, and fusion proteins or engineered chimeric antigen receptor (CAR)-T cells are the basis of these new therapies (Batlevi et al. 2016). Combination of these with well-established therapies for, e.g., hematological malignancies, increases efficacy however also is associated with severe infectious complications. The introduction of these modern drugs is continuously generating an increasing number of clinical conditions that are associated with an increased risk of severe/opportunistic/recurrent infections, reactivation of latent viruses, and appearance of secondary autoimmune phenomena. The resulting immunological deficiencies may involve innate immunity, adaptive T- and B-cell immunity, or combinations of the three. The patients at risk thus are a heterogeneous population and include, beside HIV and hematological malignancies, malignant solid tumors, hematopoietic stem cell transplant (HSCT) recipients, solid organ transplant (SOT) recipients, patients on immunosuppressive or immunomodulatory treatment for systemic autoimmune and inflammatory diseases, and other minor conditions. When considering a single clinical condition treated with a single modern therapeutic measure, the number of patients is small who might develop (severe) infectious complications. However, the ever-increasing type of conditions treated with the ever-increasing number of new drugs results in an ever-increasing number of patients at risk for severe infectious complications. Particularly two subgroups of patients with secondary susceptibility to severe infections might profit from therapies with human immunoglobulin concentrates: (a) patients with secondary hypogammaglobulinemias showing an impaired vaccination response and (b) patients developing autoimmune conditions while on therapy for B-cell malignancies, prevention of GvHD, or multiple sclerosis (e.g., following alemtuzumab treatment). Low level of circulating IgG is not an indication for therapy in such conditions. In contrast, recurrent/opportunistic infections and a proven failure of specific antibody production after vaccination are indications for replacement therapy.

In summary, the evolution of new clinical conditions complicated by susceptibility to severe/recurrent/opportunistic infections is rapid, and the number of patients at risk is steadily increasing. IgG therapies might have clinical role in those therapies which directly or indirectly target the B-cell lineage and plasma cells.

13.3.4 The Combination for Improved Clinical Success of Polyclonal IgG Concentrates with Modern Drugs Targeting Immune Cells

There is an increased body of literature that reports the successful combination of polyclonal IgGs with modern drugs that target immune cells. These combinations should not be confounded with combinations where the immunosuppressive effect of a modern therapy has to be corrected by passive immunization (see above). The most reports relate to IVIG in combination with rituximab, bortezomib, or tocilizumab either for desensitization prior to solid organ transplantation (SOT) or posttransplant immunosuppression in highly sensitized patients (Jeong et al. 2016; Jordan et al. 2016; Perez et al. 2017; Ruangkanchanasetr et al. 2014; Vo et al. 2015). IVIG in combination with rituximab has further been used in peripheral neuropathies (Oktem et al. 2016) and in a few other conditions. Usually only severe, refractory cases are receiving combination therapies, and hence the number of treated patients is small.

13.3.5 On the Edge Between Polyclonal and Recombinant Products

The "fragment crystallizable" (Fc) together with the hinge region of immunoglobulin molecules mediates the effector functions of the molecules. For IgG the Fc-fragment accomplishes the binding to the Fcγ receptors and the binding of the complement component C1q (initiation of the classical pathway of complement). The hinge region is the site where complement components C3 and C4 are bound. Already in the first report on immunomodulatory potential of polyclonal immunoglobulin preparations, an important role for the Fc-fragments was recognized (cited from (Imbach et al. 1981): "*In one patient with acute ITP 0.5 g of a pepsin-treated gammaglobulin [F(ab')$_2$]/kg body-weight/day on 3 consecutive days did not influence platelet count, whilst a single dose of 0.4 g of Ig-SRK/kg body-weight raised counts from 1.7 to 5 × 10^9/L within 6 h and to 12 × 10^9/L within 18 h.*" Interestingly enough, there exists one single study using Fc-fragment of IgG to treat ITP (Debré et al. 1993). The study was successful, was never repeated, and, nevertheless, together with other in vitro or in vivo studies, kept alive the interest about the relevance in immunomodulation by Fc- fragments, the F(ab)- fragments, or the intact IgG molecules. In a series of very elegant studies a research group around Jeffrey Ravetch, The Rockefeller University, New York, from 2001 onward (Samuelsson et al. 2001) added and continuously refined their concept how Fc-fragments might take a role in immunomodulation: terminal sialic acid-guided interaction with inhibitory Fcγ receptors being the key event (Kaneko et al. 2006; Schwab and Nimmerjahn 2013; Schwab et al. 2015). A recent publication describes a robust, controlled sialylation process to generate tetra-Fc–sialylated IVIG and its tenfold enhanced anti-inflammatory effect in a mouse model of collagen antibody-induced arthritis using a prophylactic dose (Washburn et al. 2015). The above concept is based on mice experiments, and results are discussed controversially due to conflicting findings from other groups (Bazin et al. 2006; Campbell et al. 2014; Crispin et al. 2013; Guhr et al. 2011; Käsermann et al. 2012; Leontyev et al. 2012; Leontyev et al. 2012; Othy et al. 2014; von Gunten et al. 2014; Yu et al. 2013; Schneider et al. 2017). In humans an exclusive role of terminal sialic acid-guided interaction with inhibitory Fcγ receptors as anti-inflammatory/immunomodulatory principle remains open. The mechanism of action of IgG concentrates might involve such interaction however; it is likely that this interaction is not sufficient to explain the anti-inflammatory/immunomodulatory potential of polyclonal normal IgG concentrates. Nevertheless, in humans terminal sialylation of Fc-fragments might be involved in some immunoregulatory processes. As an example, in pregnancy partial suppression of the maternal immune system is required to ensure tolerance of the fetus (Trowsdale and Betz 2006). In successful pregnancies, an increase in IgG Fc-linked

N-glycan galactosylation and sialylation and decrease after delivery were observed (Jansen et al. 2016). How far this and no other changes in glycans during pregnancy is responsible for tolerance remains open.

The interest in the biological role of Fc-fragments of IgG and their N-glycosylation is unbowed. The aim is to reproduce effector mechanism of polyclonal IgG at lower doses, and this has opened out into generation of engineered forms of Fc-fragments and their N-glycans. Multimerized recombinant Fc is one of the options. Momenta Pharmaceuticals is, among others, working on a trimeric Fc structure, and the start of a phase I study is planned for 2017 (Ortiz et al. 2016). Another avenue is pursued by Gliknik. GL-2045 is a stradomer, a multimeric IgG2 hinge-Fc in preclinical safety studies. The hinge region allows the binding of complement C3 and C4 and is an inhibitor of complement-mediated cytotoxicity (Zhou et al. 2017). HexaGard™ is a hexameric IgG1Fc with IgM tailpiece [L309C/H310L], i.e., is a biomimetic substitute of IVIG for triggering inhibitory receptors involved in controlling unwanted inflammation in autoimmune disease (http://www.lstmed.ac.uk/news-events/events/hexagard-a-biomimetic-of-intravenous-immunoglobulin-ivig-for-the-treatment-of; accessed July 2017). UCB Celltech is working on a hexameric, hybrid IgG1/4Fc IgM tailpiece. A subject-blind, investigator-blind, randomized, placebo-controlled, first-in-human study evaluates the safety/tolerability and pharmacokinetics of single ascending intravenous and subcutaneous doses of UCB7858 in healthy subjects (https://clinicaltrials.gov/ct2/show/NCT02879877; accessed July 2017). Argenex has created a monomeric IgG1Fc with high affinity for FcRn (ARGX-113). ARGX-113 is in phase II trials in myasthenia gravis and ITP. ARGX-113 enhances degradation of circulating disease-causing autoimmune antibodies by competing for binding to the Fc receptor of the newborn (FcRn), an MHC class I-like Fc receptor (Yu and Lennon 1999). FcRn is the receptor on endothelial cell that recirculates IgG and prolongs the half-lives in circulation to above 2 days (except IgG3) (Andersen and Sandlie 2009). FcRn is also the receptor for transplacental passage of IgG from mother to fetus (Firan et al. 2001). A more broad review regarding these new developments was published recently (Zürcher et al. 2016). More recently engineered IgG Fc domains that bind C1q but not effector Fcγ receptors mediated the clearance of target cells with kinetics and efficacy comparable to those of the FcγR-dependent effector functions, while they circumvented certain adverse reactions associated with FcγR engagement (Lee et al. 2017).

Beside the avenue of anti-inflammation/immunomodulation, even host defense was addressed by engineered Fc-fractions. Lysibodies are IgG Fc fusions with lysin-binding domains targeting *Staphylococcus aureus* cell wall carbohydrates for effective phagocytosis (Raz et al. 2017). Lysibodies target bacterial structures conserved over the evolution and thus escape mutations have a lesser chance for success.

In summary, innovative clinical trials with polyclonal normal IgG are not shining on the horizon. A considerable effort is taken to elucidate the biologic role of the Fc-fraction of IgG. For this purpose various, often multimeric, Fc-fragments with altered glycosylation are engineered. Some of these have entered phase II studies.

References

Andersen JT, Sandlie I. The versatile MHC class I-related FcRn protects IgG and albumin from degradation: implications for development of new diagnostics and therapeutics. Drug Metab Pharmacokinet. 2009;24:318–32.

Batlevi CL, Matsuki E, Brentjens RJ, Younes A. Novel immunotherapies in lymphoid malignancies. Nat Rev Clin Oncol. 2016;13:25–40.

Baumstark JS, Laffin RJ, Bardawil WA. A preparative method for the separation of 7S gamma globulin from human serum. Arch Biochem Biophys. 1964;108:514–22.

Bazin R, Lemieux R, Tremblay T. Reversal of immune thrombocytopenia in mice by cross-linking human immunoglobulin G with a high-affinity monoclonal antibody. Br J Haematol. 2006;135:97–100.

Berger M, Cupps TR, Fauci AS. Immunoglobulin replacement therapy by slow subcutaneous infusion. Ann Intern Med. 1980;93:55–6.

Bowman JM, Friesen AD, Pollock JM, Taylor WE. WinRho: Rh immune globulin prepared by ion exchange for intravenous use. Can Med Assoc J. 1980;123:1121–7.

Bruton OC. Agammaglobulinemia. Pediatrics. 1952;9:722–8.

Campbell IK, Miescher S, Branch DR, Mott PJ, Lazarus AH, Han D, Maraskovsky E, Zürcher AW, Neschadim A, Leontyev D, McKenzie BS, Käsermann F. Therapeutic effect of IVIG on inflammatory arthritis in mice is dependent on the Fc portion and independent of sialylation or basophils. J Immunol. 2014;192:5031–8.

Cohn EJ, Oncley JL, Strong LE, Hughes WL, Armstrong SH. Chemical, clinical and immunological studies on the product of human plasma fractionation. I. The characterization of the protein fractions of human plasma. J Clin Invest. 1944;23:417–32.

Crispin M, Yu X, Bowden TA. Crystal structure of sialylated IgG Fc: implications for the mechanism of intravenous immunoglobulin therapy. Proc Natl Acad Sci U S A. 2013;110:E3544–6.

Cunningham-Rundles C, Siegal FP, Smithwick EM, Cunningham-Rundles S, Lion-Boule A, O'Malley J, Barandun S, Good RA. Efficacy of intravenous immunoglobulin in primary humoral immunodeficiency disease. Ann Intern Med. 1984;101:435–9.

Debré M, Bonnet MC, Fridman WH, Carosella E, Philippe N, Reinert P, Vilmer E, Kaplan C, Teillaud JL, Griscelli C. Infusion of Fcg fragments for treatment of children with acute immune thrombocytopenic purpura. Lancet. 1993;342:945–9.

Diep BA, Le VTM, Badiou C, Le HN, Pinheiro MG, Duong AH, Wang X, Dip EC, Aguiar-Alves F, Basuino L, Marbach H, Mai TT, Sarda MN, Kajikawa O, Matute-Bello G, Tkaczyk C, Rasigade JP, Sellman BR, Chambers HF, Lina G. IVIG-mediated protection against necrotizing pneumonia caused by MRSA. Sci Transl Med. 2016;8:357ra124.

Fahey JL, Horbett AP. Human gamma globulin fractionation on anion exchange cellulose columns. J Biol Chem. 1959;234:2645–51.

Farag N, Mahran L, Abou-Aisha K, El-Azizi M. Assessment of the efficacy of polyclonal intravenous immunoglobulin G (IVIG) against the infectivity of clinical isolates of methicillin-resistant *Staphylococcus aureus* (MRSA) in vitro and in vivo. Eur J Clin Microbiol Infect Dis. 2013;32:1149–60.

Firan M, Bawdon R, Radu C, Ober RJ, Eaken D, Antohe F, Ghetie V, Ward ES. The MHC class I-related receptor, FcRn, plays an essential role in the maternofetal transfer of g-globulin in humans. Int Immunol. 2001;13:993–1002.

Foster J, Cole M. Oral immunoglobulin for preventing necrotizing enterocolitis in preterm and low birth-weight neonates. Cochrane Database Syst Rev. 2004;1:CD001816.
Friesen AD, Bowman JM, Bees WC. Column ion exchange chromatographic production of human immune serum globulin for intravenous use. Vox Sang. 1985;48:201–12.
Guhr T, Bloem J, Derksen NI, Wuhrer M, Koenderman AH, Aalberse RC, Rispens T. Enrichment of sialylated IgG by lectin fractionation does not enhance the efficacy of immunoglobulin G in a murine model of immune thrombocytopenia. PLoS One. 2011;6:e21246.
Hoppe HH, Mester T, Hennig W, Krebs HJ. Prevention of Rh-immunization. Modified production of IgG anti-Rh for intravenous application by ion exchange chromatography (IEC). Vox Sang. 1973;25:308–16.
Imbach P, Barandun S, D'Apuzzo V, Baumgartner C, Hirt A, Morell A, Rossi E, Schoeni M, Vest M, Wagner HP. High-dose intravenous gammaglobulin for idiopathic thrombocytopenic purpura in childhood. Lancet. 1981;1:1228–31.
Jansen BC, Bondt A, Reiding KR, Lonardi E, de Jong CJ, Falck D, Kammeijer GS, Dolhain RJ, Rombouts Y, Wuhrer M. Pregnancy-associated serum N-glycome changes studied by high-throughput MALDI-TOF-MS. Sci Rep. 2016;6:23296.
Jeong JC, Jambaldorj E, Kwon HY, Kim MG, Im HJ, Jeon HJ, In JW, Han M, Koo TY, Chung J, Song EY, Ahn C, Yang J. Desensitization using bortezomib and high-dose immunoglobulin increases rate of deceased donor kidney transplantation. Medicine (United States). 2016;95:e2635.
Jordan SC, Choi J, Kahwaji J, Vo A. Progress in desensitization of the highly HLA sensitized patient. Transplant Proc. 2016;48:802–5.
Kaneko Y, Nimmerjahn F, Ravetch JV. Anti-inflammatory activity of immunoglobulin G resulting from Fc sialylation. Science. 2006;313:670–3.
Käsermann F, Boerema DJ, Rüegsegger M, Hofmann A, Wymann S, Zürcher AW, Miescher S. Analysis and functional consequences of increased Fab-sialylation of intravenous immunoglobulin (IVIG) after lectin fractionation. PLoS One. 2012;7:e37243.
Kempf C, Morgenthaler JJ. Exclusion of infectious agents. Morell, A. and Späth, P. Novartis Pharma AG, ZLB, 14–21. 1999. Basel, Novartis Pharma AG, ZLB. Sandoglobulin Human normal Immunoglobulin (i.v.), Product monograph.
Lee CH, Romain G, Yan W, Watanabe M, Charab W, Todorova B, Lee J, Triplett K, Donkor M, Lungu OI, Lux A, Marshall N, Lindorfer MA, Goff OR, Balbino B, Kang TH, Tanno H, Delidakis G, Alford C, Taylor RP, Nimmerjahn F, Varadarajan N, Bruhns P, Zhang YJ, Georgiou G. IgG Fc domains that bind C1q but not effector Fcg receptors delineate the importance of complement-mediated effector functions. Nat Immunol. 2017;18(8):889–98. [Epub ahead of print].
Leontyev D, Katsman Y, Branch DR. Mouse background and IVIG dosage are critical in establishing the role of inhibitory Fcg receptor for the amelioration of experimental ITP. Blood. 2012;119:5261–4.
Leontyev D, Katsman Y, XZ MA, Miescher S, Käsermann F, Branch DR. Sialylation-independent mechanism involved in the amelioration of murine immune thrombocytopenia using intravenous gammaglobulin. Transfusion. 2012;52:1799–805.
Liu YY, Wang Y, Walsh TR, Yi LX, Zhang R, Spencer J, Doi Y, Tian G, Dong B, Huang X, Yu LF, Gu D, Ren H, Chen X, Lv L, He D, Zhou H, Liang Z, Liu JH, Shen J. Emergence of plasmid-mediated colistin resistance mechanism MCR-1 in animals and human beings in China: a microbiological and molecular biological study. Lancet Infect Dis. 2016;16:161–8.
Longet S, Miled S, Lötscher M, Miescher SM, Zürcher AW, Corthésy B. Human plasma-derived polymeric IgA and IgM antibodies associate with secretory component to yield biologically active secretory-like antibodies. J Biol Chem. 2013;288:4085–94.
Longet S, Vonarburg C, Lötscher M, Miescher S, Zürcher A, Corthésy B. Reconstituted human polyclonal plasma-derived secretory-like IgM and IgA maintain barrier function of epithelial cells infected with an enteropathogen. J Biol Chem. 2014;289:21617–26.
Macías-Abraham C, Sánchez Segura M, Insua Arregui C, García Nieblas MC, Hernández Flores G, Arce Hernández A, Merlín Linares JC, Martínez Triana R. Tratamiento con inmunoglobulina G subcutánea en enfermos con inmunodeficiencias primarias: resultados preliminares del

estudio multicentrico cubano – [Treatment with subcutaneous immunoglobulin G in patients with primary immunodeficiencies: preliminary results of cuban multicenter study]. Rev Cuba Hematol Imunol Hemoterapia. 2016;32:364–74.

Nitschmann H, Kistler P, Lergier W. Vereinfachtes Verfahren zur Gewinnung von humanem albumin und g-globulin aus Blutplasma mittels Alkoholfällung – [Simplified method for isolation of human albimin and g-globulin from plasma using the ethnol precipitation method]. Helv Chim Acta. 1954;37:866–73.

Oktem A, Akay BN, Boyvat A, Kundakci N, Erdem C, Bostanc-¦ S, Sanli H, Kocyigit P. Long-term results of rituximab-intravenous immunoglobulin combination therapy in patients with epidermolysis bullosa acquisita resistant to conventional therapy. J Dermatol Treat. 2016;28:50–4.

Oncley JL, Melin M, Richert DA, Cameron JW, Gross PM. The separation of the antibodies, isoagglutinins, prothrombin, plasminogen and b1-lipoprotein into subfractions of human plasma. J Am Chem Soc. 1949;71:541–50.

Ortiz DF, Lansing JC, Rutitzky L, Kurtagic E, Prod'homme T, Choudhury A, Washburn N, Bhatnagar N, Beneduce C, Holte K, Prenovitz R, Child M, Killough J, Tyler S, Brown J, Nguyen S, Schwab I, Hains M, Meccariello R, Markowitz L, Wang J, Zouaoui R, Simpson A, Schultes B, Capila I, Ling L, Nimmerjahn F, Manning AM, Bosques CJ. Elucidating the interplay between IgG-Fc valency and FcgR activation for the design of immune complex inhibitors. Sci Transl Med. 2016;8:365ra158.

Othy S, Topcu S, Saha C, Kothapalli P, Lacroix-Desmazes S, Käsermann F, Miescher S, Bayry J, Kaveri SV. Sialylation may be dispensable for reciprocal modulation of helper T cells by intravenous immunoglobulin. Eur J Immunol. 2014;44:2059–63.

Park DH, Kang GB, Kang DE, Hong JW, Lee MG, Kim KY, Han JW. A new manufacturing process to remove thrombogenic factors (II, VII, IX, X, and XI) from intravenous immunoglobulin gamma preparations. Biologicals. 2017;45:1–8.

Perez EE, Orange JS, Bonilla F, Chinen J, Chinn IK, Dorsey M, El-Gamal Y, Harville TO, Hossny E, Mazer B, Nelson R, Secord E, Jordan SC, Stiehm ER, Vo AA, Ballow M. Update on the use of immunoglobulin in human disease: a review of evidence. J Allergy Clin Immunol. 2017;139:S1–S46.

Peter JG, Heckmann JM, Novitzky N. Recommendations for the use of immunoglobulin therapy for immunomodulation and antibody replacement. S Afr Med J. 2014;104:796.

Raz A, Serrano A, Lawson C, Thaker M, Alston T, Bournazos S, Ravetch JV, Fischetti VA. Lysibodies are IgG Fc fusions with lysin binding domains targeting *Staphylococcus aureus* wall carbohydrates for effective phagocytosis. Proc Natl Acad Sci U S A. 2017;114:4781–6.

Rentsch M. Method for producing an IgM preparation for intravenous application. United States patent 6 136 312. Rotkreuzstifung Zentrallaboratorium Blutspendedienst SRK and Rotkreuzstiftung Zentrallaboratorium Blutspendedienst SRK. 09/269746(US 6136312). 24-10-2000. Bern, Switzerland. 23-4-1997.

Ruangkanchanasetr P, Satirapoj B, Termmathurapoj S, Namkhanisorn K, Suaywan K, Nimkietkajorn V, Luesutthiviboon L. Intensive plasmapheresis and intravenous immunoglobulin for treatment of antibody-mediated rejection after kidney transplant. Exp Clin Transplant. 2014;12:328–33.

Samuelsson A, Towers TL, Ravetch JV. Anti-inflammatory activity of IVIG mediated through the inhibitory Fc receptor. Science. 2001;291:484–6.

Schneider C, Wicki S, Graeter S, Timcheva TM, Keller CW, Quast I, Leontyev D, Djoumerska-Alexieva IK, Käsermann F, Jakob SM, Dimitrova PA, Branch DR, Cummings RD, Lünemann JD, Kaufmann T, Simon HU, von Gunten S. IVIG regulates the survival of human but not mouse neutrophils. Sci Rep. 2017;7:1296.

Schnoz M, Ryser DH, Barandun S, Eckmann L. Prophylaxe und Therapie mit Immunoglobulin SRK – [Prophylaxis and therapy with immunoglobulin SRC]. Helv Chir Acta. 1979;46:111–3.

Schwab I, Lux A, Nimmerjahn F. Pathways responsible for human autoantibody and therapeutic intravenous IgG activity in humanized mice. Cell Rep. 2015;13:610–20. Article Number 2065.

Schwab I, Nimmerjahn F. Intravenous immunoglobulin therapy: how does IgG modulate the immune system? Nat Rev Immunol. 2013;13:176–89.

Shapiro RS, Wasserman RL, Bonagura V, Gupta S. Emerging paradigm of primary immunodeficiency disease: individualizing immunoglobulin dose and delivery to enhance outcomes. J Clin Immunol. 2017;37:190–6.
Späth PJ, Granata G, La Marra F, Kuijpers TW, Quinti I. On the dark side of therapies with immunoglobulin concentrates: the adverse events. Front Immunol. 2015;6:11.
Späth PJ, Schneider C, von Gunten S. Clinical use and therapeutic potential of IVIG/SCIG, plasma-derived IgA or IgM, and other alternative immunoglobulin preparations. Arch Immunol Ther Exp. 2017;65:215–31.
Stein MR, Wasserman RL, Moy J, Lumry W, Grunebaum E, Nemet A, Roifman CM, Sussman G. Efficacy, safety, and tolerability of IVIG-SN in patients with primary immunodeficiency. LymphoSign J. 2015;2:21–9.
Tejada-Strop A, Costafreda MI, Dimitrova Z, Kaplan GG, Teo CG. Evaluation of potencies of immune globulin products against hepatitis A. JAMA Intern Med. 2017;177:430–2.
Trowsdale J, Betz AG. Mother's Little helpers: mechanisms of maternal-fetal tolerance. Nat Immunol. 2006;7:241–6.
Vo AA, Choi J, Kim I, Louie S, Cisneros K, Kahwaji J, Toyoda M, Ge S, Haas M, Puliyanda D, Reinsmoen N, Peng A, Villicana R, Jordan SC. A phase I/II trial of the interleukin-6 receptor specific humanized monoclonal (tocilizumab) + intravenous immunoglobulin in difficult to desensitize patients. Transplantation. 2015;99:2356–63.
von Gunten S, Shoenfeld Y, Blank M, Branch DR, Vassilev T, Käsermann F, Bayry J, Kaveri S, Simon HU. IVIG pluripotency and the concept of Fc-sialylation: challenges to the scientist. Nat Rev Immunol. 2014;14:349.
Washburn N, Schwab I, Ortiz D, Bhatnagar N, Lansing JC, Medeiros A, Tyler S, Mekala D, Cochran E, Sarvaiya H, Garofalo K, Meccariello R, Meador JW III, Rutitzky L, Schultes BC, Ling L, Avery W, Nimmerjahn F, Manning AM, Kaundinya GV, Bosques CJ. Controlled tetra-Fc sialylation of IVIg results in a drug candidate with consistent enhanced anti-inflammatory activity. Proc Natl Acad Sci U S A. 2015;112:E1297–306.
Ye S, Zeng R, Jiang P, Hou M, Liu F, Wang Z, Du X, Yuan J, Chen Y, Cao H, Ma L, Li C. Concentrations of antibodies against b-amyloid 40/42 monomer and oligomers in Chinese intravenous immunoglobulins. J Pharm Biomed Anal. 2017;138:277–82.
Yoon KL, Lee HY, JJ Y, Lee JY, Han MY, Kim KY, Huh J. Multicenter, single-arm, phase IV study of combined aspirin and high-dose "IVIG-SN" therapy for pediatric patients with Kawasaki disease. Korean Circ J. 2017;47:209–14.
Young MK, Bertolini J, Kotharu P, Maher D, Cripps AW. Do Australian immunoglobulin products meet international measles antibody titer standards? Hum Vaccin Immunother. 2017;13:607–12.
Yu Z, Lennon VA. Mechanism of intravenous immune globulin therapy in antibody-mediated autoimmune diseases. N Engl J Med. 1999;340:227–8.
Yu X, Vasiljevic S, Mitchell DA, Crispin M, Scanlan CN. Dissecting the molecular mechanism of IVIg therapy: the interaction between serum IgG and DC-SIGN is independent of antibody glycoform or Fc domain. J Mol Biol. 2013;425:1253–8.
Zhou H, Olsen H, So E, Mérigeon E, Rybin D, Owens J, LaRosa G, Block DS, Strome SE, Zhang X. A fully recombinant human IgG1 Fc multimer (GL-2045) inhibits complement-mediated cytotoxicity and induces iC3b. Blood Adv. 2017;1:504.
Zürcher AW, Spirig R, Baz Morelli A, Käsermann F. IVIG in autoimmune disease – potential next generation biologics. Autoimmun Rev. 2016;15:781–5.

Part III

Immune Thrombocytopenia: The First Immunomodulatory IgG Treatment

Updates in Immune Thrombocytopenia: Terminology, Immunomodulation and Platelet Stimulation, and Clinical Guidelines and Management

14

Cindy Neunert

14.1 Introduction

ITP results from antibody-mediated platelet destruction as well as decreased production. Recently our understanding of the pathophysiology of ITP has expanded, increasing therapeutic options. This section will outline new terminology, describe the pathophysiology, and highlight treatment options and guidelines for management.

14.2 ITP Terminology

In 2008 an International Working Group (IWG) consisting of ITP experts provided consensus regarding the terminology to be used in reference to patients with ITP (Rodeghiero et al. 2009). While the primary purpose of this document was to establish uniform research outcomes, much of the terminology applies to clinical care. The highlights of this are outlined below:

- *Diagnosis*: Now based on a platelet count of $<100 \times 10^9$/L, given that healthy individuals may have platelet counts between 100 and 150 $\times 10^9$/L with low likelihood of progression (Rodeghiero et al. 2009)
- *Disease Duration*:
  - Newly diagnosed—diagnosis until 3 months
  - Persistent—between 3 and 12 months
  - Chronic—greater than 12 months

C. Neunert, MD, MSCS
Columbia University Medical Center, 3959 Broadway, CHN 10-03, New York, NY 10032, USA
e-mail: cn2401@cumc.columbia.edu

P. Imbach (ed.), *Antibody Therapy*, https://doi.org/10.1007/978-3-319-68038-5_14

- *Severe ITP*: Patients who have clinically relevant bleeding defined as the presence of bleeding symptoms either at presentation or subsequent new bleeding symptoms which require therapeutic intervention with a different platelet-enhancing agent or an increased dose of current medication. Patients can present with emergency bleeding events. These include life-threatening bleeding such as intracranial hemorrhage, abdominal bleeding, and/or bleeding in the setting of trauma. Physicians should consider symptoms and history in order to promptly recognize and manage these events.
- *Refractory ITP*: Patients who have failed splenectomy or relapsed following splenectomy *and* have severe ITP or have a risk of bleeding that in the opinion of the physician requires therapy
- *Response Criteria*:
  - Complete response—any platelet count 100 × 10^9/L AND resolution of bleeding
  - Response—any platelet count 30 < 100 × 10^9/L AND at least doubling of the baseline count and resolution of bleeding
  - No response—any platelet count <30 × 10^9/L OR less than doubling of the baseline count and resolution of bleeding
- *Limitations to Definitions:*
  - No established bleeding score to determine exact definition of severe disease based on bleeding symptoms alone (Neunert and Arnold 2015)
  - Definition of refractory requiring that patients have undergone and failed splenectomy may not apply to certain populations such as children or those with a contraindication to splenectomy
  - The need to account for the variable time to response for different treatments
  - The need to account for therapies which require ongoing treatment (such as TPO-RA) compared to those that are given at a single time point (such as IVIg)

14.3 Immunomodulation and Platelet Stimulation

14.3.1 Pathophysiology of ITP

The earliest understanding of ITP came from the experiments of Dr. Harrington. In 1950 Dr. Harrington injected himself with blood from a patient with ITP (Harrington et al. 1951). He had a rapid decline in his platelet count, giving some of the first evidence that ITP was a blood disorder. Later it was understood that this "blood factor" was antibodies interacting with the surface of the platelets and causing them to be removed from circulation by Fc gamma receptors on splenic macrophages (van Leeuwen et al. 1982). More recently, however, we have also come to appreciate the highly complex process that appears to be disrupted in patients with ITP. These take on two distinct pathways: reduced tolerance to self and increased immune activation (Panitsas et al. 2004; McKenzie et al. 2013; Olsson et al. 2003).

- *Reduced Tolerance to Self*
  - Reduced T regulatory cells
  - Reduced B cell inhibitory Fc receptors
- *Increased Immune Activation*
  - Increased Th1/Th2 ratio
  - Increased Th17 cells
  - Direct increased in cytotoxic T cells against platelets

14.3.2 Immunomodulation

These discoveries have increased our therapeutic options with immunomodulatory medications. Table 14.1 outlines therapies available for ITP, their predominant mechanism of action, and available clinical data (Cuker and Neunert 2016).

Table 14.1 Immunomodulatorytreatment for ITP

Agent	Mechanism of action	Dosing	Response data
First-line immunotherapy			
Corticosteroids	Upregulation of anti-inflammatory proteins Downregulation of inflammatory proteins	Prednisone: 1 mg/kg/day for 21 days followed by a taper Dexamethasone: 40 mg/day for 4 days × 2–4 weekly cycles	
Intravenous Immunoglobulin (IVIg)	Fc receptor blockage Synergistic effects of innate and adaptive immunity	0.8–1.0 g/kg × 1	
Anti-D immunoglobulin	Rh red cell sensitization causing Fc receptor competition	50–75 mcg/kg × 1	
Second-line immunotherapy			
Splenectomy	Removal of site of platelet destruction	N/A	60–80%
Rituximab	Anti-CD20 monoclonal antibody	375 mg/m^2/dose weekly × 4 doses	60% overall 40% complete
Third-line immunotherapy			
6-Mercaptopurine	Inhibits purine nucleotide synthesis	50–75 mg/m^2 Qday	83%
Azathioprine	Inhibits purine nucleotide synthesis	1–2 mg/kg Qday (max 150 mg/day)	40–60%
Cyclosporin A	Inhibits calcineurin blocking transcription of cytokine genes	2.5–3 mg/kg BID (titrate to level of 100–200 ng/mL)	30–60%

(continued)

Table 14.1 (continued)

Agent	Mechanism of action	Dosing	Response data
Cyclophosphamide	Cross-links DNA causing inhibition of DNA replication Mechanism in ITP unclear	0.3–1.0 g/m^2/dose every 2–4 weeks × 1–3 doses and then 50–200 orally after response can tapered to 50 mg daily	24–85%
Vincristine	Binds to tubulin and inhibits cell division	Vincristine: 1–2 mg IV weekly × 3–6 doses	10–75%
Vinblastine		Vinblastine: 10 mg IV weekly × 3 weeks	
Dapsone	Blockade myeloperoxidase Mechanism unclear in ITP	75–100 mg Qday	40–75%
Mycophenolate mofetil	Inhibits inosine-5′-monophosphate dehydrogenase and impairs T and B lymphocyte proliferation	250–1000 mg BID	11–80%
Danazol	Unclear in ITP	50–800 mg/d orally divided into 2–4 doses per day	10–70%

14.3.3 Platelet Stimulation

It has more recently been shown that IgG from patients with ITP binds to and suppresses megakaryocyte production (Chang et al. 2003; McMillan et al. 2004). Megakaryocytes in the bone marrow also demonstrate abnormal changes consistent with apoptosis and inflammation (Houwerzijl et al. 2004). These discoveries lead to the development of thrombopoietin receptor agonists (TPO-RAs), which stimulate platelet production.

There are two current TPO-RAs that have been widely studied in adult and pediatric trials, eltrombopag and romiplostim, each outlined below.

- *Eltrombopag*
  - 25–75 mg PO Qday (titrated based on platelet count)
  - Results of mean platelet counts during clinical trial (Saleh et al. 2013)

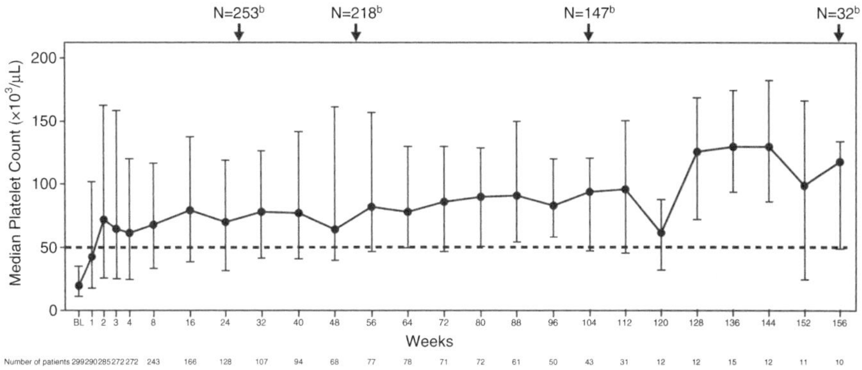

- *Romiplostim*
  - 1–10 mcg/kg SC weekly (titrated based on platelet count)
  - Results of mean platelet counts during clinical trial (Kuter et al. 2013)

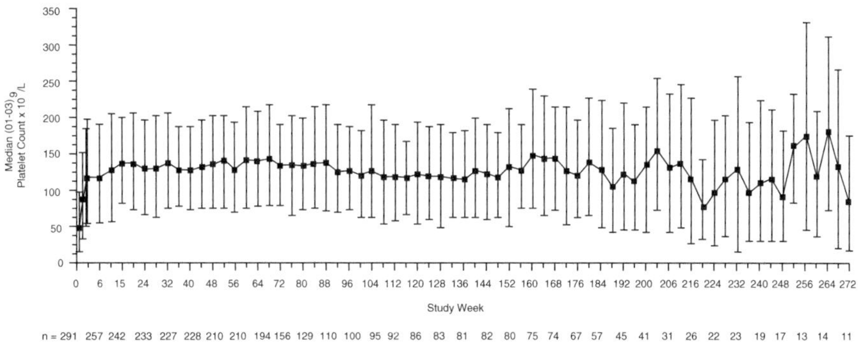

- *Major Adverse Events of the TPO-RAs*
  - Thrombocytosis, bone marrow reticulin, and thrombosis can occur with both medications.
  - Hepatic toxicity can occur with eltrombopag.
  - Rebound thrombocytopenia and bleeding can be seen with drug discontinuation.

14.4 Clinical Guidelines and Update on Management

Current clinical practice guidelines exist for the management of ITP (Neunert et al. 2011; Provan et al. 2010). Most guidelines reference treatment for patients with newly diagnosed ITP who require first-line therapy and then additional guidance for those who develop more long-standing ITP and/or become refractory to first-line therapy. General management for adult and pediatric patients is outlined below:

- *Newly Diagnosed ITP in Adults*
  - Treatment should be considered for patients with a platelet count $<30 \times 10^9/L$, and treatment is rarely needed for patients with a platelet count $>50 \times 10^9/L$.
  - Longer courses ($\geq$21 days with a taper) of corticosteroids are the preferred first-line treatment.

    Physicians should be aware of the side effects associated with long-term corticosteroid use including but not limited to mood disorders, diabetes, hypertension, weight gain, osteoporosis, and cataracts.
  - IVIg can be given along with corticosteroids if a more rapid increase in the platelet count is required.
  - IVIg and anti-D immunoglobulin can be used if there is a contraindication to corticosteroids.
- *Newly Diagnosed ITP in Pediatrics*
  - The majority of children with no or mild bleeding only do not require treatment regardless of the platelet count.
  - If treatment is necessary, patients can be treated with IVIg, anti-D immunoglobulin, or corticosteroids.
  - IVIg or anti-D immunoglobulin is preferred if a more rapid increase in the platelet count is required.
- *Persistent, Chronic, and Refractory ITP in Adults*
  - Further treatment is not necessary for asymptomatic patients with a platelet count $>30 \times 10^9/L$ unless there is concern about additional risk factors for bleeding or impaired health-related quality of life.
  - Splenectomy should be considered for all adults who have failed corticosteroids and/or additional treatment regimens.
  - TPO-RAs can be considered in patients who fail splenectomy, have a contraindication to splenectomy, and/or have failed at least one additional therapy.
  - Rituximab can be considered for patients who have failed at least one additional therapy.
- *Persistent, Chronic, and Refractory ITP in Pediatrics*
  - Rituximab may be considered as an alternative to splenectomy in children and for those who fail splenectomy and/or who have significant ongoing bleeding despite treatment with at least one additional therapy.
  - High-dose dexamethasone may be considered as an alternative to splenectomy in children and adolescents and for those who fail splenectomy and/or who have significant ongoing bleeding despite treatment with at least one additional therapy.

  - Splenectomy can be considered for children and adolescents with chronic or persistent ITP who have significant or persistent bleeding, lack of responsiveness to other therapies, and/or impaired quality of life.
  - Splenectomy and interventions with potentially serious complications should be delayed for at least 12 months when feasible.
- *Management Considerations*
  - Anti-D immunoglobulin should not be given to patients with significant anemia and requires a patient to be Rh+ in order to be effective. An average 2.0 g decline in hemoglobin is seen following use. There have also been cases of fatal intravascular hemolysis and disseminated intravascular coagulopathy following use (Gaines 2005).
  - There is no evidence to support the specific platelet count threshold for treatment in adult patients with ITP.
  - The ideal type, duration, and method of corticosteroid administration for newly diagnosed adults with ITP are currently controversial with no difference in long-term outcomes between prednisone and dexamethasone (Mithoowani et al. 2016).
  - Additional immunosuppressive agents (outlined in the section above) can be considered for patients with refractory disease; however, the data on these agents is minimal.
  - More recent evidence, not available at the time of guideline development, supports the use of TPO-RAs in children with chronic disease (Grainger et al. 2015; Tarantino et al. 2016; Bussel et al. 2011, 2015).
  - The decision to treat and therapy selected should always involve consideration of the patient preferences, bleeding symptoms, quality of life, and comorbidities.

References

Bussel JB, Buchanan GR, Nugent DJ, et al. A randomized, double-blind study of romiplostim to determine its safety and efficacy in children with immune thrombocytopenia. Blood. 2011;118(1):28–36.

Bussel JB, de Miguel PG, Despotovic JM, et al. Eltrombopag for the treatment of children with persistent and chronic immune thrombocytopenia (PETIT): a randomised, multicentre, placebo-controlled study. Lancet Haematol. 2015;2(8):e315–25.

Chang M, Nakagawa PA, Williams SA, et al. Immune thrombocytopenic purpura (ITP) plasma and purified ITP monoclonal autoantibodies inhibit megakaryocytopoiesis in vitro. Blood. 2003;102(3):887–95.

Cuker A, Neunert CE. How I treat refractory immune thrombocytopenia. Blood. 2016;128(12):1547–54.

Gaines AR. Disseminated intravascular coagulation associated with acute hemoglobinemia or hemoglobinuria following Rh(0)(D) immune globulin intravenous administration for immune thrombocytopenic purpura. Blood. 2005;106(5):1532–7.

Grainger JD, Locatelli F, Chotsampancharoen T, et al. Eltrombopag for children with chronic immune thrombocytopenia (PETIT2): a randomised, multicentre, placebo-controlled trial. Lancet. 2015;386(10004):1649–58.

Harrington WJ, Minnich V, Hollingsworth JW, Moore CV. Demonstration of a thrombocytopenic factor in the blood of patients with thrombocytopenic purpura. J Lab Clin Med. 1951;38(1):1–10.

Houwerzijl EJ, Blom NR, van der Want JJ, et al. Ultrastructural study shows morphologic features of apoptosis and para-apoptosis in megakaryocytes from patients with idiopathic thrombocytopenic purpura. Blood. 2004;103(2):500–6.

Kuter DJ, Bussel JB, Newland A, et al. Long-term treatment with romiplostim in patients with chronic immune thrombocytopenia: safety and efficacy. Br J Haematol. 2013;161(3):411–23.

McKenzie CG, Guo L, Freedman J, Semple JW. Cellular immune dysfunction in immune thrombocytopenia (ITP). Br J Haematol. 2013;163(1):10–23.

McMillan R, Wang L, Tomer A, Nichol J, Pistillo J. Suppression of in vitro megakaryocyte production by antiplatelet autoantibodies from adult patients with chronic ITP. Blood. 2004;103(4):1364–9.

Mithoowani S, Gregory-Miller K, Goy J, et al. High-dose dexamethasone compared with prednisone for previously untreated primary immune thrombocytopenia: a systematic review and meta-analysis. Lancet Haematol. 2016;3(10):e489–e96.

Neunert C, Arnold DM. Severe bleeding events in adults and children with primary immune thrombocytopenia: a systematic review: reply. J Thromb Haemost: JTH. 2015;13(8):1522–3.

Neunert C, Lim W, Crowther M, et al. The American Society of Hematology 2011 evidence-based practice guideline for immune thrombocytopenia. Blood. 2011;117(16):4190–207.

Olsson B, Andersson PO, Jernas M, et al. T-cell-mediated cytotoxicity toward platelets in chronic idiopathic thrombocytopenic purpura. Nat Med. 2003;9(9):1123–4.

Panitsas FP, Theodoropoulou M, Kouraklis A, et al. Adult chronic idiopathic thrombocytopenic purpura (ITP) is the manifestation of a type-1 polarized immune response. Blood. 2004;103(7):2645–7.

Provan D, Stasi R, Newland AC, et al. International consensus report on the investigation and management of primary immune thrombocytopenia. Blood. 2010;115(2):168–86.

Rodeghiero F, Stasi R, Gernsheimer T, et al. Standardization of terminology, definitions and outcome criteria in immune thrombocytopenic purpura of adults and children: report from an international working group. Blood. 2009;113(11):2386–93.

Saleh MN, Bussel JB, Cheng G, et al. Safety and efficacy of eltrombopag for treatment of chronic immune thrombocytopenia: results of the long-term, open-label EXTEND study. Blood. 2013;121(3):537–45.

Tarantino MD, Bussel JB, Blanchette VS, et al. Romiplostim in children with immune thrombocytopenia: a phase 3, randomised, double-blind, placebo-controlled study. Lancet. 2016;388(10039):45–54.

van Leeuwen EF, van der Ven JT, Engelfriet CP, von dem Borne AE. Specificity of autoantibodies in autoimmune thrombocytopenia. Blood. 1982;59(1):23–6.

15 Health-Related Quality of Life in Patients with Immune Thrombocytopenia

Robert J. Klaassen and Nancy L. Young

15.1 Introduction

I walked into the examination room to see my second patient of the day—five other families were quietly sitting in the waiting room awaiting their turn. She was a 15-year-old girl with immune thrombocytopenia (ITP) diagnosed just over 1 year ago. Her platelet count ranged from 20 to 30 × 10^9/l, but she had not required any emergency department visits or had any significant bleeding events over the past 6 months. All in all she seemed stable, so my plan was to continue with the current treatment approach of "watch and wait".

I was about to wrap up the visit when I noticed that she was looking dejected and asked her how she was doing. She explained that she had been very active in rugby before the diagnosis, and now she had no energy and spent most of her time on the couch. I had, on multiple occasions, previously reassured her that she could fully engage in all non-contact sports, but she still felt restricted and run down. Because of this interaction, I changed my plan and discuss in detail the many second-line treatment options available for chronic ITP.

This clinical example illustrates that patients' perceptions contribute an essential component of the history which in turn has a central bearing on the treatment plan. It also shows that elucidating this information in the clinic setting often occurs by chance. In this chapter, we will discuss options for a more intentional and systematic approach, using quality of life assessment tools.

R.J. Klaassen, MD (✉)
Division of Hematology/Oncology, Department of Pediatrics, University of Ottawa, Children's Hospital of Eastern Ontario, 401 Smyth, Ottawa, ON, Canada, K1H 8L1
e-mail: rklaassen@cheo.on.ca

N.L. Young, PhD
School of Rural and Northern Health, Laurentian University, Sudbury, ON, Canada

P. Imbach (ed.), *Antibody Therapy*, https://doi.org/10.1007/978-3-319-68038-5_15

15.2 What Is Quality of Life and Health-Related Quality of Life (HRQoL)?

Quality of life (QOL) has been defined by the World Health Organisation as "an individuals' perception of their position in life in the context of the culture and value systems in which they live and in relation to their goals, expectations, standards and concerns" (WHOQOL Group 1993). They organised QOL into six domains: physical, psychological, level of independence, social relationships, environmental and spiritual/religion/personal beliefs. A more concise way of looking at QOL is the gap between our expectations and our experience (Calman 1984). Further narrowing the concept is the term health-related quality of life (HRQOL), which excludes some of the domains that are generally not influenced by health services, such as spiritual beliefs and finances (which may be relevant depending on the local health care system). In many instances, the terms are used interchangeably, but we will focus this chapter on HRQOL.

15.3 Why Do We Need to Measure HRQOL?

Clinicians intuitively know that HRQOL is important in medical decision-making; this is an essential component of the "art of medicine". At the start of this chapter, I provided an example of a patient who "on paper" did not fulfil the criteria for going on to second-line (potentially curative) therapy for ITP. It was only when I started delving into her perception about her disease that I became aware of the impact of her illness on her HRQOL. I have other patients with the exact same clinical phenotype, who were perfectly content and did not recommend a change in course of their treatment.

The problem with this ad hoc approach to evaluating HRQOL is that important deficits in HRQOL can easily be missed, especially when dealing with poorly communicative teenagers. A less perceptive clinician, or any one of us on a busy day, may have walked out of the room without any further discussion. The alternative, especially in the research setting, is to systematically collect data on HRQOL, typically using patient-reported outcome measures (PROs). This allows for a more standardised approach to looking at HRQOL and provides numeric comparisons over time and between patients.

15.4 Types of Measures

Two general types of measures can be used to measure HRQOL: (1) generic and (2) disease specific, each having their own advantages and disadvantages (Eiser and Jenney 2007). Generic HRQOL tools can be used across disease groups and can even be administered to "healthy" populations (Varni et al. 2003). This allows for comparisons between different patient populations using the healthy population as a reference. Because these tools can be used in many different settings, they are well known to clinicians and are therefore easier to understand, with the resulting scores being easy to interpret. Examples include the medical outcomes study short-form survey (SF 36) https://campaign.optum.com/optum-outcomes.html (Ware 2004), which is commonly used in adults and the Pediatric Quality of Life Inventory (PedsQL) http://www.pedsql.org/ in children (Varni et al. 2003).

Disease-specific HRQOL tools have the advantage of including specific questions related to the disease states that are not covered by generic tools, such as ITP-related questions as in "I worried about my platelet count…" which is included in the Kids ITP Tools (KIT) http://www.flintbox.com/public/project/3044 (Barnard et al. 2003) but is obviously not present in the PedsQL. The main advantage of this particular method of questioning is that a very detailed picture of the patients HRQOL can be obtained, which is more sensitive to change over time (Klaassen et al. 2007). The disadvantage of these tools is that comparisons between disease groups are not possible, and since they are less well known, interpretation of the scores may be less intuitive.

In general, both types of measures have unique value and should be included, when possible. A generic tool will provide the broad perspective that allows comparison to other groups and the healthy population, whereas the disease-specific tool allows a more detailed picture of the patient's perception of their disease. The respondent burden in a particular study or clinical setting must also be considered and may require a choice be made to use one or the other approach.

The two available disease-specific measures routinely used in ITP include the KIT for children (Klaassen et al. 2013) and the ITP-PAQ for adults (Mathias et al. 2007). Since these tools are crucial to the full understanding of HRQOL in this disease, I will describe them in more detail.

15.4.1 The Kids' ITP Tools (KIT)

The KIT was initially developed in North America specifically for children with ITP and their parents (Barnard et al. 2003) and later refined (Klaassen et al. 2007; Klaassen and Young 2010) and cross-culturally validated for other regions of the world (Klaassen et al. 2013). It has three versions: one for the child (child self-report), where the child is asked to focus on what he/she thought about and did; another for the parent to complete on behalf of the child (parent proxy report), where the parent is asked to focus on their child's HRQOL; and finally one for the parent complete about themselves (parent impact report) to capture the HRQOL experience of the parent. All of the versions consist of 26 questions with the total score ranging from 0 (worst) to 100 (best) HRQOL. There are no subscales. Data supporting the validity, reliability and responsiveness of KIT has been published (Klaassen et al. 2007). The KIT has been cross-culturally translated into 24 languages in 21 countries.

15.4.2 ITP-Patient-Administered Questionnaire (ITP-PAQ)

The ITP-PAQ is a questionnaire developed for use in adults with chronic ITP to measure HRQOL, consisting of 44 items grouped into 10 scales: Physical Symptoms

(6 items), Bother-Physical Health (3), Fatigue/Sleep (4), Activity (2), Fear (5), Psychological Health (5), Work (4), Social Activity (4), Women's Reproductive Health (6) and Overall Quality of Life (5) (Mathias et al. 2007, 2009). No summary score is calculated. Each scale is scored from 0 to 100, with higher scores representing better HRQOL. It was found to be valid with moderate correlation to the SF-36 and was able to differentiate ITP patients on treatment from those off treatment (McMillan et al. 2008). The ITP-PAQ can be used to describe the burden of illness as well as an outcome measure to assess the efficacy or effectiveness of ITP treatments.

15.5 Study Results

15.5.1 Paediatric

HRQOL has been assessed in a number of paediatric studies with intriguing results—a review of 90 children with ITP found no correlation between the KIT, the platelet count and bleeding scores, clearly indicating that quality of life is perceived differently by the patient and family from the platelet count and bleeding (Neunert et al. 2009). A further analysis of 217 children failed to find a difference in self-reported KIT scores between children who received treatment compared to those who were simply observed (Grainger et al. 2013). This same study found that parents proxy-reported scores were significantly lower for children with newly diagnosed ITP who were treated vs. not treated (mean KIT scores of 48 and 64, respectively, $p = 0.03$) (Grainger et al. 2013). This raises the possibility that treatment may be detrimental to patients' HRQOL, or conversely when parents perceive that their child's HRQOL is low, they elect to treat their child.

Of interest, multiple randomised trials of the thrombopoietin receptor agonist (TPO RA) drugs have failed to show a significant improvement in HRQOL, based on self-report or proxy report, when compared to placebo in a sample that demonstrated significant improvements in the platelet count during the same period (Bussel et al. 2015; Tarantino et al. 2016). The main reason for this finding was that there was almost as much improvement in the placebo arm as the treatment arm, pointing to the impact of participating in a clinical trial that lessens over the course of the study. One pilot study of Romiplostim did show a significant improvement in parental burden in the treatment arm compared to placebo (change of +24 vs. −6, $p = 0.008$) (Klaassen et al. 2011).

The one consistent finding across all studies is that patients with newly diagnosed ITP have lower HRQOL scores than patients with chronic ITP (Grainger et al. 2013; Mokhtar et al. 2014) and that scores steadily increase with time after initial diagnosis as many patients go into remission, and the patients and their family adjust to the disease. Those patients who continue to have disease on follow up understandably report lower HRQOL scores compared to those patients who go into remission (Fig. 15.1) (Flores et al. 2017; Heitink-Polle et al. 2014).

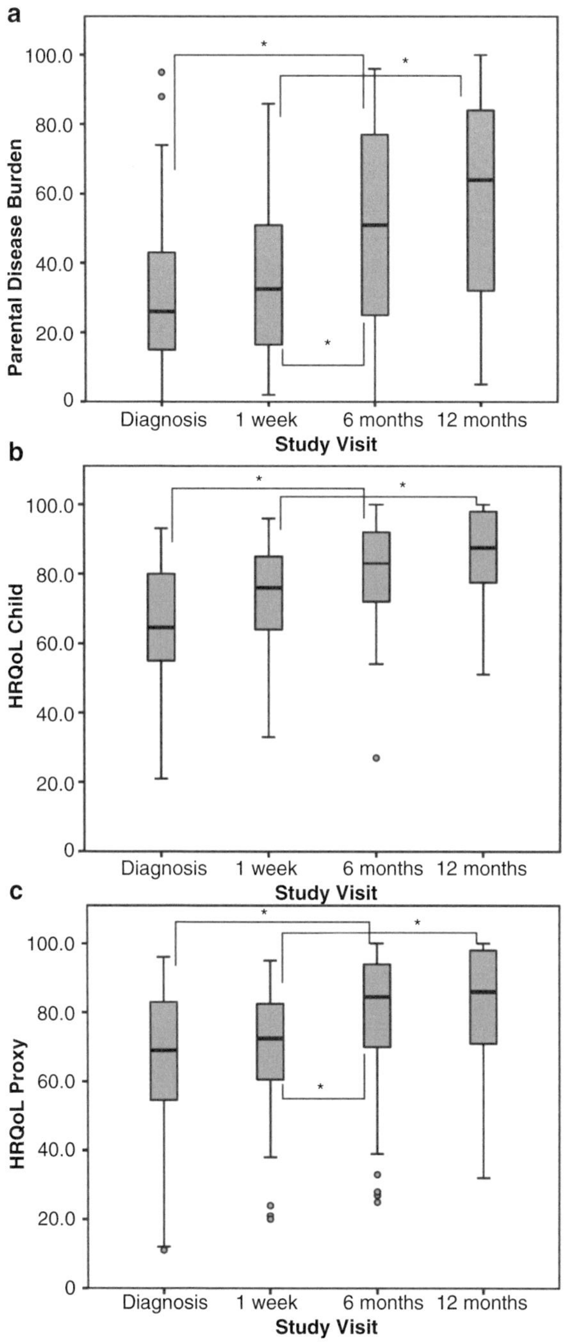

Fig. 15.1 Change in KIT scores for parent (**a**), child (**b**) and proxy (**c**) questionnaires from diagnosis through 12 months (parent, $p = 0.009$; child, $p < 0.0005$; proxy $p = 0.001$). Asterisks denote statistically significant improvement in score from six pairwise comparisons ($p < 0.008$; 0.05/6). Adapted from Flores et al. (2017)

15.5.2 Adult

Adults with ITP have consistently been shown to have lower HRQOL when compared to the healthy population in studies measuring the SF36 in China, the USA, the UK and Italy (Fig. 15.2) (Efficace et al. 2016; McMillan et al. 2008; Snyder et al. 2008; Zhou et al. 2007) and the EQ-5D in the USA, the UK, France, the Netherlands and Spain (Sanz et al. 2011; Snyder et al. 2008). In particular, between five and seven of the eight domains of the SF36 were significantly lower, with only bodily pain not affected (which makes sense clinically). General health, role physical (the ability to get things done), vitality (energy) and social functioning were the domains consistently discrepant across studies from the control population, pointing to the impact of ITP on overall functioning (McMillan et al. 2008; Snyder et al. 2008; Zhou et al. 2007). When compared to other patient populations, ITP patients had worse SF36 scores than patients with hypertension, arthritis and cancer, similar scores to diabetes and higher scores than patients with congestive heart failure or missing a limb.

As opposed to the situation in paediatrics, adult therapeutic studies have clearly shown that second-line therapies result in significant improvements in HRQOL when compared to placebo (George et al. 2009; Kuter et al. 2010; Sanz et al. 2011). An analysis of two phase 3 randomised placebo-controlled European studies of romiplostim that incorporated the EQ-5D, a health utility-based measure which can be used in economic evaluation, showed a significant

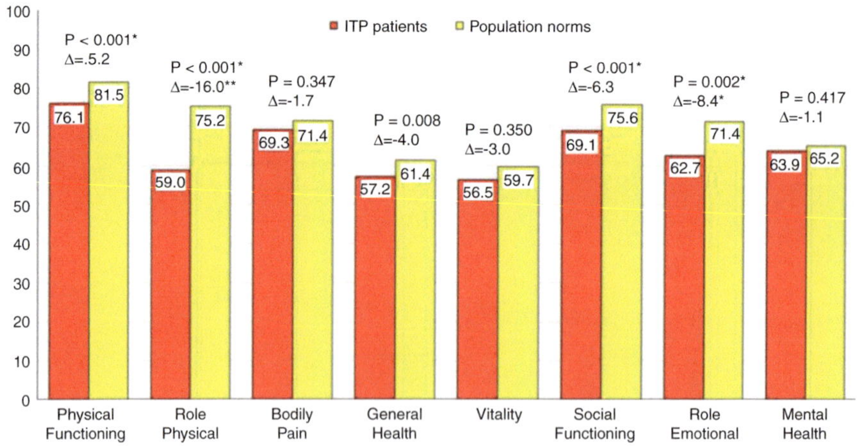

Fig. 15.2 Adjusted comparisons of SF-36 scales between pITP patients (overall population) and general population norms. Legend Δ mean differences were adjusted for age, sex, education, geographic area and marital status: *The score difference exceeds the minimally important difference (i.e. 8 points); **The score difference exceeds twice the minimally important difference; # statistically significant after Bonferroni adjustment (adjusted alpha = 0.05/8 = 0.00625). Adapted from Efficace et al. (2016)

improvement over 6 months in the index score (0.05 vs. −0.03, $p = 0.015$) but did not achieve significance with the visual analogue score (6.42 vs. 0.48, $p = 0.066$). Using the disease-specific measure ITP-PAQ, an analysis of two American randomised placebo-controlled trials, again of romiplostim, showed significant improvement in seven of ten scales (Symptoms, Bother, Activity, Fear, Psychological Health, Social Activity and Women's Reproductive Health) when compared to placebo (George et al. 2009). This was confirmed in an open-label comparison of romiplostim to standard of care, which showed statistically significant improvement in six scales (Symptoms, Bother, Activity, Fear, Psychological Health, Social Activity) and Overall QOL for patients given romiplostim. Eltrombopag has much less adult QOL data available, with the landmark NEJM published in 2007 showing no change in SF36 scores. This is likely due to the fact that they did not incorporate a disease-specific tool into their trials (Bussel et al. 2007).

15.6 Fatigue

A specific mention needs to be made of the issue of fatigue in ITP, since this is an important symptom that has been reported in numerous studies in spite of the lack of a clear pathogenic link to ITP (Efficace et al. 2016; Newton et al. 2011). A large combined US and UK study published in 2011 of 653 adults using the Fatigue Impact Scale (FIS) found significantly increased rates of fatigue when compared to the healthy population (UK 39%, USA 22% with FIS score ≥40 vs. 2.5%, respectively; $p < 0.0001$) (Newton et al. 2011). This was confirmed in an Italian ITP study which used the Multidimensional Fatigue Inventory (MFI) and again found significantly worse general, mental and physical fatigue as well as reduced activity (p for all dimensions <0.001) (Efficace et al. 2016). Children experience fatigue as well, with a study that administered the Fatigue Scale-Child, Adolescent and Parent (FS-C, A, P) to 102 children with ITP showing that children as young as seven experienced significantly more fatigue than the healthy population (Grace et al. 2016).

ITP patients have been complaining about this symptom long before it was documented in the literature but was often dismissed by clinicians as unrelated to their disease. A review article on the topic by Hill et al. proposed a pathogenic model (Fig. 15.3) linking ITP with peripheral inflammation, bruising and activity restrictions, anaemia and iron deficiency, tied in with social factors and cognitive/behavioural issues all contributing to fatigue (Hill and Newland 2015). Going forward, assessment of fatigue needs to be included in the arsenal of patient-reported outcomes for this illness.

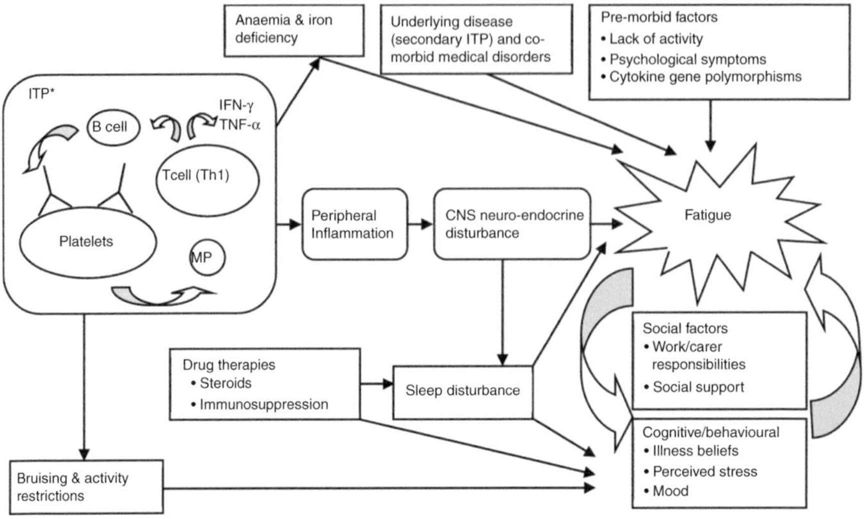

Fig. 15.3 Model of the pathogenesis of ITP-associated fatigue. ITP, immune thrombocytopenia; B cell, autoantibody-producing B lymphocytes; T cell Th1, T lymphocytes with a T helper 1 polarisation; TNF-α, tumour necrosis factor alpha; IFN-γ, interferon gamma; MP, microparticles; CNS, central nervous system. *T cells can attack platelets directly, secrete pro-inflammatory cytokines and drive formation of autoreactive B cells. This results in antibody- and complement-mediated platelet destruction. Platelet microparticles are prothrombotic and able to activate the pro-inflammatory complement pathway. Adapted from Hill and Newland (2015)

15.7 Implementing HRQOL Tools in Clinical Practice

All of this leads to the recommendation proposed at the start of the chapter: How do we implement a more intentional and systematic approach, using HRQOL assessment tools? Unfortunately, most of the available HRQOL tools were developed for the research setting and need to be further assessed in the clinic to determine if they can be used for clinical decision-making. A number of investigators have been focusing on this task, with the International Society of Quality of Life releasing a user's guide in 2015 for the implementation of patient-reported outcomes in clinical practice http://www.isoqol.org/research-publications/isoqol-publications. Older literature has not clearly shown that using these tools in the clinic has influenced the management of patients' problems (Greenhalgh 2009), but fortunately that early work has clarified different strategies to make this successful in the future. With the widespread implementation of electronic health records by many clinicians, the reality of integrating HRQOL tools into routine clinical practice has become tantalisingly close.

Returning to my patient described in the introduction, after our discussion of possible second-line ITP therapies, she elected to receive a course of rituximab. Fortunately she experienced no significant side effects, and a few months later, she was in remission with a respectable platelet count. Clinically she felt much better and was smiling with renewed energy. A fortunate outcome that should hopefully become more commonplace with the systematic integration of HRQOL tools into the clinic.

References

Barnard D, Woloski M, Feeny D, McCusker P, Wu J, David M, Bussel J, Lusher J, Wakefield C, Henriques S, Blanchette V. Development of disease-specific health-related quality-of-life instruments for children with immune thrombocytopenic purpura and their parents. J Pediatr Hematol Oncol. 2003;25(1):56–62.

Bussel JB, Cheng G, Saleh MN, Psaila B, Kovaleva L, Meddeb B, Kloczko J, Hassani H, Mayer B, Stone NL, Arning M, Provan D, Jenkins JM. Eltrombopag for the treatment of chronic idiopathic thrombocytopenic purpura. N Engl J Med. 2007;357(22):2237–47.

Bussel JB, de Miguel PG, Despotovic JM, Grainger JD, Sevilla J, Blanchette VS, Krishnamurti L, Connor P, David M, Boayue KB, Matthews DC, Lambert MP, Marcello LM, Iyengar M, Chan GW, Chagin KD, Theodore D, Bailey CK, Bakshi KK. Eltrombopag for the treatment of children with persistent and chronic immune thrombocytopenia (PETIT): a randomised, multicentre, placebo-controlled study. Lancet Haematol. 2015;2(8):e315–25.

Calman KC. Quality of life in cancer patients—an hypothesis. J Med Ethics. 1984;10(3):124–7.

Efficace F, Mandelli F, Fazi P, Santoro C, Gaidano G, Cottone F, Borchiellini A, Carpenedo M, Simula MP, Di Giacomo V, Bergamaschi M, Vincelli ID, Rodeghiero F, Ruggeri M, Scaramucci L, Rambaldi A, Cascavilla N, Forghieri F, Petrungaro A, Ditonno P, Caocci G, Cirrincione S, Mazzucconi MG. Health-related quality of life and burden of fatigue in patients with primary immune thrombocytopenia by phase of disease. Am J Hematol. 2016;91(10):995–1001.

Eiser C, Jenney M. Measuring quality of life. Arch Dis Child. 2007;92(4):348–50.

Flores A, Klaassen RJ, Buchanan GR, Neunert CE. Patterns and influences in health-related quality of life in children with immune thrombocytopenia: a study from the Dallas ITP Cohort. Pediatr Blood Cancer. 2017;64(8):e26405.

George JN, Mathias SD, Go RS, Guo M, Henry DH, Lyons R, Redner RL, Rice L, Schipperus MR. Improved quality of life for romiplostim-treated patients with chronic immune thrombocytopenic purpura: results from two randomized, placebo-controlled trials. Br J Haematol. 2009;144(3):409–15.

Grace R, Despotovic J, Bennett C, Klaassen RJ. Fatigue in pediatric immune thrombocytopenia (ITP): baseline prevalence in patients starting second line therapies in the first ITP consortium of North America research study (ICON1). Pediatr Blood Cancer. 2016;63(S1):S20. Ref Type: Abstract.

Grainger JD, Young NL, Blanchette VS, Klaassen RJ. Quality of life in immune thrombocytopenia following treatment. Arch Dis Child. 2013;98(11):895–7.

Greenhalgh J. The applications of PROs in clinical practice: what are they, do they work, and why? Qual Life Res. 2009;18(1):115–23.

Heitink-Polle KM, Haverman L, Annink KV, Schep SJ, de HM, Bruin MC. Health-related quality of life in children with newly diagnosed immune thrombocytopenia. Haematologica. 2014;99(9):1525–31.

Hill QA, Newland AC. Fatigue in immune thrombocytopenia. Br J Haematol. 2015;170(2):141–9.

Klaassen RJ, Blanchette V, Burke TA, Wakefield C, Grainger JD, Gaedicke G, Riedlinger A, Dufort G, Citrin E, Reguerre Y, Pellier I, Curtis C, Young NL. Quality of life in childhood immune thrombocytopenia: international validation of the kids' ITP tools. Pediatr Blood Cancer. 2013;60(1):95–100.

Klaassen RJ, Blanchette VS, Barnard D, Wakefield CD, Curtis C, Bradley CS, Neufeld EJ, Buchanan GR, Silva MP, Chan AK, Young NL. Validity, reliability, and responsiveness of a

new measure of health-related quality of life in children with immune thrombocytopenic purpura: the kids' ITP tools. J Pediatr. 2007;150(5):510–5.
Klaassen RJ, Mathias SD, Buchanan G, Bussel J, Deuson R, Young NL, Collier A, Bomgaars L, Blanchette V. Pilot study of the effect of romiplostim on child health-related quality of life (HRQoL) and parental burden in immune thrombocytopenia (ITP). Pediatr Blood Cancer. 2011;58(3):395–8.
Klaassen RJ, Young NL. Health-related quality of life outcomes for patients with immune thrombocytopenic purpura. Ann Hematol. 2010;89(1):51–4.
Kuter DJ, Rummel M, Boccia R, Macik BG, Pabinger I, Selleslag D, Rodeghiero F, Chong BH, Wang X, Berger DP. Romiplostim or standard of care in patients with immune thrombocytopenia. N Engl J Med. 2010;363(20):1889–99.
Mathias SD, Bussel JB, George JN, McMillan R, Okano GJ, Nichol JL. A disease-specific measure of health-related quality of life for use in adults with immune thrombocytopenic purpura: its development and validation. Health Qual Life Outcomes. 2007;5:11.
Mathias SD, Gao SK, Rutstein M, Snyder CF, Wu AW, Cella D. Evaluating clinically meaningful change on the ITP-PAQ: preliminary estimates of minimal important differences. Curr Med Res Opin. 2009;25(2):375–83.
McMillan R, Bussel JB, George JN, Lalla D, Nichol JL. Self-reported health-related quality of life in adults with chronic immune thrombocytopenic purpura. Am J Hematol. 2008;83(2):150–4.
Mokhtar GM, Farid SM, Shaker NM, Farrag KE. Health-related quality of life of Egyptian children with immune thrombocytopenia and their parents. J Pediatr Hematol Oncol. 2014;36(3):194–9.
Neunert CE, Buchanan GR, Blanchette V, Barnard D, Young NL, Curtis C, Klaassen RJ. Relationships among bleeding severity, health-related quality of life, and platelet count in children with immune thrombocytopenic purpura. Pediatr Blood Cancer. 2009;53(4):652–4.
Newton JL, Reese JA, Watson SI, Vesely SK, Bolton-Maggs PH, George JN, Terrell DR. Fatigue in adult patients with primary immune thrombocytopenia. Eur J Haematol. 2011;86(5):420–9.
Sanz MA, Aledort L, Mathias SD, Wang X, Isitt JJ. Analysis of EQ-5D scores from two phase 3 clinical trials of romiplostim in the treatment of immune thrombocytopenia (ITP). Value Health. 2011;14(1):90–6.
Snyder CF, Mathias SD, Cella D, Isitt JJ, Wu AW, Young J. Health-related quality of life of immune thrombocytopenic purpura patients: results from a web-based survey. Curr Med ResOpin. 2008;24(10):2767–76.
Tarantino MD, Bussel JB, Blanchette VS, Despotovic J, Bennett C, Raj A, Williams B, Beam D, Morales J, Rose MJ, Carpenter N, Nie K, Eisen M. Romiplostim in children with immune thrombocytopenia: a phase 3, randomised, double-blind, placebo-controlled study. Lancet. 2016;388(10039):45–54.
Varni JW, Burwinkle TM, Seid M, Skarr D. The PedsQL 4.0 as a pediatric population health measure: feasibility, reliability, and validity. Ambul Pediatr. 2003;3(6):329–41.
Ware JE. SF-36 health survey update. In: Maruish ME, editor. The use of psychological testing for treatment planning and outcome assessment, vol. 3. 3rd ed. Mahwah: Lawrence Erlbaum Associates; 2004. p. 693–718.
WHOQOL Group. Study protocol for the World Health Organization project to develop a Quality of Life assessment instrument (WHOQOL). Qual Life Res. 1993;2(2):153–9.
Zhou Z, Yang L, Chen Z, Chen X, Guo Y, Wang X, Dong X, Wang T, Zhang L, Qiu Z, Yang R. Health-related quality of life measured by the Short Form 36 in immune thrombocytopenic purpura: a cross-sectional survey in China. Eur J Haematol. 2007;78(6):518–23.

ITP in Childhood: Predictors of Disease Duration

16

Carolyn M. Bennett

16.1 Introduction

Immune thrombocytopenia (ITP) is an acquired autoimmune disorder characterized by increased platelet destruction and decreased platelet production resulting in isolated thrombocytopenia (Harrington et al. 1951; McMillan et al. 2004; Zufferey et al. 2017). ITP may present at any age, including infancy, but the natural history in children usually differs from adults (Imbach et al. 2006; Kuhne et al. 2011). Most adults with ITP have an insidious onset of disease without a preceding viral illness and develop chronic disease that persists beyond 6–12 months, while the majority of children will have self-limited thrombocytopenia that resolves completely within weeks to months of presentation (Provan et al. 2010; Kuhne et al. 2003; Grimaldi-Bensouda et al. 2016; Stasi et al. 1995). At the time of diagnosis, the patients who will experience spontaneous remission cannot be distinguished reliably from those who will have chronic disease.

ITP is diagnosed clinically based on the presence of bleeding signs or symptoms and isolated thrombocytopenia in the absence of other physical or laboratory abnormalities or other causes of thrombocytopenia (Kuhne et al. 2003). The bleeding manifestations are variable but most often include mucocutaneous bleeding such as bruising, petechiae, oral purpura, epistaxis, and menorrhagia (in females) (Kuhne et al. 2011; Neunert et al. 2008). While the skin and mucous membrane findings can be impressive, many children have surprisingly little bleeding despite profound thrombocytopenia (Kuhne et al. 2003). While severe bleeding such as intracranial hemorrhage is rare, it can occur unpredictably without evidence of trauma or other

C.M. Bennett, MD, MSc
Emory University School of Medicine, Atlanta, GA, USA

Aflac Cancer and Blood Disorder Center, Children's Healthcare of Atlanta, 5461 Meridian Mark Road, Suite 400, Atlanta, GA 30342, USA
e-mail: carolyn.bennett@choa.org

P. Imbach (ed.), *Antibody Therapy*, https://doi.org/10.1007/978-3-319-68038-5_16

inciting event and may cause serious morbidity and mortality (Kuhne et al. 2003; Psaila et al. 2009).

The majority of children with ITP will have spontaneous disease resolution within weeks to months of presentation (Imbach et al. 2006). About 20–30% of children will have persistent thrombocytopenia beyond 6 months of diagnosis. However, in contrast to adults with ITP, a significant proportion of children with persistent ITP at 6 months will have disease resolution by 1 year (Imbach et al. 2006). The long-term remission rate is high, and in most children with chronic ITP, the outcome is favorable (Rosthoj et al. 2012; Donato et al. 2009; Watts 2004; Akbayram et al. 2011). Only about 5–10% of children who present with ITP will have clinically significant chronic ITP that requires treatment (Bennett and Tarantino 2009; Aronis et al. 1994).

Since serious bleeding is unusual and spontaneous resolution common, children with newly diagnosed ITP are often observed closely without treatment (Neunert et al. 2011; Provan et al. 2010). Pharmacologic therapy can be reserved for patients with significant or troublesome bleeding. Patients with chronic ITP who have mild to moderate thrombocytopenia and minimal bleeding may be managed with close observation alone or with standard first-line ITP therapies: corticosteroids, intravenous immune globulin, or anti-D immune globulin (in patients who are Rh positive and have intact spleens) (Neunert et al. 2011; Provan et al. 2010; Blanchette et al. 1994; Andrew et al. 1992; Papagianni et al. 2011; Blanchette et al. 1993; Imbach et al. 1985). The small but significant group of children with severe thrombocytopenia and bleeding present a difficult therapeutic challenge. Second-line therapies include splenectomy (Rijcken et al. 2014; Montalvo et al. 2014; Kuhne 2013), immunosuppressive therapy, (rituximab, azathioprine, 6-mercaptopurine, mycophenolate mofetil) (Rao et al. 2005; Provan et al. 2006; Saleh et al. 2000; Bennett et al. 2005; Sobota et al. 2009; Hilgartner et al. 1970), and thrombopoietin-receptor agonists (eltrombopag, romiplostim) (Tarantino et al. 2016; Grainger et al. 2015). Only eltrombopag and romiplostim are FDA approved for the treatment of chronic ITP. While splenectomy is effective in children with ITP, it is often avoided in this age group because of the lifelong risk of overwhelming bacterial sepsis (Ahmed et al. 2016; Aronis et al. 2004; Kuhne et al. 2007). Immunosuppressive therapies may be used as splenectomy sparing treatments but are not effective in many patients. Thrombopoietin-receptor agonists may show higher efficacy, but long-term treatment is usually necessary to maintain adequate platelet counts. There is no standard of care for children with severe, symptomatic ITP, and treatment decisions are usually based on patient preference, age, activity level, provider experience, anecdotal evidence, expert opinion, and consensus guidelines.

While the long-term outcome for most children with ITP is favorable, during periods of severe thrombocytopenia, there can be significant patient and family anxiety about the ongoing risk of bleeding. Many children with chronic ITP have activity restrictions which impact quality of life negatively. The ability to predict disease course reliably would be helpful for families to manage anxiety and improve quality of life. The identification of predictors of chronic disease in children with ITP would be extremely beneficial to providers and families in making treatment decisions. Patients with a high likelihood of disease remission could be spared unnecessary and potentially harmful treatment.

16.2 Challenges

The design of a prospective clinical trial with adequate power requires ample patient numbers. Since chronic ITP is a rare disease, generating the numbers necessary for a clinical trial at a single center is difficult. However, large multicenter studies are challenging and expensive to complete. Hence, the majority of studies investigating prognostic factors in ITP are prospective observational studies or retrospective studies and while these are valuable in forwarding our knowledge of the natural history of ITP, they have limitations. A large proportion of patients in prospective long-term observational studies may be lost to follow-up, thereby limiting the analysis and subsequent conclusions. In small single-center studies, the findings may not be generalizable to all populations. In the many published ITP studies over the last decades, widely discrepant criteria are used to evaluate patient characteristics, define chronic disease, measure responses, and report outcomes. The resulting heterogeneity complicates the interpretation of results and their application into clinical practice. The International Working Group in ITP has recommended standardization of terminology for diagnosis and management of ITP with the goal of bringing harmonization to ITP research (Rodeghiero et al. 2009). The new definitions for ITP diagnosis were based on the high rate of spontaneous remission in children with ITP, even after 12 months. The recommendations were to define three phases of ITP: newly diagnosed ITP (up to 3 months from diagnosis), persistent ITP (from 3–12 months), and chronic ITP (lasting more than 12 months). While this standardization may be helpful for future study design and interpretation, it does not aid in comparing older studies of chronic ITP in childhood to more recent ones. There is also heterogeneity in the parameters that are studied. Predictors of interest in one study may not be included in the data collection of another, so the results cannot be compared across studies. For example, in a recent systemic review and meta-analysis of 54 articles published from 1975 to 2013, many potentially interesting predictors such as antinuclear antibody titer were only reported in a handful of studies and common baseline measurements such as mean presenting platelet counts were only reported in 18 of 54 articles (Heitink-Polle et al. 2014). Hopefully, with the development of new multicenter groups and the growth of established registries, future studies will take a more harmonized approach. Despite these challenges, the current body of evidence defining predictors of ITP outcome is valuable for disease management and patient quality of life.

16.3 Biomarker Predictors of Chronic ITP

The majority of recent studies that evaluate potential predictors of chronic disease are retrospective or prospective observational studies. There is one recent randomized controlled trial that investigated potential predictors of chronic disease at

12 months after diagnosis. Table 16.1 summarizes the results of a selected list of recent studies that have investigated predictors of chronic ITP.

In a multicenter, prospective study of children with newly diagnosed ITP conducted by Nordic ITP study group, the following characteristics at diagnosis were associated with chronic disease at 6 months post diagnosis: insidious onset of symptoms (>2 weeks duration), older age (>10 years), no history of prior infection, absence of wet purpura, female gender, and platelet count $>5 \times 10^9$/l (Zeller et al. 2005). Insidious onset of disease was the strongest predictor of chronic disease (Zeller et al. 2005). The Intercontinental Cooperative ITP Study Group Registry I, a large multicenter, international, prospective observational study of 2540 children with newly diagnosed ITP, found that older age at diagnosis and higher presenting platelet count increased the risk of chronic ITP at 6 months post diagnosis (Kuhne et al. 2003). Infants under 1 year of age had the lowest likelihood of chronicity (Kuhne et al. 2003). In the ICIS Registry II study, a prospective observational study of 1239 children with newly diagnosed ITP, data were analyzed at 12 and 24 months to investigate factors that were associated with ITP duration (Bennett et al. 2016). In a multivariate analysis of these data, younger children, particularly children under 1 year of age were less likely to develop chronic disease (Bennett et al. 2017). Gender, platelet count, and bleeding severity at diagnosis were not significant predictors of chronicity in the multivariate analysis (Bennett et al. 2017).

Numerous retrospective studies have reported a significant associations between chronic ITP (measured at 6 or 12 months) and various biomarkers, most notably older age, insidious onset of symptoms, higher platelet count, negative history of prior infection or immunization, the absence of mucosal bleeding, and female gender, all measured at diagnosis (Donato et al. 2009; Akbayram et al. 2011; Chotsampancharoen et al. 2017; ElAlfy et al. 2010; Glanz et al. 2008). A recent systematic review and meta-analysis reported that older age (>11 years), higher platelet count ($\geq 20 \times 10^9$/l), insidious onset of symptoms, no history of prior infection or vaccination, and female gender were predictive of chronic ITP (Heitink-Polle et al. 2014). Bleeding at diagnosis, a predictor of short ITP duration in some studies, was not significant in the systemic review (Heitink-Polle et al. 2014).

Other laboratory findings have been studied less frequently but may be important to include inclusion in future studies. Two studies have found significantly lower absolute lymphocyte counts at diagnosis in patients developing chronic disease (Deel et al. 2013; Ahmed et al. 2010). Antinuclear antibody testing has been studied infrequently. In the meta-analysis and systemic review, there were three studies which reported association between ANA positivity at diagnosis and chronic disease (Heitink-Polle et al. 2014). Other measures such as hemoglobin, platelet antibodies, bone marrow results, and mean platelet volume did not consistently predict chronic disease (Heitink-Polle et al. 2014).

Table 16.1 Selected list of studies evaluating predictors of chronic ITP in children

Year	Type of study	Duration of ITP (months)	Patients enrolled *n*	Patients with outcome data *n*	Patients with cITP *n* (%)	Features measured at diagnosis of ITP	Significant predictors of cITP	Ref
2003	Prospective Observational Multicenter	6	2540	1742	651 (37.4)	Age Gender Platelet count Onset Prior infection Bleeding	Older age Higher platelet count (in children over 1 year of age only) Infants <1 year have lowest risk of cITP	(Kuhne et al. 2003)
2004	Prospective Observational Multicenter	6	506	423	106 (25.1)	Age Gender Platelet count onset Prior infection Bleeding treatment Season	Insidious onset Age ≥8 years No prior infection Girls ages >7 years with insidious onset of symptoms have high risk of cITP	(Zeller et al. 2005)
2004	Prospective Observational Multicenter	6	63	60	16 (26.6)	Age Gender Platelet count Prior infection Bleeding treatment Fcγ-receptor gene polymorphisms	Higher platelet count ($>10 \times 10^9$/l) No prior infection FCGR2B 232I/T polymorphism	(Bruin et al. 2004)

(continued)

Table 16.1 (continued)

Year	Type of study	Duration of ITP (months)	Patients enrolled *n*	Patients with outcome data *n*	Patients with cITP *n* (%)	Features measured at diagnosis of ITP	Significant predictors of cITP	Ref
2006	Retrospective Single center	6	79	72	19 (26.3)	Age Gender Platelet count Onset of symptoms bleeding API Season	No prior infection insidious onset	(Roganovic and Letica-Crepulja 2006)
2008	Retrospective Population-based Multicenter	6	259	257	60 (23)	Age Gender Platelet count Prior infection Bleeding site Treatment	Older age (>10 years) Higher platelet count (>20 × 10^9/l) No mucosal bleeding No prior infection absence of mucosal bleeding Patients older than 10 years and with platelets >20 × 10^9/l had highest risk of chronic disease	(Glanz et al. 2008)

2009	Prospective Matched pair Multicenter	6	2605	1984	630 (31.8)	Age Gender Platelet count Prior infection Treatment	Older age Higher platelet ($>20 \times 10^9$/l) No prior infection Children treated with IVIG were less likely to have chronic disease	(Tamminga et al. 2009)
2009	Retrospective Multicenter	6	1683	1418	404 (28.5)	Age Gender Platelet count Prior infection Bleeding severity Type of purpura Treatment Seasonal incidence	Older age (>9 years) Higher platelet count ($>10 \times 10^9$/l) No prior infection Infants have lowest risk of chronic disease	(Donato et al. 2009)
2010	Retrospective Multicenter	6	409	344	120 (34.9)	Age Gender Platelet count Onset Prior infection Bleeding severity Bleeding site Treatment	Older age (>10 years) Higher platelet count ($>20 \times 10^9$/l) Insidious onset No mucosal bleeding No prior infection	(ElAlfy et al. 2010)

(continued)

Table 16.1 (continued)

Year	Type of study	Duration of ITP (months)	Patients enrolled *n*	Patients with outcome data *n*	Patients with cITP *n* (%)	Features measured at diagnosis of ITP	Significant predictors of cITP	Ref
2010	Retrospective Multicenter	6	625	475	270 (56.8)	Age Gender Platelet count Bleeding site Bleeding severity	Older age (≥8 years) Male gender	(Bansal et al. 2010)
2011	Retrospective Single center	6	260	260	69	Age Gender Platelet count Onset Prior infection Treatment Season Bleeding	Older age (>10 years) No prior infection Higher platelet count	(Akbayram et al. 2011)
2013	Retrospective	3 6 12	472	312	Not reported	Age Gender Platelet count Onset Prior infection Bleeding Treatment	Older age (≥10 years) Insidious onset	(Revel-Vilk et al. 2013)

2014	Systemic review & Meta-analysis	6 12	N/A	N/A	N/A	Age Gender Platelet count Prior infection Onset Bleeding Treatment Hemoglobin White blood cells Antinuclear antibody (ANA) Platelet antibody Bone marrow parameters Genetic factors	Older age (≥11 years) Female gender Higher platelet count No prior infection Insidious onset ANA positivity Treatment with corticosteroids and IVIG Treatment with IVIG alone was protective	(Heitink-Polle et al. 2014)
2016	Prospective Observational	12 24	1239	705[a] 383[b]	286[a] 152[b]	Age Gender Platelet counts Bleeding severity Treatment	Older age (≥10 years) Less bleeding (significant at 12 months only) Combination therapy with IVIG and corticosteroids protective	(Bennett et al. 2016)

(continued)

Table 16.1 (continued)

Year	Type of study	Duration of ITP (months)	Patients enrolled *n*	Patients with outcome data *n*	Patients with cITP *n* (%)	Features measured at diagnosis of ITP	Significant predictors of cITP	Ref
2016	Randomized controlled trial (2009–2015)	12	100 patients observation only		10.4	Age Gender Platelet count Onset Prior infection Bleeding Leukocyte count Lymphocyte count Treatment response	Age (>10 years) Insidious onset No mucosal bleeding Lower leukocyte count Lower lymphocyte count Absence of complete response to IVIG at 1 week was associated with cITP cITP not lower in IVIG arm	(Heitink-Polle et al. 2016)
			100 patients IVIG		10.2			
2017	Retrospective Single center	12	417	405	113	Age Gender Platelet count Treatment Onset of symptoms Bleeding Prior infection	Older age (>5 years) Insidious onset Platelet count at 4 weeks post diagnosis of at least $\geq 100 \times 10^9$/l was associated ITP resolution by 12 months	(Chotsampancharoen et al. 2017)

cITP chronic ITP

[a]705 patients had outcome data at 12 months; 286 of these had cITP

[b]383 patients had outcome data at 24 months; 152 of these had cITP

16.4 Treatment-Related Factors

Management of children with newly diagnosed ITP consists of close observation versus treatment with IVIG or corticosteroids. Two recent guidelines support the use of careful observation over treatment in asymptomatic children with newly diagnosed ITP (Neunert et al. 2011; Provan et al. 2010). However, several observational and retrospective studies suggested a lower risk of chronic ITP in children treated with IVIG. In a matched pair analysis of the ICIS I Registry data, children initially treated with IVIG were more likely to have ITP resolution than children who received no therapy (Tamminga et al. 2009). In the meta-analysis, 14 studies assessed the association between initial treatment with IVIG and chronic disease (Heitink-Polle et al. 2014). This analysis showed significantly less chronic ITP in patients treated with IVIG at diagnosis (Heitink-Polle et al. 2014). In the ICIS Registry II study, treatment with IVIG at diagnosis was not protective against the development of chronic ITP, but interestingly, combination therapy with IVIG and corticosteroids was associated with a lower risk of chronic disease (Bennett et al. 2017). In contrast, the meta-analysis reported a higher risk of chronic ITP in patients who received a combination of IVIG and methylprednisolone at diagnosis (Heitink-Polle et al. 2014).

The initial findings of a phase 3, multicenter, randomized, controlled clinical trial evaluating the efficacy of IVIG treatment versus close observation in children with newly diagnosed ITP were presented at the annual meeting of the American Society of Hematology in 2016 and appear to have settled this issue. In this study, the rate of chronic ITP did not differ significantly between the IVIG treated group and the observation only group (Heitink-Polle et al. 2016). However, in patients randomized to receive IVIG, recovery rates were higher in the first 3 months after diagnosis, and bleeding was less common than in the observation group (Heitink-Polle et al. 2016). The study also investigated biomarker predictors of chronic disease and found that the following features at diagnosis were associated with a higher risk of developing chronic disease: older age, longer duration of symptoms, no mucosal bleeding, lower leukocyte count, and lower lymphocyte count (Heitink-Polle et al. 2016). This study supports prior retrospective studies showing the significance of lymphocyte and leukocyte counts in the development of chronic ITP (see above). In the IVIG group, the absence of complete response at 1 week was associated with development of chronic ITP (Heitink-Polle et al. 2016).

16.5 Genetic Factors

With the development of modern genetic methods, novel approaches are being used to identify markers of disease outcome and potential therapeutic targets. Several studies have utilized genetic approaches to investigate factors that might be involved in the pathogenesis of ITP and might predict outcome or treatment response.

In a gene expression profile of whole blood samples of patients with newly diagnosed and chronic ITP, children with chronic disease showed significant upregulation of interferon-regulated genes (Sood et al. 2008) and overexpression of *VNN1*, a gene involved in the oxidative stress pathway (Zhang et al. 2011).

Functional variants of inflammatory cytokine genes and low-affinity Fcγ receptor (FcγR) genes have been implicated in autoimmune disease. In a pilot study of 37 children with chronic ITP and 218 controls, genotyping was performed on common variants in the regulatory regions of cytokines (*TNF*, *LTA*, *IL1RN*, *IL1A*, *IL4*, *IL6*, *IL10*) and structural variants of the low-affinity FcγRs (*FCGR2A*, *FCGR3A*, *FCGR3B*) (Foster et al. 2001). Two combinations of genotypes, *TNF* and *FCGR3A*, were significantly associated with chronic ITP (Foster et al. 2001). In a prospective study of newly diagnosed ITP patients, the FCGR2B-232I/T polymorphism was overrepresented in patients who developed chronic disease (Bruin et al. 2004). In the systemic review and meta-analysis of predictors of chronic ITP, 18 articles reported allele frequencies of 29 different genes, but only two allele frequencies showed significantly higher risks for chronic ITP: TGF-B1 cod 25 allele A and IL-4 intron 3 allele RP1 (Heitink-Polle et al. 2014). In recent study using whole genome sequencing of genes associated with cellular immunity in patients with chronic ITP, two genes *IFNA17* (interferon alpha 17) and *IFNLR1* (interferon-lambda receptor 1) which are involved in T-cell function showed an increased frequency in children with chronic ITP compared to controls (Despotovic et al. 2015).

In a 2010 review of genetic studies in pediatric ITP, Bergmann et al. assessed the feasibility, advantages and disadvantages of potential genetic approaches in studying pediatric ITP including linkage studies, genome-wide association studies, comparative genomics, candidate gene approaches, and pharmacogenetics studies and reviewed the current literature of genetic factors associated with pediatric ITP (Bergmann et al. 2010). This report may be referenced for a more in-depth review of genetic studies in childhood ITP that is beyond the scope of this chapter.

16.6 Discussion

ITP in children is typically a self-limited disorder that resolves within several weeks to months after the onset of symptoms. While the risk of clinically significant bleeding is low and the outcome is favorable in the majority of patients, children with severe thrombocytopenia require close observation and activity restrictions, which often contribute to patient and parental anxiety and negatively impact quality of life.

Chronic ITP in childhood has a benign course in the majority of cases and may resolve with or without therapy even several years from onset (Aronis et al. 1994). A small but significant group of patients will have severe, chronic ITP that requires ongoing treatment to prevent or treat bleeding. At diagnosis, it is not possible to distinguish patients who will have a short ITP duration from those who will have chronic disease. Identifying reliable prognostic factors at diagnosis that predict ITP outcome would be invaluable for clinicians and families to guide treatment decisions and ultimately improve quality of life.

Despite the limitations of current research, there is a considerable body of evidence to support these predictors of chronic ITP in children which are present at initial diagnosis: older age, higher platelet count, longer duration of symptoms, female gender, absence of a preceding infection, lower leukocyte count, and lower lymphocyte count. However, in a randomized clinical trial measuring the effect of IVIG treatment on the development of chronic disease, female gender, higher platelet count, and the absence of a prior infection or immunization were not significant predictive factors. Therefore, based on this new evidence, these biomarkers may not be strongly predictive of chronic disease in childhood ITP after all.

Several prior studies demonstrated a potentially protective effect of IVIG treatment at diagnosis against the development of chronic ITP (Blanchette et al. 1993; Tamminga et al. 2009). These findings were interesting and had potential clinical significance in the treatment of newly diagnosed children. The recent randomized, controlled clinical trial showed that the rate of chronic ITP was no different in the IVIG group compared to observation alone. However, this study did show that in the IVIG group, recovery rates were higher during the first 3 months, and bleeding was less frequent than in the observation group.

The prospective observational ICIS II registry study indicated that combination therapy with both IVIG and corticosteroids led to a lower risk of chronic ITP, but the large number of patients lost to follow-up was problematic in this study and may have impacted the analysis. By contrast, in a meta-analysis and systematic review, a significantly higher risk for chronic ITP was found in patients treated with IVIG and corticosteroids in combination, but only a univariate analysis could be performed, so confounding and bias may have influenced the results.

Based on the current somewhat contradictory evidence, it would be inappropriate to recommend up front pharmacologic therapy to young children with newly diagnosed ITP solely to prevent the development of chronic disease, given that most children have spontaneous disease resolution and no clinically significant bleeding. However, treatment with IVIG alone or in combination with corticosteroids might be beneficial to selected patients with clinically significant bleeding.

Various candidate genes and genetic pathways have been implicated in the development of autoimmune disease, including ITP, but to date, there is no convincing reproducible evidence for any genetic markers of ITP outcome. Large multicenter studies are necessary to discover genes or genetic pathways involved in the development of chronic ITP.

Conclusions

While great progress has been made in discovering risk factors which determine ITP outcome, important questions and challenges remain. The current predictors present at ITP diagnosis, specifically younger age, shorter duration of symptoms, higher leukocyte count, and higher lymphocyte count, can be applied to newly diagnosed patients to help determine the likelihood of short disease duration, and these patients can be managed with close observation and treated only if bleeding. Unfortunately, the current predictors are not adequate in identifying those patients who will ultimately develop clinically significant chronic disease. Future studies utilizing large ITP registries and genetic approaches are needed to discover novel biomarkers that reliably predict ITP course.

References

Ahmed R, Devasia AJ, Viswabandya A, Lakshmi KM, Abraham A, Karl S, Mathai J, Jacob PM, Abraham D, Srivastava A, et al. Long-term outcome following splenectomy for chronic and persistent immune thrombocytopenia (ITP) in adults and children: splenectomy in ITP. Ann Hematol. 2016;95(9):1429–34.

Ahmed I, Rajpurkar M, Thomas R, Chitlur M. Initial lymphocyte count and the development of persistent/chronic immune thrombocytopenic purpura. Pediatr Blood Cancer. 2010;55(3):508–11.

Akbayram S, Dogan M, Ustyol L, Akgun C, Peker E, Bilici S, Caksen H, Oner AF. The clinical outcome of 260 pediatric ITP patients in one center. Clin Appl Thromb Hemost. 2011;17(6):E30–5.

Andrew M, Blanchette VS, Adams M, Ali K, Barnard D, Chan KW, DeVeber LB, Esseltine D, Israels S, Korbrinsky N, et al. A multicenter study of the treatment of childhood chronic idiopathic thrombocytopenic purpura with anti-D. J Pediatr. 1992;120(4 Pt 1):522–7.

Aronis S, Platokouki H, Avgeri M, Pergantou H, Keramidas D. Retrospective evaluation of long-term efficacy and safety of splenectomy in chronic idiopathic thrombocytopenic purpura in children. Acta Paediatr. 2004;93(5):638–42.

Aronis S, Platokouki H, Mitsika A, Haidas S, Constantopoulos A. Seventeen years of experience with chronic idiopathic thrombocytopenic purpura in childhood. Is therapy always better? Pediatr Hematol Oncol. 1994;11(5):487–98.

Bansal D, Bhamare TA, Trehan A, Ahluwalia J, Varma N, Marwaha RK. Outcome of chronic idiopathic thrombocytopenic purpura in children. Pediatr Blood Cancer. 2010;54(3):403–7.

Bennett CM, Neunert C, Grace RF, Buchanan G, Imbach P, Vesely SK, Kuhne T. Predictors of remission in children with newly diagnosed immune thrombocytopenia: data from the Intercontinental Cooperative ITP Study Group Registry II participants. Pediatr Blood Cancer. 2017. https://doi.org/10.1002/pbc.26736 [Epub ahead of print].

Bennett CM, Rogers ZR, Kinnamon DD, Bussel JB, Mahoney DH, Abshire TC, Sawaf H, Moore TB, Loh ML, Glader BE et al. Prospective phase 1/2 study of rituximab in childhood and adolescent chronic immune thrombocytopenic purpura. In: 18th Annual Meeting of the American-Society-of-Pediatric-Hematology-Oncology: May 13–17 2005; Washington, DC; 2005. p. 2639–42.

Bennett CM, Tarantino M. Chronic immune thrombocytopenia in children: epidemiology and clinical presentation. Hematol Oncol Clin North Am. 2009;23(6):1223–38.

Bergmann AK, Grace RF, Neufeld EJ. Genetic studies in pediatric ITP: outlook, feasibility, and requirements. Ann Hematol. 2010;89(Suppl 1):S95–103.

Blanchette V, Imbach P, Andrew M, Adams M, McMillan J, Wang E, Milner R, Ali K, Barnard D, Bernstein M, et al. Randomised trial of intravenous immunoglobulin G, intravenous anti-D, and oral prednisone in childhood acute immune thrombocytopenic purpura. Lancet. 1994;344(8924):703–7.

Blanchette VS, Luke B, Andrew M, Sommerville-Nielsen S, Barnard D, de Veber B, Gent M. A prospective, randomized trial of high-dose intravenous immune globulin G therapy, oral prednisone therapy, and no therapy in childhood acute immune thrombocytopenic purpura. J Pediatr. 1993;123(6):989–95.

Bruin M, Bierings M, Uiterwaal C, Revesz T, Bode L, Wiesman ME, Kuijpers T, Tamminga R, de Haas M. Platelet count, previous infection and FCGR2B genotype predict development of chronic disease in newly diagnosed idiopathic thrombocytopenia in childhood: results of a prospective study. Br J Haematol. 2004;127(5):561–7.

Chotsampancharoen T, Sripornsawan P, Duangchoo S, Wongchanchailert M, McNeil E. Predictive factors for resolution of childhood immune thrombocytopenia: experience from a single tertiary center in Thailand. Pediatr Blood Cancer. 2017;64(1):128–34.

Deel MD, Kong M, Cross KP, Bertolone SJ. Absolute lymphocyte counts as prognostic indicators for immune thrombocytopenia outcomes in children. Pediatr Blood Cancer. 2013;60(12):1967–74.

Despotovic JM, Polfus LM, Flanagan JM, Bennett CM, Lambert MP, Neunert C, Kumar M, Klaassen RJ, Thornburg C, Jeng M, et al. Genes influencing the development and severity of chronic ITP identified through whole exome sequencing. Blood. 2015;126(23):3.

Donato H, Picon A, Martinez M, Rapetti MC, Rosso A, Gomez S, Rossi N, Bacciedoni V, Schvartzman G, Riccheri C, et al. Demographic data, natural history, and prognostic factors of idiopathic thrombocytopenic purpura in children: a multicentered study from Argentina. Pediatr Blood Cancer. 2009;52(4):491–6.

ElAlfy M, Farid S, Abdel Maksoud A. Predictors of chronic idiopathic thrombocytopenic purpura. Pediatr Blood Cancer. 2010;54(7):959–62.

Foster CB, Zhu S, Erichsen HC, Lehrnbecher T, Hart ES, Choi E, Stein S, Smith MW, Steinberg SM, Imbach P, et al. Polymorphisms in inflammatory cytokines and Fcgamma receptors in childhood chronic immune thrombocytopenic purpura: a pilot study. Br J Haematol. 2001;113(3):596–9.

Glanz J, France E, Xu S, Hayes T, Hambidge S. A population-based, multisite cohort study of the predictors of chronic idiopathic thrombocytopenic purpura in children. Pediatrics. 2008;121(3):e506–12.

Grainger JD, Locatelli F, Chotsampancharoen T, Donyush E, Pongtanakul B, Komvilaisak P, Sosothikul D, Drelichman G, Sirachainan N, Holzhauer S, et al. Eltrombopag for children with chronic immune thrombocytopenia (PETIT2): a randomised, multicentre, placebo-controlled trial. Lancet. 2015;386(10004):1649–58.

Grimaldi-Bensouda L, Nordon C, Michel M, Viallard JF, Adoue D, Magy-Bertrand N, Durand JM, Quittet P, Fain O, Bonnotte B, et al. Immune thrombocytopenia in adults: a prospective cohort study of clinical features and predictors of outcome. Haematologica. 2016;101(9):1039–45.

Harrington WJ, Minnich V, Hollingsworth JW, Moore CV. Demonstration of a thrombocytopenic factor in the blood of patients with thrombocytopenic purpura. J Lab Clin Med. 1951;38(1):1–10.

Heitink-Polle KM, Nijsten J, Boonacker CW, de Haas M, Bruin MC. Clinical and laboratory predictors of chronic immune thrombocytopenia in children: a systematic review and meta-analysis. Blood. 2014;124(22):3295–307.

Heitink-Polle KMJ, Uiterwaal CSPM, Porcelijn L, Tamminga RYJ, Smiers FJ, van Woerden NL, Wesseling J, Laarhoven AG, de Haas M, Bruin MCA. Treatment with Intravenous Immunoglobulin Does Not Prevent Chronic Immune Thrombocytopenia in Children: Results of a Randomized Controlled Trial. Blood. 2016;128(22):866.

Hilgartner MW, Lanzkowsky P, Smith CH. The use of azathioprine in refractory idiopathic thrombocytopenic purpura in children. Acta Paediatr Scand. 1970;59(4):409–15.

Imbach P, Kuhne T, Muller D, Berchtold W, Zimmerman S, Elalfy M, Buchanan GR. Childhood ITP: 12 months follow-up data from the prospective registry I of the Intercontinental Childhood ITP Study Group (ICIS). Pediatr Blood Cancer. 2006;46(3):351–6.

Imbach P, Wagner HP, Berchtold W, Gaedicke G, Hirt A, Joller P, Mueller-Eckhardt C, Muller B, Rossi E, Barandun S. Intravenous immunoglobulin versus oral corticosteroids in acute immune thrombocytopenic purpura in childhood. Lancet. 1985;2(8453):464–8.

Kuhne T. Update on the Intercontinental Cooperative ITP Study Group (ICIS) and on the pediatric and Adult Registry on Chronic ITP (PARC ITP). Pediatr Blood Cancer. 2013;60(Suppl 1):S15–8.

Kuhne T, Berchtold W, Michaels LA, Wu R, Donato H, Espina B, Tamary H, Rodeghiero F, Chitlur M, Rischewski J, et al. Newly diagnosed immune thrombocytopenia in children and adults: a comparative prospective observational registry of the Intercontinental Cooperative Immune Thrombocytopenia Study Group. Haematologica. 2011;96(12):1831–7.

Kuhne T, Blanchette V, Buchanan GR, Ramenghi U, Donato H, Tamminga RY, Rischewski J, Berchtold W, Imbach P. Splenectomy in children with idiopathic thrombocytopenic purpura: a prospective study of 134 children from the Intercontinental Childhood ITP Study Group. Pediatr Blood Cancer. 2007;49(6):829–34.

Kuhne T, Buchanan GR, Zimmerman S, Michaels LA, Kohan R, Berchtold W, Imbach P, Intercontinental Childhood ITPSG, Intercontinental Childhood ITPSG. A prospective comparative study of 2540 infants and children with newly diagnosed idiopathic thrombocytopenic purpura (ITP) from the Intercontinental Childhood ITP Study Group. J Pediatr. 2003;143(5):605–8.

McMillan R, Wang L, Tomer A, Nichol J, Pistillo J. Suppression of in vitro megakaryocyte production by antiplatelet autoantibodies from adult patients with chronic ITP. Blood. 2004;103(4):1364–9.

Montalvo J, Velazquez D, Pantoja JP, Sierra M, Lopez-Karpovitch X, Herrera MF. Laparoscopic splenectomy for primary immune thrombocytopenia: clinical outcome and prognostic factors. J Laparoendosc Adv Surg Tech A. 2014;24(7):466–70.

Neunert CE, Buchanan GR, Imbach P, Bolton-Maggs PH, Bennett CM, Neufeld EJ, Vesely SK, Adix L, Blanchette VS, Kuhne T, et al. Severe hemorrhage in children with newly diagnosed immune thrombocytopenic purpura. Blood. 2008;112(10):4003–8.

Neunert C, Lim W, Crowther M, Cohen A, Solberg L Jr, Crowther MA. American Society of H: The American Society of Hematology 2011 evidence-based practice guideline for immune thrombocytopenia. Blood. 2011;117(16):4190–207.

Papagianni A, Economou M, Tragiannidis A, Karatza E, Tsatra I, Gombakis N, Athanassiadou-Piperopoulou F, Athanasiou-Metaxa M. Standard-dose intravenous anti-D immunoglobulin versus intravenous immunoglobulin in the treatment of newly diagnosed childhood primary immune thrombocytopenia. J Pediatr Hematol Oncol. 2011;33(4):265–9.

Provan D, Moss AJ, Newland AC, Bussel JB. Efficacy of mycophenolate mofetil as single-agent therapy for refractory immune thrombocytopenic purpura. Am J Hematol. 2006;81(1):19–25.

Provan D, Newland A, Norfolk D, Bolton-Maggs P, Lilleyman J, Greer I, May A, Murphy M, Ouwehand W, Watson S, et al. Guidelines for the investigation and management of idiopathic thrombocytopenic purpura in adults, children and in pregnancy. Br J Haematol. 2003;120(4):574–96.

Provan D, Stasi R, Newland AC, Blanchette VS, Bolton-Maggs P, Bussel JB, Chong BH, Cines DB, Gernsheimer TB, Godeau B, et al. International consensus report on the investigation and management of primary immune thrombocytopenia. Blood. 2010;115(2):168–86.

Psaila B, Petrovic A, Page LK, Menell J, Schonholz M, Bussel JB. Intracranial hemorrhage (ICH) in children with immune thrombocytopenia (ITP): study of 40 cases. Blood. 2009;114(23):4777–83.

Rao VK, Dugan F, Dale JK, Davis J, Tretler J, Hurley JK, Fleisher T, Puck J, Straus SE. Use of mycophenolate mofetil for chronic, refractory immune cytopenias in children with autoimmune lymphoproliferative syndrome. Br J Haematol. 2005;129(4):534–8.

Revel-Vilk S, Yacobovich J, Frank S, Ben-Ami T, Yechieli M, Shkalim V, Lebel A, Semo-Oz R, Tamary H. Age and duration of bleeding symptoms at diagnosis best predict resolution of childhood immune thrombocytopenia at 3, 6, and 12 months. J Pediatr. 2013;163(5):1335–1339 e1331–1332.

Rijcken E, Mees ST, Bisping G, Krueger K, Bruewer M, Senninger N, Mennigen R. Laparoscopic splenectomy for medically refractory immune thrombocytopenia (ITP): a retrospective cohort study on longtime response predicting factors based on consensus criteria. Int J Surg. 2014;12(12):1428–33.

Rodeghiero F, Stasi R, Gernsheimer T, Michel M, Provan D, Arnold DM, Bussel JB, Cines DB, Chong BH, Cooper N, et al. Standardization of terminology, definitions and outcome criteria in immune thrombocytopenic purpura of adults and children: report from an international working group. Blood. 2009;113(11):2386–93.

Roganovic J, Letica-Crepulja M. Idiopathic thrombocytopenic purpura: a 15-year natural history study at the Children's Hospital Rijeka, Croatia. Pediatr Blood Cancer. 2006;47(5 Suppl):662–4.

Rosthoj S, Rajantie J, Treutiger I, Zeller B, Tedgard U, Henter JI, NOPHO ITP Working Group. Duration and morbidity of chronic immune thrombocytopenic purpura in children: five-year follow-up of a Nordic cohort. Acta Paediatr. 2012;101(7):761–6.

Saleh MN, Gutheil J, Moore M, Feinberg B, Bunch P, Butler J, Lavelle P, Kunkel L, Benyunes K, Grillo-Lopez A, et al. A pilot study of anti-CD20 MoAb Rituximab in patients with refractory immune thrombocytopenic purpura (ITP). Blood. 2000;96(11):1086.

Sobota A, Neufeld EJ, Lapsia S, Bennett CM. Response to mercaptopurine for refractory autoimmune cytopenias in children. Pediatr Blood Cancer. 2009;52(1):80–4.

Sood R, Wong W, Gotlib J, Jeng M, Zehnder JL. Gene expression and pathway analysis of immune thrombocytopenic purpura. Br J Haematol. 2008;140(1):99–103.

Stasi R, Stipa E, Masi M, Cecconi M, Scimo MT, Oliva F, Sciarra A, Perrotti AP, Adomo G, Amadori S, et al. Long-term observations of 208 adults with chronic idiopathic thrombocytopenic purpura. Am J Med. 1995;98(5):436–42.

Tamminga R, Berchtold W, Bruin M, Buchanan GR, Kuhne T. Possible lower rate of chronic ITP after IVIG for acute childhood ITP an analysis from registry I of the Intercontinental Cooperative ITP Study Group (ICIS). Br J Haematol. 2009;146(2):180–4.

Tarantino MD, Bussel JB, Blanchette VS, Despotovic J, Bennett C, Raj A, Williams B, Beam D, Morales J, Rose MJ, et al. Romiplostim in children with immune thrombocytopenia: a phase 3, randomised, double-blind, placebo-controlled study. Lancet. 2016;388(10039):45–54.

Watts RG. Idiopathic thrombocytopenic purpura: a 10-year natural history study at the Children's Hospital of Alabama. Clin Pediatr (Phila). 2004;43(8):691–702.

Zeller B, Rajantie J, Hedlund-Treutiger I, Tedgard U, Wesenberg F, Jonsson AG, Henter JI, Rosthoj S, Grp NIW, Five Natl Study G. Childhood idiopathic thrombocytopenic purpura in the Nordic countries: epidemiology and predictors of chronic disease. Acta Paediatr. 2005;94(2):178–84.

Zhang B, Lo C, Shen L, Sood R, Jones C, Cusmano-Ozog K, Park-Snyder S, Wong W, Jeng M, Cowan T, et al. The role of vanin-1 and oxidative stress-related pathways in distinguishing acute and chronic pediatric ITP. Blood. 2011;117(17):4569–79.

Zufferey A, Kapur R, Semple JW. Pathogenesis and therapeutic mechanisms in immune thrombocytopenia (ITP). J Clin Med. 2017;6(2):16.

Immune Functions of Platelets

17

Rick Kapur and John W. Semple

17.1 General Introduction

Platelets are anucleate and small cellular fragments (~2–4 μM in diameter) derived from bone marrow-resident megakaryocytes (~50–100 μM in diameter) and are known to be indispensable for the regulation of hemostasis (Semple et al. 2011). Platelet generation is a complex and highly regulated process (Machlus and Italiano 2013), and recently it has been suggested that also the lung may be an important site for the production of platelets (Lefrancais et al. 2017). This may perhaps reflect the diverse nature of platelets, and indeed a recent body of work has revealed that platelets are involved in several other functional processes beyond hemostasis, in both health and disease (Kapur et al. 2015b; Semple et al. 2011; Youssefian et al. 2002; McMorran et al. 2009; Wong et al. 2013; Clark et al. 2007; Sreeramkumar et al. 2014; Boilard et al. 2010; Kapur and Semple 2016a, b). These non-hemostatic functions will be discussed in this chapter generally outlined as "Platelets and Pathogens," reflecting the ability of platelets to battle

R. Kapur
Division of Hematology and Transfusion Medicine, Lund University, BMC C14, Klinikgatan 26, Lund 221 84, Sweden

J.W. Semple (✉)
Division of Hematology and Transfusion Medicine, Lund University, BMC C14, Klinikgatan 26, Lund 221 84, Sweden

Keenan Research Centre for Biomedical Science, St. Michael's Hospital, Toronto, ON, Canada

The Toronto Platelet Immunobiology Group, St. Michael's Hospital, Toronto, ON, Canada

Canadian Blood Services, Toronto, ON, Canada

Departments of Pharmacology, Medicine, and Laboratory Medicine and Pathobiology, University of Toronto, Toronto, ON, Canada
e-mail: John_w.semple@med.lu.se

P. Imbach (ed.), *Antibody Therapy*, https://doi.org/10.1007/978-3-319-68038-5_17

invading pathogens, and "Platelet-Target Cell Communication," illustrating how platelets use sophisticated channels in order to communicate with a variety of effector cells.

17.2 Platelets and Pathogens

17.2.1 Pathogen Recognition

Platelets initiate their antimicrobial host defense through sensing the threat of invading pathogens or damage during inflammation, via their immune receptors called pattern recognition receptors. These include immunoglobulin or complement receptors and Toll-like receptors (TLRs) (Semple et al. 2011). These receptors directly bind invading pathogens and microbes, including their derived materials. Pathogens first encounter TLRs on professional phagocytes, such as neutrophils, dendritic cells (DCs), or macrophages (Semple et al. 2011; Janeway 1992; Janeway and Medzhitov 2002). The expression of TLRs 1–9 has been described on human as well as on murine platelets, demonstrating a functional role for some of these TLRs (Semple et al. 2011). For instance, TLR4 was shown to mediate lipopolysaccharide (LPS, a gram-negative endotoxin)-induced thrombocytopenia and TNF-α production in vivo (Andonegui et al. 2005; Cognasse et al. 2005; Aslam et al. 2006; Semple et al. 2007; Patrignani et al. 2006; Stahl et al. 2006; Zhang et al. 2009a). Also, TLR4-knockout mice displayed decreased circulating platelet counts and reticulated platelets, suggesting TLR4 to be of importance in platelet production (Andonegui et al. 2005; Jayachandran et al. 2007). Triggering of TLR2 on human platelets by Pam_3CSK_4, a synthetic ligand mimicking bacterial lipopeptide, enabled a thromboinflammatory response via activation of phosphoinositide 3-kinase (Blair et al. 2009). Platelet TLR2 and TLR4 were also involved in a setting of periodontitis, which is associated with an increased risk for cardiovascular diseases (Assinger et al. 2012). The periodontopathogens (*A. actinomycetemcomitans* and *P. gingivalis*) upregulated the expression of CD40L, known to mediate thrombotic and inflammatory processes, on human platelets via TLR2 and TLR4 (Assinger et al. 2012). Additionally, platelet TLR3 was shown to respond to poly I:C, indicating an effect on innate immune responses when detecting viral dsRNA (Anabel et al. 2014). Platelet TLR7, on the other hand, mediated host survival and platelet counts during infection with encephalomyocarditis virus (EMCV) in mice, independently of thrombosis (Koupenova et al. 2014). In contrast to the sensing of external danger signals, platelet TLR9 appears to be more important as a sensor for internal signals. It was shown that platelet TLR9 was functional in a setting of oxidative stress, through stimulation of platelet activation, granule secretion, aggregation in vitro, and thrombosis in vivo (Panigrahi et al. 2013). Notably, thrombocytopenia was shown to impair the host defense during pulmonary infection with the gram-positive bacteria *S. pneumoniae* in mice (van den Boogaard et al. 2015);

however, platelet activation by *S. pneumoniae* was subsequently shown to occur independently of TLR signaling (de Stoppelaar et al. 2016), indicating a different recognition mechanism of *S. pneumoniae* by platelets. Taken together, besides their hemostatic functions, platelets play a role as pathogen sensors in the blood circulation.

17.2.2 Pathogen Retainment

Platelets can harbor pathogens on their plasma membrane as well as internally (Youssefian et al. 2002; Flaujac et al. 2010), such as viruses (Assinger 2014; Flaujac et al. 2010), bacteria (Yeaman 2010a, b; Kerrigan and Cox 2010), and parasites (McMorran et al. 2009). Platelets were also involved in acute and chronic hepatic disease due to hepatitis B virus, via upregulating virus-specific CD8+ T cells and nonspecific inflammatory cells into the liver (Aiolfi and Sitia 2015). Interestingly, activated platelets were shown to surround or encapsulate the bacterium *Staphylococcus aureus*, forcing the pathogens into clusters resulting in restricted bacterial growth (Kraemer et al. 2011). This mechanism was dependent upon secretion of the antimicrobial peptide β-defensin and signaling through neutrophil extracellular trap (NET) formation (Kraemer et al. 2011). NETs have now been suggested to be involved in both infectious and noninfectious pathologies including thrombosis and coagulopathy, tumor growth, cardiac fibrosis, transfusion-related acute lung injury, sickle cell disease, storage of red blood cells, and diabetes (Fuchs et al. 2010; Thomas et al. 2012; Demers et al. 2012; Fuchs et al. 2013; Chen et al. 2014; Caudrillier et al. 2012; Wong et al. 2015; Martinod et al. 2016; Demers et al. 2016; Martinod et al. 2017; Jorch and Kubes 2017). Bacteria (methicillin-resistant *S. aureus* and *Bacillus cereus*) were also trapped on hepatic Kupffer cells, via engaging platelet adhesion receptor GP1b (Wong et al. 2013). In that study, infected GP1bα-deficient mice suffered more endothelial cell and Kupffer cell damage, resulting in more vascular leakage and rapid mortality (Wong et al. 2013). Activation of platelets during sepsis can contribute to disseminated intravascular coagulation, resulting in blood vessel occlusion, increased ischemia, and multiple organ failure, and it can also contribute to stimulation of pro- and anti-inflammatory cytokine production (de Stoppelaar et al., de Stoppelaar et al. 2014). This platelet activation is evident from increased surface P-selectin expression (Gawaz et al. 1997; Russwurm et al. 2002) and increased levels of triggering receptor expressed on myeloid cell-like transcript-1 (Washington et al. 2009) or PF-4 in mice (de Stoppelaar et al. 2013). Sepsis patients with platelet counts $<50 \times 10^9$/L, however, displayed a dysregulated host response which included increased endothelial cell activation without differences in coagulation activation (Claushuis et al. 2016). In addition, during sepsis neutrophils were also shown to be activated by platelet TLR4, enabling the release of NETs, which trapped bacteria in blood vessels of the liver and lungs (Clark et al. 2007). It was suggested that platelets can act as circulatory sentinel cells, sensing infectious agents and presenting them to neutrophils and/or the reticuloendothelial system (Aslam et al. 2006; Semple et al. 2007; Patrignani et al. 2006; Stahl et al. 2006; Zhang et al. 2009a). On one hand platelet-dependent NET formation may have its beneficial effects as bacteria are entangled in NETs; on the other hand, it may also be detrimental to the host. When neutrophils are activated by LPS and come into contact with the endothelium, there is little injury; however, if bound neutrophils encounter platelets with bound LPS, neutrophils are activated resulting in NET formation accompanied by release of reactive oxygen species, which damages the underlying endothelium (Clark et al. 2007). Furthermore, it has been reported that neutrophils are able to scan platelets for activation in the bloodstream via P-selectin ligand signaling, enhancing inflammation (Sreeramkumar et al. 2014). Platelet P-selectin, soluble or cellular, was also described to stimulate NET formation in mice through binding to neutrophil P-selectin glycoprotein ligand-1 (PSGL-1) (Etulain et al. 2015). Also in a setting of diabetes, in which neutrophils are more susceptible to NET formation, NETs were found to impair wound healing. It was therefore suggested that cleaving NETs or inhibiting their formation may be an effective approach to improve wound healing and reduce inflammation in diabetes (Wong et al. 2015).

17.2.3 Pathogen Elimination

Platelets have not only been implicated in detecting and retaining bacteria; they also appear to be involved in the clearance of bacterial infections. For instance, in infective endocarditis, thrombin-stimulated platelets were shown to facilitate the clearance of *streptococci* (Dankert et al. 1995). Additionally, in murine *P. gingivalis* infection, platelet TLR2 was implicated in the generation of platelet-neutrophil aggregates (Blair et al. 2009), and later it was demonstrated that phagocytosis of periodontopathogens by neutrophils occurred via platelets, TLR2, and plasma factors (Assinger et al. 2011). Also, platelets could redirect the course of the bacteria *Listeria monocytogenes* from less immunogenic phagocytes toward the more immunologically active $CD8\alpha^+$ dendritic cells in the spleen, using a mechanism dependent upon GP1b and complement component C3 (Verschoor et al. 2011). Furthermore, McMorran and colleagues elegantly demonstrated that activated platelets can kill the malarial parasite *Plasmodium* inside the red blood cell (McMorran et al. 2009). In a follow-up study, they elucidated that this platelet-mediated killing of *Plasmodium* was dependent upon platelet factor 4 (PF4 or CXCL4) and the erythrocyte Duffy-antigen receptor (Fy) (McMorran et al. 2012). This implies that Duffy-negative individuals, thus lacking Fy, would be incapable of eliminating this intraerythrocytic malarial parasite through activated platelets. In apparent contrast, however, a recent study reported that there is no evidence to support *Plasmodium* killing by platelets and that platelets do not contribute to a protective immune response which clears the *Plasmodium* infection, but that they activate a pathogenic response to *Plasmodium* using platelet CD40 (Gramaglia et al. 2017).

17.2.4 Pathogen Evasion

As a countermeasure, viruses and bacteria are able to evade these immune responses elicited by platelets. This can be supported by the fact that acute viral or bacterial infections often result in low platelet counts or thrombocytopenia. This has frequently been observed in the autoimmune bleeding disorder immune thrombocytopenia (ITP) (Cines et al. 2014). The pathogenesis of infection-induced platelet destruction is incompletely understood, but several mechanisms have been suggested. These include molecular mimicry between platelet antigens and viral/bacterial antigens, which triggers cross-reactive autoantibody production (Zhang et al. 2009b; Wright et al. 1996; Takahashi et al. 2004; Li et al. 2005; Chia et al. 1998). In addition, ITP patients infected with the gram-negative bacteria *Helicobacter pylori* displayed an elevation of their platelet counts following *Helicobacter pylori*-eradication therapy (Asahi et al. 2008). Similarly, the gram-negative bacterial endotoxin LPS also enhanced antiplatelet antibody-mediated phagocytosis of platelets in vitro (Semple et al. 2007), as well as an increased platelet clearance in vivo upon coinjection of antiplatelet antibodies and LPS in mice (Tremblay et al. 2007). Furthermore, C-reactive protein (CRP), an acute phase protein which rapidly increases during acute bacterial and viral infections and therefore is clinically used as a biomarker for acute infections and inflammation, was found to strongly enhance antibody-mediated platelet destruction both in vitro and in vivo in mice (Kapur et al. 2015a). CRP was also found to be elevated in pediatric ITP, and treatment with IVIg was correlated with increased platelet counts, decreased levels of CRP, and reduced clinical bleeding severity (Kapur et al. 2015a). Interestingly, an increased CRP value at diagnosis appeared to be predictive for slower platelet count recovery after 3 months (Kapur et al. 2015a). This finding was validated in a cohort of newly diagnosed adult ITP patients, in which increased CRP levels at diagnosis were shown to negatively predict recovery of platelet counts after steroid treatment (Rama Kishore et al. 2017).

17.3 Platelet-Target Cell Communication

17.3.1 Release of Mediators

Platelets can also elicit immune response through release of several mediators including platelet CD40L, which is released upon platelet activation giving rise to soluble CD40L (sCD40L) in circulation (Henn et al. 2001). Platelet-derived CD40L can also enhance CD8+ T-cell responses upon infection with *Listeria monocytogenes* (Elzey et al. 2008; Iannacone et al. 2005) and bind to dendritic cells (DCs) impairing differentiation, suppressing proinflammatory DC cytokines (IL-12p70 and TNF), and increasing the production of the anti-inflammatory cytokine IL-10 by DCs (Kissel et al. 2006). Furthermore, activated platelets were described to enhance lymphocyte adhesion to endothelial cells (Diacovo et al. 1998) and facilitate lymphocyte homing in high endothelial venules (Diacovo et al. 1996). Additionally, platelets are able to stimulate B-cell differentiation and Ab class switching via their CD40L (von Hundelshausen and Weber 2007; Elzey et al. 2003). Several other signaling pathways have been linked to platelet activation via the CD40L-CD40 axis, including NF-κB (Hachem et al. 2012; Malaver et al. 2009; Spinelli et al. 2010; Gambaryan et al. 2010; Karim et al. 2013; Liu et al. 2002), illustrating that platelets are well equipped for modulating adaptive immune responses via their CD40L and/or their secreted sCD40L.

Platelets can secrete a multitude of different cytokines and chemokines, most of them located within different granules, which may differently impact hemostasis and wound repair on one hand (Mazzucco et al. 2010), but they may also affect proinflammatory or anti-inflammatory immune reactions on the other hand (Assoian et al. 1983). TGF-β levels, for instance, seem regulated by platelets in an autoimmune setting of ITP, as low levels of TGF-β were observed during active ITP while those levels normalized again upon successful treatment of ITP which increased the platelet counts and normalized the T-regulatory cell numbers (Andersson et al. 2000, 2002). The platelet α granules contain a large variety of soluble immune factors, like chemokines, which include PF (CXCL4), RANTES (CCL5), β-thromboglobulin (β-TG, an isoform of CXCL7), and MIP-1α (CCL3) (Blair and Flaumenhaft 2009). These chemokines are released upon platelet activation and elicit diverse immunomodulatory responses. PF-4, for example, renders monocytes resistant to apoptosis and enhances their differentiation into macrophages (Gleissner 2012). Besides that, PF-4 can stimulate neutrophil adhesion to unstimulated endothelial cells and release content from platelet granules (Petersen et al. 1999). In contrast, platelet-derived β-TGs, which are proteolytic products of inactive precursors, can either stimulate or inhibit neutrophil activity (Brandt et al. 2000). On the other hand, PF4 can negatively regulate Th17 differentiation, thereby limiting murine cardiac allograft rejection (Shi et al. 2014a). Also, platelet-derived MIP-1α can enhance histamine release from basophils (Alam et al. 1992) and is chemotactic for T cells (Schall et al. 1993). In addition, platelet can also release IL-33 which was found to induce eosinophilic airway inflammation (Takeda et al. 2016).

17.3.2 Microparticle Shedding

Platelet microparticles (also referred to as microvesicles) are small extracellular vesicles produced by budding of the cytoplasmic membrane. Originally, they were described as "dust" released from activated platelets which supported thrombin generation, even without the presence of intact platelets (Wolf 1967). Generally, the size of microparticles ranges from ~100 to 1000 nm in diameter, although the majority are ~200 nm. Microparticles are distinct from exosomes, which are ~50–100 nm in diameter and originating via exocytosis from multivesicular bodies (Buzas et al. 2014). Platelets are potent producers of microparticles, as compared to other cell types, as was demonstrated by the high abundance of platelet microparticles in circulation using cryotransmission electron microscopy and gold nanospheres conjugated to antibodies against the platelet CD41 (Arraud et al. 2014). Microparticle formation is associated with increased levels of intracellular calcium, cytoskeletal rearrangement, and membrane phosphatidylserine (PS) exposure (Morel et al. 2011), which supports coagulation considering its anionic properties, but platelet microparticles express modest levels of tissue factor (TF) and seem to be less procoagulant than their monocyte-derived counterparts, which express PS as well as TF (Owens and Mackman 2011). The proteasome also appears to be important for microparticle formation, as the proteasome inhibitor bortezomib was found to reduce platelet microparticle release following stimulation with thrombin, LPS, or ADP (Gupta et al. 2014). Examination of platelet activation under physiological flow conditions revealed elongated membrane tendrils (up to 250 μM) emerging from platelets, so-called flow-induced protrusions (FLIPRs) (Tersteeg et al. 2014). FLIPRs also expose PS, recruit monocytes and neutrophils, and appear to shed off PS+ microparticles (Tersteeg et al. 2014). In contrast, however, PS- microparticles have also been described in body fluids (Arraud et al. 2014; Connor et al. 2010; Perez-Pujol et al. 2007; Cloutier et al. 2013), demonstrating the complexity of platelet microparticle production. Platelet microparticles have been described in various inflammatory conditions, in which platelets become activated (Nurden 2011; Reid and Webster 2012), and clinically they may be associated with disease progression. For example, in blood and synovial fluid of patients suffering from rheumatoid arthritis (RA), platelet microparticles were found to be elevated (Boilard et al. 2010; Gyorgy et al. 2012; Rousseau et al. 2015; Gitz et al. 2014; Boilard et al. 2012). Moreover, in vivo depletion of platelets in a murine RA model was shown to attenuate the inflammation (Boilard et al. 2010; Mott and Lazarus 2013). As microparticles are observed in sterile, as well as under inflammatory, conditions, it remains unclear how exactly platelet microparticle formation is regulated. Multiple signaling pathways may be leading up to platelet activation and triggering the production of platelet microparticles, such as via apoptosis, high shear forces, or platelet surface receptors. The disease setting, at least partly, influences how microparticles are shedded, as in RA the collagen receptor glycoprotein VI (GPVI) becomes activated, while in sepsis microparticles are produced via TLR4 signaling via LPS (Boilard et al. 2010; Brown and McIntyre 2011). Both these signals, however, are accompanied by increased IL-1 levels, indicating a common proinflammatory source. Additionally, microparticles can be formed by signaling through immune complexes, made up of bacterial components and well-conserved epitopes expressed by influenza viruses, engaging the platelet FcγRIIA (Boilard et al. 2014; Sun et al. 2013).

From a functional perspective, platelet microparticles can facilitate communication of platelets with other cells and thereby regulate immune functions, as platelet microparticles can contain a heterogeneous cargo consisting of various cytokines and chemokines (e.g., IL-1, RANTES), potent lipid mediators (e.g., thromboxane A_2), enzymes (e.g., inducible NO synthase), surface receptors (e.g., CD40L), auto-antigens (e.g., citrullinated fibrinogen), nucleic acids (e.g., microRNA), transcription factors (e.g., PPARγ, RuvB-like2, STAT3, STAT5a), or respiratory competent mitochondria (Laffont et al. 2013; Cloutier et al. 2013; Nurden 2011; Reid and Webster 2012; Boudreau et al. 2014; Ray et al. 2008; Garcia et al. 2005). As the microparticles can express PS and surface receptors, they interact with other cells via integrin and through the PS-binding proteins lactadherin (Dasgupta et al. 2009) and developmental endothelial locus-1 (Del-1) (Dasgupta et al. 2012). These proteins appear to be involved in the clearance of microparticles and the interaction with other cells, as Del-1 −/− and lactadherin −/− mice appear to have a high degree of microparticles in their plasma (Dasgupta et al. 2009, 2012). Transcription factors transported within platelet microparticles can enable transcellular effects, such as PPARγ, which was packed inside platelet microparticles and transferred to monocytes where it conveyed transcellular effects (Ray et al. 2008). Platelet-derived microparticles were also shown to inhibit IL-17 and IFN-γ production by T-regulatory cells (Tregs) and stimulate Treg stability during inflammation, in a P-selectin-dependent manner (Dinkla et al. 2016). Currently, however, more research is required to establish the nature of the specific signals which lead to the internalization of microparticles by the recipient target cells. Microparticles appear to be important biomarkers in inflammatory disorders, but further delineation of their function, mechanisms of generation, and routing are warranted, in order to better understand their role in health and disease (Melki et al. 2017).

17.3.3 RNA Transfer

Platelets are known to express and secrete many different molecules during platelet activation, and they do so via distinct mechanisms (Blair and Flaumenhaft 2009; Italiano et al. 2008; Sehgal and Storrie 2007; White and Rompietti 2007). Despite being anucleate, platelets have been shown to express significant amounts of RNA, including mRNAs (e.g., (pre)mature RNA), structural and catalytic RNAs (e.g., ribosomal and tRNA), regulatory RNAs (e.g., microRNA), and non-coding RNA (e.g., antisense RNA) (Rowley et al. 2011, 2012; Lood et al. 2010; Healy et al. 2006; Goodall et al. 2010; Simon et al. 2014; Edelstein et al. 2013; Ple et al. 2012; McManus et al. 2013; Freedman et al. 2010; Raghavachari et al. 2007; Risitano et al. 2012; Clancy and Freedman 2014; Laffont et al. 2013; Gidlof et al. 2013; Landry et al. 2009; Rondina and Weyrich 2015). Moreover, platelets also possess the molecular machinery which allows them to translate mRNA into proteins and to transfer RNA to recipient cells, such as platelet microRNA-223 which is transferred to human umbilical vein endothelial cells (Risitano et al. 2012; Clancy and Freedman 2014; Laffont et al. 2013; Gidlof et al. 2013; Rondina and Weyrich 2015). Intercellular transfer of platelet RNA to target cells can occur via platelet microparticles, as described earlier. However, the content of platelet RNA transcript does not fully match to the platelet proteome content (Burkhart et al. 2012). The role of platelet mRNA and its impact on platelet function in both health and disease is currently actively being investigated (Schubert et al. 2014).

17.3.4 Platelet MHC Class I Signaling

Platelets harbor two different types of MHC class I molecules: platelet plasma membrane bound and intracellularly (Shulman et al. 1962). The MHC class I molecules on the platelet plasma membrane are mainly adsorbed from plasma. The platelet-membrane MHC class I molecules appear to be somewhat instable, as can passively dissociate from the platelet during storage or can be eluted from the membrane upon chloroquine diphosphate or acid treatment, without affecting the platelet-membrane integrity (Blumberg et al. 1984; Kao et al. 1986; Kao 1987, 1988; Neumuller et al. 1993; Ghio et al. 1999; Gouttefangeas et al. 2000). Interestingly, denatured MHC class I can elicit faulty interactions with CD8+ T cells, energizing CTLs, following transfusions. For instance, allogeneic platelet MHC class I molecules are incapable of stimulating CTL-mediated cytotoxicity on their own (Gouttefangeas et al. 2000) but can mediate an immunosuppressive-like reaction to transfused blood cells. CBA mice transfused with allogeneic BALB/c platelets accepted donor-specific skin grafts, in contrast to non-transfused recipients (Aslam et al. 2008). This implies that allogeneic platelets may inhibit T-cell-mediated cytotoxicity reactions, like skin graft rejections. Intracellular platelet MHC class I, on the other hand, is associated with α granules and generally consists of intact integral membrane proteins associated with β2-microglobulin (Zufferey et al. 2014). It was also demonstrated that platelets contain the entire proteasome system, including TAP molecules, but the endoplasmic reticulum is absent. Interestingly, the proteasome function was found to be critical for thrombopoiesis (Shi et al. 2014b). In syngeneic settings, platelet activation can lead to expression of nascent MHC class I molecules, which are capable of presenting antigens to CD8+ T cells. Activated platelets were shown to present malarial peptides to malaria-specific T cells, resulting in enhanced immunity against the parasite (Chapman et al. 2012). Therefore, the type of platelet MHC class I, bound to the platelet plasma membrane or intracellularly, will determine the response toward T cells (suppression or activation).

A brief summary of the immune-sensing functions of platelets is depicted in Fig. 17.1.

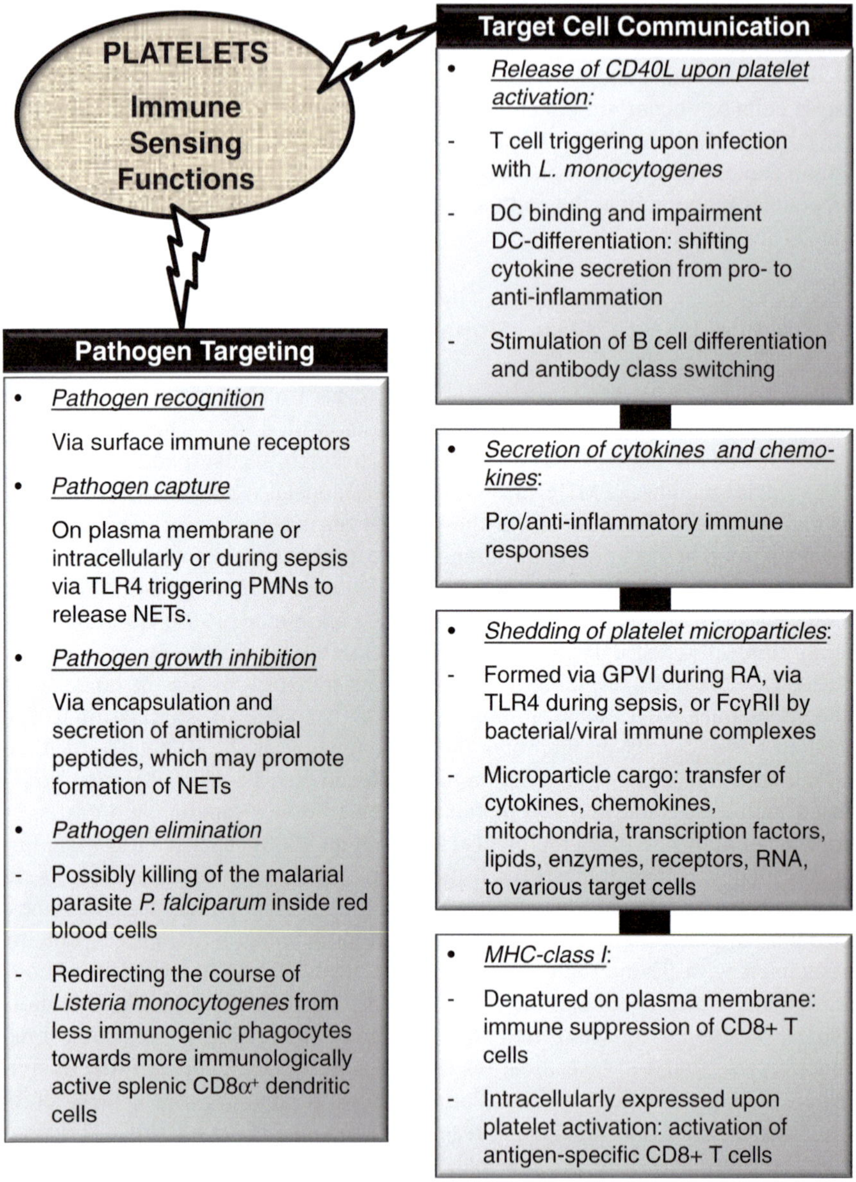

Fig. 17.1 Immune functions of platelets. The immune-sensing functions of platelets, generally depicted as pathogen targeting and target cell communication

Conclusions

Platelets have traditionally been acknowledged as master regulators of hemostasis. It has now, however, become evident that platelets are in fact much more diverse and are capable of immune-sensing functions as well. Platelets can not only enforce sophisticated protection mechanisms against invading pathogens but are also capable of impacting and regulating immune functions in a large variety of cells. They do so by utilizing numerous mechanisms, via diverse surface molecules, through secretion of several pro- and inflammatory mediators and through release of microparticles carrying a varying cargo. These relatively novel aspects have shed new light on platelet functions beyond hemostasis and will open up new avenues of research.

References

Aiolfi R, Sitia G. Chronic hepatitis B: role of anti-platelet therapy in inflammation control. Cell Mol Immunol. 2015;12(3):264–8.

Alam R, Forsythe PA, Stafford S, Lett-Brown MA, Grant JA. Macrophage inflammatory protein-1 alpha activates basophils and mast cells. J Exp Med. 1992;176:781–6.

Anabel AS, Eduardo PC, Pedro Antonio HC, Carlos SM, Juana NM, Honorio TA, Nicolas VS, Sergio Roberto AR. Human platelets express Toll-like receptor 3 and respond to poly I:C. Hum Immunol. 2014;75:1244–51.

Andersson PO, Olsson A, Wadenvik H. Reduced transforming growth factor-beta1 production by mononuclear cells from patients with active chronic idiopathic thrombocytopenic purpura. Br J Haematol. 2002;116:862–7.

Andersson PO, Stockelberg D, Jacobsson S, Wadenvik H. A transforming growth factor-beta1-mediated bystander immune suppression could be associated with remission of chronic idiopathic thrombocytopenic purpura. Ann Hematol. 2000;79:507–13.

Andonegui G, Kerfoot SM, McNagny K, Ebbert KV, Patel KD, Kubes P. Platelets express functional Toll-like receptor-4. Blood. 2005;106:2417–23.

Arraud N, Linares R, Tan S, Gounou C, Pasquet JM, Mornet S, Brisson AR. Extracellular vesicles from blood plasma: determination of their morphology, size, phenotype and concentration. J Thromb Haemost. 2014;12:614–27.

Asahi A, Nishimoto T, Okazaki Y, Suzuki H, Masaoka T, Kawakami Y, Ikeda Y, Kuwana M. Helicobacter pylori eradication shifts monocyte Fcgamma receptor balance toward inhibitory FcgammaRIIB in immune thrombocytopenic purpura patients. J Clin Invest. 2008;118:2939–49.

Aslam R, Speck ER, Kim M, Crow AR, Bang KW, Nestel FP, Ni H, Lazarus AH, Freedman J, Semple JW. Platelet Toll-like receptor expression modulates lipopolysaccharide-induced thrombocytopenia and tumor necrosis factor-alpha production in vivo. Blood. 2006;107:637–41.

Aslam R, Speck ER, Kim M, Freedman J, Semple JW. Transfusion-related immunomodulation by platelets is dependent on their expression of MHC Class I molecules and is independent of white cells. Transfusion. 2008;48:1778–86.

Assinger A. Platelets and infection – an emerging role of platelets in viral infection. Front Immunol. 2014;5:649.

Assinger A, Laky M, Badrnya S, Esfandeyari A, Volf I. Periodontopathogens induce expression of CD40L on human platelets via TLR2 and TLR4. Thromb Res. 2012;130:e73–8.

Assinger A, Laky M, Schabbauer G, Hirschl AM, Buchberger E, Binder BR, Volf I. Efficient phagocytosis of periodontopathogens by neutrophils requires plasma factors, platelets and TLR2. J Thromb Haemost. 2011;9:799–809.

Assoian RK, Komoriya A, Meyers CA, Miller DM, Sporn MB. Transforming growth factor-beta in human platelets. Identification of a major storage site, purification, and characterization. J Biol Chem. 1983;258:7155–60.

Blair P, Flaumenhaft R. Platelet alpha-granules: basic biology and clinical correlates. Blood Rev. 2009;23:177–89.

Blair P, Rex S, Vitseva O, Beaulieu L, Tanriverdi K, Chakrabarti S, Hayashi C, Genco CA, Iafrati M, Freedman JE. Stimulation of Toll-like receptor 2 in human platelets induces a thromboinflammatory response through activation of phosphoinositide 3-kinase. Circ Res. 2009;104:346–54.

Blumberg N, Masel D, Mayer T, Horan P, Heal J. Removal of HLA-AB antigens from platelets. Blood. 1984;63:448–50.

Boilard E, Blanco P, Nigrovic PA. Platelets: active players in the pathogenesis of arthritis and SLE. Nat Rev Rheumatol. 2012;8:534–42.

Boilard E, Nigrovic PA, Larabee K, Watts GF, Coblyn JS, Weinblatt ME, Massarotti EM, Remold-O'Donnell E, Farndale RW, Ware J, Lee DM. Platelets amplify inflammation in arthritis via collagen-dependent microparticle production. Science. 2010;327:580–3.

Boilard E, Pare G, Rousseau M, Cloutier N, Dubuc I, Levesque T, Borgeat P, Flamand L. Influenza virus H1N1 activates platelets through FcgammaRIIA signaling and thrombin generation. Blood. 2014;123:2854–63.

Boudreau LH, Duchez AC, Cloutier N, Soulet D, Martin N, Bollinger J, Pare A, Rousseau M, Naika GS, Levesque T, Laflamme C, Marcoux G, Lambeau G, Farndale RW, Pouliot M, Hamzeh-Cognasse H, Cognasse F, Garraud O, Nigrovic PA, Guderley H, Lacroix S, Thibault L, Semple JW, Gelb MH, Boilard E. Platelets release mitochondria serving as substrate for bactericidal group IIA-secreted phospholipase A2 to promote inflammation. Blood. 2014;124:2173–83.

Brandt E, Petersen F, Ludwig A, Ehlert JE, Bock L, Flad HD. The beta-thromboglobulins and platelet factor 4: blood platelet-derived CXC chemokines with divergent roles in early neutrophil regulation. J Leukoc Biol. 2000;67:471–8.

Brown GT, McIntyre TM. Lipopolysaccharide signaling without a nucleus: kinase cascades stimulate platelet shedding of proinflammatory IL-1beta-rich microparticles. J Immunol. 2011;186:5489–96.

Burkhart JM, Vaudel M, Gambaryan S, Radau S, Walter U, Martens L, Geiger J, Sickmann A, Zahedi RP. The first comprehensive and quantitative analysis of human platelet protein composition allows the comparative analysis of structural and functional pathways. Blood. 2012;120:e73–82.

Buzas EI, Gyorgy B, Nagy G, Falus A, Gay S. Emerging role of extracellular vesicles in inflammatory diseases. Nat Rev Rheumatol. 2014;10:356–64.

Caudrillier A, Kessenbrock K, Gilliss BM, Nguyen JX, Marques MB, Monestier M, Toy P, Werb Z, Looney MR. Platelets induce neutrophil extracellular traps in transfusion-related acute lung injury. J Clin Invest. 2012;122:2661–71.

Chapman LM, Aggrey AA, Field DJ, Srivastava K, Ture S, Yui K, Topham DJ, Baldwin WM III, Morrell CN. Platelets present antigen in the context of MHC class I. J Immunol. 2012;189:916–23.

Chen G, Zhang D, Fuchs TA, Manwani D, Wagner DD, Frenette PS. Heme-induced neutrophil extracellular traps contribute to the pathogenesis of sickle cell disease. Blood. 2014;123:3818–27.

Chia WK, Blanchette V, Mody M, Wright JF, Freedman J. Characterization of HIV-1-specific antibodies and HIV-1-crossreactive antibodies to platelets in HIV-1-infected haemophiliac patients. Br J Haematol. 1998;103:1014–22.

Cines DB, Cuker A, Semple JW. Pathogenesis of immune thrombocytopenia. Presse Med. 2014;43:e49–59.

Clancy L, Freedman JE. New paradigms in thrombosis: novel mediators and biomarkers platelet RNA transfer. J Thromb Thrombolysis. 2014;37:12–6.

Clark SR, Ma AC, Tavener SA, McDonald B, Goodarzi Z, Kelly MM, Patel KD, Chakrabarti S, McAvoy E, Sinclair GD, Keys EM, Allen-Vercoe E, Devinney R, Doig CJ, Green FH, Kubes P. Platelet TLR4 activates neutrophil extracellular traps to ensnare bacteria in septic blood. Nat Med. 2007;13:463–9.

Claushuis TA, van Vught LA, Scicluna BP, Wiewel MA, Klein Klouwenberg PM, Hoogendijk AJ, Ong DS, Cremer OL, Horn J, Franitza M, Toliat MR, Nurnberg P, Zwinderman AH, Bonten MJ, Schultz MJ, van der Poll T. Thrombocytopenia is associated with a dysregulated host response in critically ill sepsis patients. Blood. 2016;127:3062–72.

Cloutier N, Tan S, Boudreau LH, Cramb C, Subbaiah R, Lahey L, Albert A, Shnayder R, Gobezie R, Nigrovic PA, Farndale RW, Robinson WH, Brisson A, Lee DM, Boilard E. The exposure of autoantigens by microparticles underlies the formation of potent inflammatory components: the microparticle-associated immune complexes. EMBO Mol Med. 2013;5:235–49.

Cognasse F, Hamzeh H, Chavarin P, Acquart S, Genin C, Garraud O. Evidence of Toll-like receptor molecules on human platelets. Immunol Cell Biol. 2005;83:196–8.

Connor DE, Exner T, Ma DD, Joseph JE. The majority of circulating platelet-derived microparticles fail to bind annexin V, lack phospholipid-dependent procoagulant activity and demonstrate greater expression of glycoprotein Ib. Thromb Haemost. 2010;103:1044–52.

Dankert J, van der Werff J, Zaat SA, Joldersma W, Klein D, Hess J. Involvement of bactericidal factors from thrombin-stimulated platelets in clearance of adherent viridans streptococci in experimental infective endocarditis. Infect Immun. 1995;63:663–71.

Dasgupta SK, Abdel-Monem H, Niravath P, Le A, Bellera RV, Langlois K, Nagata S, Rumbaut RE, Thiagarajan P. Lactadherin and clearance of platelet-derived microvesicles. Blood. 2009;113:1332–9.

Dasgupta SK, Le A, Chavakis T, Rumbaut RE, Thiagarajan P. Developmental endothelial locus-1 (Del-1) mediates clearance of platelet microparticles by the endothelium. Circulation. 2012;125:1664–72.

de Stoppelaar SF, Claushuis TA, Schaap MC, Hou B, van der Poll T, Nieuwland R, van't Veeer C. Toll-like receptor signalling is not involved in platelet response to Streptococcus pneumoniae in vitro or in vivo. PLoS One. 2016;11:e0156977.

de Stoppelaar SF, van't Veeer C, van der Poll T. The role of platelets in sepsis. Thromb Haemost. 2014;112:666–77.

de Stoppelaar SF, van't Veer C, van den Boogaard FE, Nieuwland R, Hoogendijk AJ, de Boer OJ, Roelofs JJ, van der Poll T. Protease activated receptor 4 limits bacterial growth and lung pathology during late stage Streptococcus pneumoniae induced pneumonia in mice. Thromb Haemost. 2013;110:582–92.

Demers M, Krause DS, Schatzberg D, Martinod K, Voorhees JR, Fuchs TA, Scadden DT, Wagner DD. Cancers predispose neutrophils to release extracellular DNA traps that contribute to cancer-associated thrombosis. Proc Natl Acad Sci U S A. 2012;109:13076–81.

Demers M, Wong SL, Martinod K, Gallant M, Cabral JE, Wang Y, Wagner DD. Priming of neutrophils toward NETosis promotes tumor growth. Oncoimmunology. 2016;5:e1134073.

Diacovo TG, Catalina MD, Siegelman MH, von Andrian UH. Circulating activated platelets reconstitute lymphocyte homing and immunity in L-selectin-deficient mice. J Exp Med. 1998;187:197–204.

Diacovo TG, Puri KD, Warnock RA, Springer TA, von Andrian UH. Platelet-mediated lymphocyte delivery to high endothelial venules. Science. 1996;273:252–5.

Dinkla S, van CB, van der Heijden WA, He X, Wallbrecher R, Dumitriu IE, van der Ven AJ, Bosman GJ, Koenen HJ, Joosten I. Platelet microparticles inhibit IL-17 production by regulatory T cells through P-selectin. Blood. 2016;127:1976–86.

Edelstein LC, Simon LM, Montoya RT, Holinstat M, Chen ES, Bergeron A, Kong X, Nagalla S, Mohandas N, Cohen DE, Dong JF, Shaw C, Bray PF. Racial differences in human platelet PAR4 reactivity reflect expression of PCTP and miR-376c. Nat Med. 2013;19: 1609–16.

Elzey BD, Schmidt NW, Crist SA, Kresowik TP, Harty JT, Nieswandt B, Ratliff TL. Platelet-derived CD154 enables T-cell priming and protection against Listeria monocytogenes challenge. Blood. 2008;111:3684–91.

Elzey BD, Tian J, Jensen RJ, Swanson AK, Lees JR, Lentz SR, Stein CS, Nieswandt B, Wang Y, Davidson BL, Ratliff TL. Platelet-mediated modulation of adaptive immunity. A communication link between innate and adaptive immune compartments. Immunity. 2003;19:9–19.

Etulain J, Martinod K, Wong SL, Cifuni SM, Schattner M, Wagner DD. P-selectin promotes neutrophil extracellular trap formation in mice. Blood. 2015;126:242–6.
Flaujac C, Boukour S, Cramer-Borde E. Platelets and viruses: an ambivalent relationship. Cell Mol Life Sci. 2010;67:545–56.
Freedman JE, Larson MG, Tanriverdi K, O'Donnell CJ, Morin K, Hakanson AS, Vasan RS, Johnson AD, Iafrati MD, Benjamin EJ. Relation of platelet and leukocyte inflammatory transcripts to body mass index in the Framingham heart study. Circulation. 2010;122:119–29.
Fuchs TA, Alvarez JJ, Martinod K, Bhandari AA, Kaufman RM, Wagner DD. Neutrophils release extracellular DNA traps during storage of red blood cell units. Transfusion. 2013;53:3210–6.
Fuchs TA, Brill A, Duerschmied D, Schatzberg D, Monestier M, Myers DD Jr, Wrobleski SK, Wakefield TW, Hartwig JH, Wagner DD. Extracellular DNA traps promote thrombosis. Proc Natl Acad Sci U S A. 2010;107:15880–5.
Gambaryan S, Kobsar A, Rukoyatkina N, Herterich S, Geiger J, Smolenski A, Lohmann SM, Walter U. Thrombin and collagen induce a feedback inhibitory signaling pathway in platelets involving dissociation of the catalytic subunit of protein kinase A from an NFkappaB-IkappaB complex. J Biol Chem. 2010;285:18352–63.
Garcia BA, Smalley DM, Cho H, Shabanowitz J, Ley K, Hunt DF. The platelet microparticle proteome. J Proteome Res. 2005;4:1516–21.
Gawaz M, Dickfeld T, Bogner C, Fateh-Moghadam S, Neumann FJ. Platelet function in septic multiple organ dysfunction syndrome. Intensive Care Med. 1997;23:379–85.
Ghio M, Contini P, Mazzei C, Brenci S, Barberis G, Filaci G, Indiveri F, Puppo F. Soluble HLA class I, HLA class II, and Fas ligand in blood components: a possible key to explain the immunomodulatory effects of allogeneic blood transfusions. Blood. 1999;93:1770–7.
Gidlof O, van der Brug M, Ohman J, Gilje P, Olde B, Wahlestedt C, Erlinge D. Platelets activated during myocardial infarction release functional miRNA, which can be taken up by endothelial cells and regulate ICAM1 expression. Blood. 2013;121:3908–26.
Gitz E, Pollitt AY, Gitz-Francois JJ, Alshehri O, Mori J, Montague S, Nash GB, Douglas MR, Gardiner EE, Andrews RK, Buckley CD, Harrison P, Watson SP. CLEC-2 expression is maintained on activated platelets and on platelet microparticles. Blood. 2014;124:2262–70.
Gleissner CA. Macrophage phenotype modulation by CXCL4 in atherosclerosis. Front Physiol. 2012;3:1.
Goodall AH, Burns P, Salles I, Macaulay IC, Jones CI, Ardissino D, de BB, Bray SL, Deckmyn H, Dudbridge F, Fitzgerald DJ, Garner SF, Gusnanto A, Koch K, Langford C, O'Connor MN, Rice CM, Stemple D, Stephens J, Trip MD, Zwaginga JJ, Samani NJ, Watkins NA, Maguire PB, Ouwehand WH. Transcription profiling in human platelets reveals LRRFIP1 as a novel protein regulating platelet function. Blood. 2010;116:4646–56.
Gouttefangeas C, Diehl M, Keilholz W, Hornlein RF, Stevanovic S, Rammensee HG. Thrombocyte HLA molecules retain nonrenewable endogenous peptides of megakaryocyte lineage and do not stimulate direct allocytotoxicity in vitro. Blood. 2000;95:3168–75.
Gramaglia I, Velez J, Combes V, Grau GE, Wree M, van der Heyde HC. Platelets activate a pathogenic response to blood-stage Plasmodium infection but not a protective immune response. Blood. 2017;129:1669–79.
Gupta N, Li W, Willard B, Silverstein RL, McIntyre TM. Proteasome proteolysis supports stimulated platelet function and thrombosis. Arterioscler Thromb Vasc Biol. 2014;34:160–8.
Gyorgy B, Szabo TG, Turiak L, Wright M, Herczeg P, Ledeczi Z, Kittel A, Polgar A, Toth K, Derfalvi B, Zelenak G, Borocz I, Carr B, Nagy G, Vekey K, Gay S, Falus A, Buzas EI. Improved flow cytometric assessment reveals distinct microvesicle (cell-derived microparticle) signatures in joint diseases. PLoS One. 2012;7:e49726.
Hachem A, Yacoub D, Zaid Y, Mourad W, Merhi Y. Involvement of nuclear factor kappaB in platelet CD40 signaling. Biochem Biophys Res Commun. 2012;425:58–63.
Healy AM, Pickard MD, Pradhan AD, Wang Y, Chen Z, Croce K, Sakuma M, Shi C, Zago AC, Garasic J, Damokosh AI, Dowie TL, Poisson L, Lillie J, Libby P, Ridker PM, Simon DI. Platelet expression profiling and clinical validation of myeloid-related protein-14 as a novel determinant of cardiovascular events. Circulation. 2006;113:2278–84.

Henn V, Steinbach S, Buchner K, Presek P, Kroczek RA. The inflammatory action of CD40 ligand (CD154) expressed on activated human platelets is temporally limited by coexpressed CD40. Blood. 2001;98:1047–54.
Iannacone M, Sitia G, Isogawa M, Marchese P, Castro MG, Lowenstein PR, Chisari FV, Ruggeri ZM, Guidotti LG. Platelets mediate cytotoxic T lymphocyte-induced liver damage. Nat Med. 2005;11:1167–9.
Italiano JE Jr, Richardson JL, Patel-Hett S, Battinelli E, Zaslavsky A, Short S, Ryeom S, Folkman J, Klement GL. Angiogenesis is regulated by a novel mechanism: pro- and antiangiogenic proteins are organized into separate platelet alpha granules and differentially released. Blood. 2008;111:1227–33.
Janeway CA Jr. The immune system evolved to discriminate infectious nonself from noninfectious self. Immunol Today. 1992;13:11–6.
Janeway CA Jr, Medzhitov R. Innate immune recognition. Annu Rev Immunol. 2002;20:197–216.
Jayachandran M, Brunn GJ, Karnicki K, Miller RS, Owen WG, Miller VM. In vivo effects of lipopolysaccharide and TLR4 on platelet production and activity: implications for thrombotic risk. J Appl Physiol (1985). 2007;102:429–33.
Jorch SK, Kubes P. An emerging role for neutrophil extracellular traps in noninfectious disease. Nat Med. 2017;23:279–87.
Kao KJ. Plasma and platelet HLA in normal individuals: quantitation by competitive enzyme-linked immunoassay. Blood. 1987;70:282–6.
Kao KJ. Selective elution of HLA antigens and beta 2-microglobulin from human platelets by chloroquine diphosphate. Transfusion. 1988;28:14–7.
Kao KJ, Cook DJ, Scornik JC. Quantitative analysis of platelet surface HLA by W6/32 anti-HLA monoclonal antibody. Blood. 1986;68:627–32.
Kapur R, Heitink-Polle KM, Porcelijn L, Bentlage AE, Bruin MC, Visser R, Roos D, Schasfoort RB, de HM, van der Schoot CE, Vidarsson G. C-reactive protein enhances IgG-mediated phagocyte responses and thrombocytopenia. Blood. 2015a;125:1793–802.
Kapur R, Semple JW. Platelets as immune-sensing cells. Blood Adv. 2016a;1:10–4.
Kapur R, Semple JW. The nonhemostatic immune functions of platelets. Semin Hematol. 2016b;53(Suppl 1):S2–6.
Kapur R, Zufferey A, Boilard E, Semple JW. Nouvelle cuisine: platelets served with inflammation. J Immunol. 2015b;194:5579–87.
Karim ZA, Zhang J, Banerjee M, Chicka MC, Al HR, Hamilton TR, Roche PA, Whiteheart SW. IkappaB kinase phosphorylation of SNAP-23 controls platelet secretion. Blood. 2013;121:4567–74.
Kerrigan SW, Cox D. Platelet-bacterial interactions. Cell Mol Life Sci. 2010;67:513–23.
Kissel K, Berber S, Nockher A, Santoso S, Bein G, Hackstein H. Human platelets target dendritic cell differentiation and production of proinflammatory cytokines. Transfusion. 2006;46:818–27.
Koupenova M, Vitseva O, MacKay CR, Beaulieu LM, Benjamin EJ, Mick E, Kurt-Jones EA, Ravid K, Freedman JE. Platelet-TLR7 mediates host survival and platelet count during viral infection in the absence of platelet-dependent thrombosis. Blood. 2014;124:791–802.
Kraemer BF, Campbell RA, Schwertz H, Cody MJ, Franks Z, Tolley ND, Kahr WH, Lindemann S, Seizer P, Yost CC, Zimmerman GA, Weyrich AS. Novel anti-bacterial activities of beta-defensin 1 in human platelets: suppression of pathogen growth and signaling of neutrophil extracellular trap formation. PLoS Pathog. 2011;7:e1002355.
Laffont B, Corduan A, Ple H, Duchez AC, Cloutier N, Boilard E, Provost P. Activated platelets can deliver mRNA regulatory Ago2*microRNA complexes to endothelial cells via microparticles. Blood. 2013;122:253–61.
Landry P, Plante I, Ouellet DL, Perron MP, Rousseau G, Provost P. Existence of a microRNA pathway in anucleate platelets. Nat Struct Mol Biol. 2009;16:961–6.
Lefrancais E, Ortiz-Munoz G, Caudrillier A, Mallavia B, Liu F, Sayah DM, Thornton EE, Headley MB, David T, Coughlin SR, Krummel MF, Leavitt AD, Passegue E, Looney MR. The lung is a site of platelet biogenesis and a reservoir for haematopoietic progenitors. Nature. 2017;544:105–9.

Li Z, Nardi MA, Karpatkin S. Role of molecular mimicry to HIV-1 peptides in HIV-1-related immunologic thrombocytopenia. Blood. 2005;106:572–6.
Liu F, Morris S, Epps J, Carroll R. Demonstration of an activation regulated NF-kappaB/I--kappaBalpha complex in human platelets. Thromb Res. 2002;106:199–203.
Lood C, Amisten S, Gullstrand B, Jonsen A, Allhorn M, Truedsson L, Sturfelt G, Erlinge D, Bengtsson AA. Platelet transcriptional profile and protein expression in patients with systemic lupus erythematosus: up-regulation of the type I interferon system is strongly associated with vascular disease. Blood. 2010;116:1951–7.
Machlus KR, Italiano JE Jr. The incredible journey: from megakaryocyte development to platelet formation. J Cell Biol. 2013;201:785–96.
Malaver E, Romaniuk MA, D'Atri LP, Pozner RG, Negrotto S, Benzadon R, Schattner M. NF-kappaB inhibitors impair platelet activation responses. J Thromb Haemost. 2009;7:1333–43.
Martinod K, Witsch T, Erpenbeck L, Savchenko A, Hayashi H, Cherpokova D, Gallant M, Mauler M, Cifuni SM, Wagner DD. Peptidylarginine deiminase 4 promotes age-related organ fibrosis. J Exp Med. 2017;214:439–58.
Martinod K, Witsch T, Farley K, Gallant M, Remold-O'Donnell E, Wagner DD. Neutrophil elastase-deficient mice form neutrophil extracellular traps in an experimental model of deep vein thrombosis. J Thromb Haemost. 2016;14:551–8.
Mazzucco L, Borzini P, Gope R. Platelet-derived factors involved in tissue repair-from signal to function. Transfus Med Rev. 2010;24:218–34.
McManus DD, Beaulieu LM, Mick E, Tanriverdi K, Larson MG, Keaney JF Jr, Benjamin EJ, Freedman JE. Relationship among circulating inflammatory proteins, platelet gene expression, and cardiovascular risk. Arterioscler Thromb Vasc Biol. 2013;33:2666–73.
McMorran BJ, Marshall VM, de GC, Drysdale KE, Shabbar M, Smyth GK, Corbin JE, Alexander WS, Foote SJ. Platelets kill intraerythrocytic malarial parasites and mediate survival to infection. Science. 2009;323:797–800.
McMorran BJ, Wieczorski L, Drysdale KE, Chan JA, Huang HM, Smith C, Mitiku C, Beeson JG, Burgio G, Foote SJ. Platelet factor 4 and Duffy antigen required for platelet killing of Plasmodium falciparum. Science. 2012;338:1348–51.
Melki I, Tessandier N, Zufferey A, Boilard E. Platelet microvesicles in health and disease. Platelets. 2017;28(3):1–8.
Morel O, Jesel L, Freyssinet JM, Toti F. Cellular mechanisms underlying the formation of circulating microparticles. Arterioscler Thromb Vasc Biol. 2011;31:15–26.
Mott PJ, Lazarus AH. CD44 antibodies and immune thrombocytopenia in the amelioration of murine inflammatory arthritis. PLoS One. 2013;8:e65805.
Neumuller J, Tohidast-Akrad M, Fischer M, Mayr WR. Influence of chloroquine or acid treatment of human platelets on the antigenicity of HLA and the 'thrombocyte-specific' glycoproteins Ia/IIa, IIb, and IIb/IIIa. Vox Sang. 1993;65:223–31.
Nurden AT. Platelets, inflammation and tissue regeneration. Thromb Haemost. 2011;105(Suppl 1):S13–33.
Owens AP III, Mackman N. Microparticles in hemostasis and thrombosis. Circ Res. 2011;108:1284–97.
Panigrahi S, Ma Y, Hong L, Gao D, West XZ, Salomon RG, Byzova TV, Podrez EA. Engagement of platelet toll-like receptor 9 by novel endogenous ligands promotes platelet hyperreactivity and thrombosis. Circ Res. 2013;112:103–12.
Patrignani P, Di FC, Tacconelli S, Moretta V, Baccante G, Sciulli MG, Ricciotti E, Capone ML, Antonucci I, Guglielmi MD, Stuppia L, Porreca E. Reduced thromboxane biosynthesis in carriers of toll-like receptor 4 polymorphisms in vivo. Blood. 2006;107:3572–4.
Perez-Pujol S, Marker PH, Key NS. Platelet microparticles are heterogeneous and highly dependent on the activation mechanism: studies using a new digital flow cytometer. Cytometry A. 2007;71:38–45.
Petersen F, Bock L, Flad HD, Brandt E. Platelet factor 4-induced neutrophil-endothelial cell interaction: involvement of mechanisms and functional consequences different from those elicited by interleukin-8. Blood. 1999;94:4020–8.

Ple H, Maltais M, Corduan A, Rousseau G, Madore F, Provost P. Alteration of the platelet transcriptome in chronic kidney disease. Thromb Haemost. 2012;108:605–15.
Raghavachari N, Xu X, Harris A, Villagra J, Logun C, Barb J, Solomon MA, Suffredini AF, Danner RL, Kato G, Munson PJ, Morris SM Jr, Gladwin MT. Amplified expression profiling of platelet transcriptome reveals changes in arginine metabolic pathways in patients with sickle cell disease. Circulation. 2007;115:1551–62.
Rama Kishore Y, Prashantha B, Girish M, Manaswitha B. Increased C-reactive protein levels at diagnosis negatively predict platelet count recovery after steroid-treatment in newly diagnosed adult immune thrombocytopenia patients. Thromb Res. 2017;152:61–3.
Ray DM, Spinelli SL, Pollock SJ, Murant TI, O'Brien JJ, Blumberg N, Francis CW, Taubman MB, Phipps RP. Peroxisome proliferator-activated receptor gamma and retinoid X receptor transcription factors are released from activated human platelets and shed in microparticles. Thromb Haemost. 2008;99:86–95.
Reid VL, Webster NR. Role of microparticles in sepsis. Br J Anaesth. 2012;109:503–13.
Risitano A, Beaulieu LM, Vitseva O, Freedman JE. Platelets and platelet-like particles mediate intercellular RNA transfer. Blood. 2012;119:6288–95.
Rondina MT, Weyrich AS. Regulation of the genetic code in megakaryocytes and platelets. J Thromb Haemost. 2015;13(Suppl 1):S26–32.
Rousseau M, Belleannee C, Duchez AC, Cloutier N, Levesque T, Jacques F, Perron J, Nigrovic PA, Dieude M, Hebert MJ, Gelb MH, Boilard E. Detection and quantification of microparticles from different cellular lineages using flow cytometry. Evaluation of the impact of secreted phospholipase A2 on microparticle assessment. PLoS One. 2015;10:e0116812.
Rowley JW, Oler AJ, Tolley ND, Hunter BN, Low EN, Nix DA, Yost CC, Zimmerman GA, Weyrich AS. Genome-wide RNA-seq analysis of human and mouse platelet transcriptomes. Blood. 2011;118:e101–11.
Rowley JW, Schwertz H, Weyrich AS. Platelet mRNA: the meaning behind the message. Curr Opin Hematol. 2012;19:385–91.
Russwurm S, Vickers J, Meier-Hellmann A, Spangenberg P, Bredle D, Reinhart K, Losche W. Platelet and leukocyte activation correlate with the severity of septic organ dysfunction. Shock. 2002;17:263–8.
Schall TJ, Bacon K, Camp RD, Kaspari JW, Goeddel DV. Human macrophage inflammatory protein alpha (MIP-1 alpha) and MIP-1 beta chemokines attract distinct populations of lymphocytes. J Exp Med. 1993;177:1821–6.
Schubert S, Weyrich AS, Rowley JW. A tour through the transcriptional landscape of platelets. Blood. 2014;124:493–502.
Sehgal S, Storrie B. Evidence that differential packaging of the major platelet granule proteins von Willebrand factor and fibrinogen can support their differential release. J Thromb Haemost. 2007;5:2009–16.
Semple JW, Aslam R, Kim M, Speck ER, Freedman J. Platelet-bound lipopolysaccharide enhances Fc receptor-mediated phagocytosis of IgG-opsonized platelets. Blood. 2007;109:4803–5.
Semple JW, Italiano JE Jr, Freedman J. Platelets and the immune continuum. Nat Rev Immunol. 2011;11:264–74.
Shi G, Field DJ, Ko KA, Ture S, Srivastava K, Levy S, Kowalska MA, Poncz M, Fowell DJ, Morrell CN. Platelet factor 4 limits Th17 differentiation and cardiac allograft rejection. J Clin Invest. 2014a;124:543–52.
Shi DS, Smith MC, Campbell RA, Zimmerman PW, Franks ZB, Kraemer BF, Machlus KR, Ling J, Kamba P, Schwertz H, Rowley JW, Miles RR, Liu ZJ, Sola-Visner M, Italiano JE Jr, Christensen H, Kahr WH, Li DY, Weyrich AS. Proteasome function is required for platelet production. J Clin Invest. 2014b;124:3757–66.
Shulman NR, Aster RH, Pearson HA, Hiller MC. Immunoreactions involving platelet. VI. Reactions of maternal isoantibodies responsible for neonatal purpura. Differentiation of a second platelet antigen system. J Clin Invest. 1962;41:1059–69.
Simon LM, Edelstein LC, Nagalla S, Woodley AB, Chen ES, Kong X, Ma L, Fortina P, Kunapuli S, Holinstat M, McKenzie SE, Dong JF, Shaw CA, Bray PF. Human platelet microRNA-

mRNA networks associated with age and gender revealed by integrated plateletomics. Blood. 2014;123:e37–45.
Spinelli SL, Casey AE, Pollock SJ, Gertz JM, McMillan DH, Narasipura SD, Mody NA, King MR, Maggirwar SB, Francis CW, Taubman MB, Blumberg N, Phipps RP. Platelets and megakaryocytes contain functional nuclear factor-kappaB. Arterioscler Thromb Vasc Biol. 2010;30:591–8.
Sreeramkumar V, Adrover JM, Ballesteros I, Cuartero MI, Rossaint J, Bilbao I, Nacher M, Pitaval C, Radovanovic I, Fukui Y, McEver RP, Filippi MD, Lizasoain I, Ruiz-Cabello J, Zarbock A, Moro MA, Hidalgo A. Neutrophils scan for activated platelets to initiate inflammation. Science. 2014;346:1234–8.
Stahl AL, Svensson M, Morgelin M, Svanborg C, Tarr PI, Mooney JC, Watkins SL, Johnson R, Karpman D. Lipopolysaccharide from enterohemorrhagic Escherichia coli binds to platelets through TLR4 and CD62 and is detected on circulating platelets in patients with hemolytic uremic syndrome. Blood. 2006;108:167–76.
Sun D, Popescu NI, Raisley B, Keshari RS, Dale GL, Lupu F, Coggeshall KM. Bacillus anthracis peptidoglycan activates human platelets through FcgammaRII and complement. Blood. 2013;122:571–9.
Takahashi T, Yujiri T, Shinohara K, Inoue Y, Sato Y, Fujii Y, Okubo M, Zaitsu Y, Ariyoshi K, Nakamura Y, Nawata R, Oka Y, Shirai M, Tanizawa Y. Molecular mimicry by Helicobacter pylori CagA protein may be involved in the pathogenesis of H. pylori-associated chronic idiopathic thrombocytopenic purpura. Br J Haematol. 2004;124:91–6.
Takeda T, Unno H, Morita H, Futamura K, Emi-Sugie M, Arae K, Shoda T, Okada N, Igarashi A, Inoue E, Kitazawa H, Nakae S, Saito H, Matsumoto K, Matsuda A. Platelets constitutively express IL-33 protein and modulate eosinophilic airway inflammation. J Allergy Clin Immunol. 2016;138:1395–403.
Tersteeg C, Heijnen HF, Eckly A, Pasterkamp G, Urbanus RT, Maas C, Hoefer IE, Nieuwland R, Farndale RW, Gachet C, de Groot PG, Roest M. FLow-induced PRotrusions (FLIPRs): a platelet-derived platform for the retrieval of microparticles by monocytes and neutrophils. Circ Res. 2014;114:780–91.
Thomas GM, Carbo C, Curtis BR, Martinod K, Mazo IB, Schatzberg D, Cifuni SM, Fuchs TA, von Andrian UH, Hartwig JH, Aster RH, Wagner DD. Extracellular DNA traps are associated with the pathogenesis of TRALI in humans and mice. Blood. 2012;119:6335–43.
Tremblay T, Aubin E, Lemieux R, Bazin R. Picogram doses of lipopolysaccharide exacerbate antibody-mediated thrombocytopenia and reduce the therapeutic efficacy of intravenous immunoglobulin in mice. Br J Haematol. 2007;139:297–302.
van den Boogaard FE, Schouten M, de Stoppelaar SF, Roelofs JJ, Brands X, Schultz MJ, Van't Veer C, van der Poll T. Thrombocytopenia impairs host defense during murine Streptococcus pneumoniae pneumonia. Crit Care Med. 2015;43:e75–83.
Verschoor A, Neuenhahn M, Navarini AA, Graef P, Plaumann A, Seidlmeier A, Nieswandt B, Massberg S, Zinkernagel RM, Hengartner H, Busch DH. A platelet-mediated system for shuttling blood-borne bacteria to CD8alpha+ dendritic cells depends on glycoprotein GPIb and complement C3. Nat Immunol. 2011;12:1194–201.
von Hundelshausen P, Weber C. Platelets as immune cells: bridging inflammation and cardiovascular disease. Circ Res. 2007;100:27–40.
Washington AV, Gibot S, Acevedo I, Gattis J, Quigley L, Feltz R, De La Mota A, Schubert RL, Gomez-Rodriguez J, Cheng J, Dutra A, Pak E, Chertov O, Rivera L, Morales J, Lubkowski J, Hunter R, Schwartzberg PL, McVicar DW. TREM-like transcript-1 protects against inflammation-associated hemorrhage by facilitating platelet aggregation in mice and humans. J Clin Invest. 2009;119:1489–501.
White GC, Rompietti R. Platelet secretion: indiscriminately spewed forth or highly orchestrated? J Thromb Haemost. 2007;5:2006–8.
Wolf P. The nature and significance of platelet products in human plasma. Br J Haematol. 1967;13:269–88.

Wong SL, Demers M, Martinod K, Gallant M, Wang Y, Goldfine AB, Kahn CR, Wagner DD. Diabetes primes neutrophils to undergo NETosis, which impairs wound healing. Nat Med. 2015;21:815–9.

Wong CH, Jenne CN, Petri B, Chrobok NL, Kubes P. Nucleation of platelets with blood-borne pathogens on Kupffer cells precedes other innate immunity and contributes to bacterial clearance. Nat Immunol. 2013;14:785–92.

Wright JF, Blanchette VS, Wang H, Arya N, Petric M, Semple JW, Chia WK, Freedman J. Characterization of platelet-reactive antibodies in children with varicella-associated acute immune thrombocytopenic purpura (ITP). Br J Haematol. 1996;95:145–52.

Yeaman MR. Bacterial-platelet interactions: virulence meets host defense. Future Microbiol. 2010a;5:471–506.

Yeaman MR. Platelets in defense against bacterial pathogens. Cell Mol Life Sci. 2010b;67:525–44.

Youssefian T, Drouin A, Masse JM, Guichard J, Cramer EM. Host defense role of platelets: engulfment of HIV and Staphylococcus aureus occurs in a specific subcellular compartment and is enhanced by platelet activation. Blood. 2002;99:4021–9.

Zhang G, Han J, Welch EJ, Ye RD, Voyno-Yasenetskaya TA, Malik AB, Du X, Li Z. Lipopolysaccharide stimulates platelet secretion and potentiates platelet aggregation via TLR4/MyD88 and the cGMP-dependent protein kinase pathway. J Immunol. 2009a;182:7997–8004.

Zhang W, Nardi MA, Borkowsky W, Li Z, Karpatkin S. Role of molecular mimicry of hepatitis C virus protein with platelet GPIIIa in hepatitis C-related immunologic thrombocytopenia. Blood. 2009b;113:4086–93.

Zufferey A, Schvartz D, Nolli S, Reny JL, Sanchez JC, Fontana P. Characterization of the platelet granule proteome: evidence of the presence of MHC1 in alpha-granules. J Proteome. 2014;101:130–40.

Check for updates

18 Thrombopoietin Receptor Agonists: Characteristics, Adverse Effects, and Indications

Jenny Despotovic and Amanda Grimes

18.1 Introduction

While the most commonly utilized first-line therapeutics for the treatment of immune thrombocytopenia (ITP) target the peripheral destruction of platelets, a preponderant second-line therapeutic agent targeting increased megakaryopoiesis and/or platelet production has now emerged, in the form of thrombopoietin receptor agonists (TPO-RAs). These TPO-RAs, eltrombopag and romiplostim, have been proven safe and effective in treating ITP in both children and adults and have also been approved for use in severe aplastic anemia and chronic hepatitis, with ongoing investigation in the treatment of other clinical entities as well, including myelodysplastic syndrome and acute myelogenous leukemia, chemotherapy-induced thrombocytopenia, congenital thrombocytopenia, and other diseases. This chapter will detail TPO-RA use in all of these different clinical settings.

18.2 Background

Thrombopoietin (TPO) is the major regulator of platelet production, acting largely via the JAK and STAT signaling pathways to stimulate megakaryocyte growth and platelet production (Kuter 2014). Shortly after identification and purification of TPO by five different groups in 1994 (de Sauvage et al. 1994; Lok et al. 1994; Bartley et al. 1994; Kuter et al. 1994; Kato et al. 1995), recombinant human TPO products were created and tested in immune thrombocytopenia (ITP) and other thrombocytopenic conditions. However, one of these agents resulted in the development of antibodies to the recombinant TPO protein, causing neutralization of

J. Despotovic, DO, MS • A. Grimes, MD (✉)
Pediatric Hematology/Oncology, Baylor College of Medicine/Texas Children's Hospital, 6701 Fannin Street, Houston, TX 77030, USA
e-mail: jmdespot@txch.org; abgrimes@txch.org

P. Imbach (ed.), *Antibody Therapy*, https://doi.org/10.1007/978-3-319-68038-5_18

both the recombinant TPO and endogenous TPO in some subjects, which resulted in severe thrombocytopenia (Li et al. 2001). This resulted in cessation of further development of recombinant TPO products. Development of less immunogenic second-generation TPO receptor agonists (RAs) ensued. These second-generation TPO mimetics bind to the TPO receptor at different sites, but both stimulate increased platelet production via the same mechanism as endogenous TPO. There are currently two TPO-RAs licensed for the treatment of ITP. Eltrombopag olamine is a non-peptide small-molecule TPO mimetic which activates the TPO receptor by binding to a transmembrane site on the receptor; and romiplostim is a peptide-antibody (Fc fragment) fusion protein which activates the TPO receptor by binding to its extra-cytoplasmic domain just as endogenous TPO does (Kuter 2014) (See Fig. 18.1) (Imbach and Crowther 2011). Both TPO-RAs have good efficacy and favorable safety profiles and were approved by the US Food and Drug Administration (FDA) for the treatment of chronic ITP in adults in 2008 (fda.gov 2017a, b). Eltrombopag received FDA approval for children with ITP in 2015 (fda.gov 2017a). These agents are common second-line treatment options for ITP and now have expanding roles in other thrombocytopenic conditions (Rodeghiero and Carli 2017).

18.3 Clinical Use and Pharmaceutical Considerations

Eltrombopag is approved for clinical use in children and adults with chronic ITP refractory to or recurrent after first-line therapies (including intravenous immunoglobulin [IVIG], anti-RhD immune globulin, glucocorticoids), adults with severe aplastic anemia (SAA) refractory to first-line therapies (immunosuppressive therapy) and ineligible for hematopoietic stem cell transplant (HSCT), and adults with chronic hepatitis secondary to hepatitis C virus (HCV) infection (to enable interferon therapy). Romiplostim is approved for clinical use in adults with chronic ITP refractory to or recurrent after first-line therapies.

Eltrombopag is an oral medication that is taken once daily. It should be administered on an empty stomach in order to maximize absorption. Additionally, eltrombopag binds strongly to divalent cations and cannot be taken in close proximity to a calcium-rich meal or the administration of multivitamin and/or mineral supplements (2 h before or 4 h after), as this cation binding would prevent absorption of the eltrombopag molecule. Dose should be titrated for a goal platelet count of 50,000/μL–200,000/μL, with desired platelet response typically achieved within an average of 7 weeks (Neunert et al. 2016). Eltrombopag is generally well tolerated and safe for long-term use. Romiplostim is administered via subcutaneous injection once weekly. Dosage is titrated for a goal platelet count of 50,000/μL–200,000/μL, with desired platelet response typically achieved within an average of 6 weeks (Neunert et al. 2016). Generally, romiplostim therapy is also well tolerated and safe for long-term use.

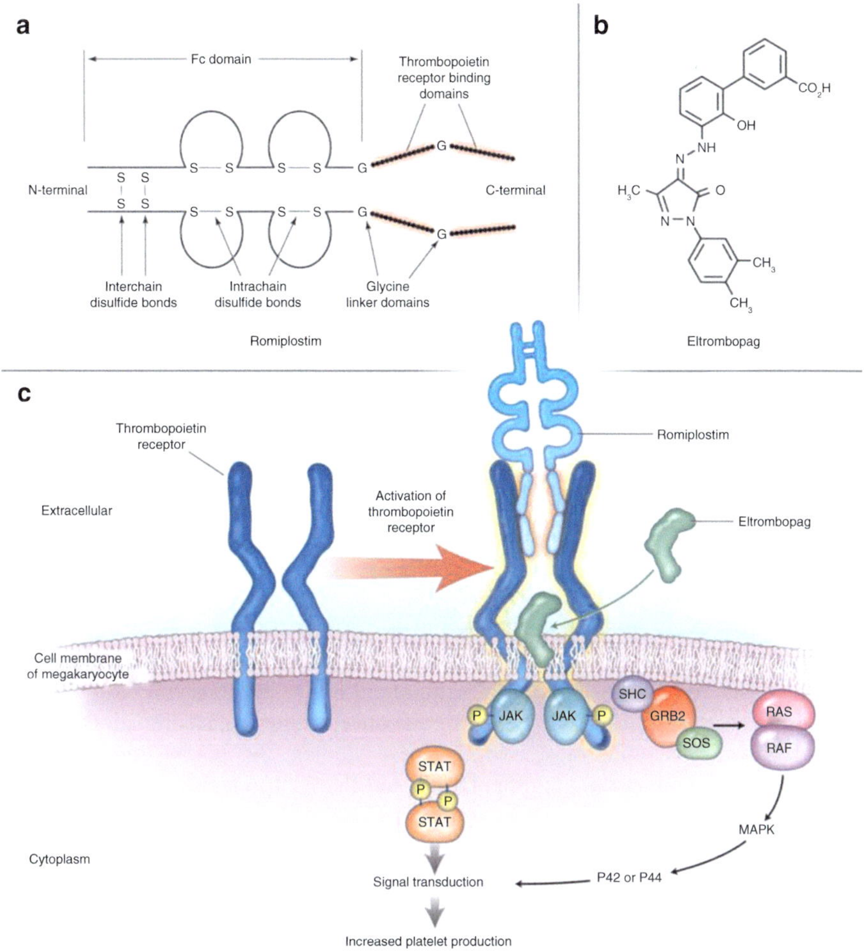

Fig. 18.1 Structure of romiplostim and eltrombopag and the cellular mechanisms of action. Panel (**a**) shows the chemical structure of romiplostim, which is composed of the Fc portion of IgG1, to which two thrombopoietin peptides consisting of 14 amino acids are coupled through glycine bridges at the C-terminal of each γ heavy chain. Panel (**b**) shows the chemical structure of eltrombopag. Panel (**c**) shows the cellular mechanisms of action of romiplostim, which binds to the thrombopoietin receptor, and of eltrombopag, which binds to the thrombopoietin receptor's transmembrane domain, thereby activating signaling that leads to increased platelet production. GRB2 denotes growth factor receptor-binding protein 2, JAK Janus kinase, MAPK mitogen-activated protein kinase, P phosphorylation, RAF rapidly accelerated fibrosarcoma kinase, RAS rat sarcoma GTPase, SHC Src homology collagen protein, and STAT signal transducer and activator of transcription. From *The New England Journal of Medicine*, Paul Imbach and Mark Crowther, Thrombopoietin-Receptor Agonists for Primary Immune Thrombocytopenia, Volume 365, Pages 734–741, Copyright © (2011) Massachusetts Medical Society. Reprinted with permission

18.4 Adverse Effects and Theoretical Risks Associated with TPO-RA Use

Overall, TPO-RAs are very well tolerated; and clinical data over the past 10–15 years demonstrate that many of the theoretical risks potentially associated with TPO-RAs have not been seen in clinical practice. However, some adverse effects of TPO-RAs have been identified, and some theoretical risks require further investigation before definitive conclusions regarding actual risk associated with TPO-RA use can be made. Providers utilizing TPO-RAs in clinical practice should therefore be aware of these risks and adverse effects. Potential risks associated with TPO-RA use include thrombotic and/or thromboembolic complications, bone marrow fibrosis, rebound thrombocytopenia, cataracts, hepatic abnormalities, development of cross-reactive antibodies, and cytogenetic abnormalities/clonal evolution.

18.4.1 Adverse Effects and Risks Associated with both TPO-RA Agents (Eltrombopag and Romiplostim)

18.4.1.1 Risk of Thrombosis

Increased risk of thrombotic complications in patients receiving TPO-RA therapy has been a significant and closely monitored concern, with most studies confirming a slightly increased risk of thrombosis among ITP patients receiving both eltrombopag and romiplostim. However, the significance of this risk has remained uncertain, given the potential biases within these studies, the preexisting increased thrombotic risk among the ITP population, and the contribution of prior therapies (i.e., splenectomy) to thrombotic risk. A recent review of industry-sponsored eltrombopag and romiplostim investigations (Rodeghiero 2016) estimated the rate of thromboembolic events to be 2.5–3.2 per 100 patient-years with eltrombopag and 4.2–7.5 per 100 patient-years with romiplostim. The rate of thromboembolic events in ITP patients treated with TPO-RAs therefore appears to be higher than that in the general population, as well as that in ITP patients not receiving TPO-RA therapy, in which there is already ~two-fold increased risk of thromboembolism at baseline, compared to the general population (Rodeghiero 2016). Notably, occurrence of thromboembolic events was associated with advanced age and comorbid risk factors (hypertension, obesity, smoking, etc.), with the majority of data reported in adult patients. Pediatric ITP patients treated with both romiplostim (Tarantino et al. 2016; Bussel et al. 2015a) and eltrombopag (Bussel et al. 2015b) reported no occurrence of thromboembolic events in initial industry trials, although two thromboembolic events in pediatric ITP patients treated at ITP Consortium of North America (ICON) sites (2.5%), both receiving eltrombopag, were later reported (Neunert et al. 2016), with overall incidence of thrombosis among pediatric ITP patients receiving TPO-RA therapy remaining very low. Thrombotic risk in ITP patients treated with TPO-RAs does not appear to correlate linearly with the platelet count and also does not appear to correlate consistently with medication dose (Rodeghiero et al. 2013; Saleh et al. 2013). The extent of thrombotic risk associated with TPO-RA therapy is still being established, with ongoing investigation needed to verify true incidence rates and/or associations while controlling for confounding variables. As these data are further clarified, providers should be aware of this risk in clinical practice and evaluate individual risk factors on a case-by-case basis when considering initiation of TPO-RA therapy. Additionally, dosage should be titrated to achieve and maintain the minimum platelet count needed to reduce the risk of bleeding (≥50,000/μL), but attempt should not be made to normalize platelet count. Care should be taken to avoid thrombocytosis, as this could potentially contribute to the risk of thrombosis.

18.4.1.2 Risk of Bone Marrow Fibrosis

Accelerated bone marrow fibrosis is another theoretical risk associated with TPO-RA therapy. Given that TPO-RAs work by stimulating megakaryopoiesis and increased platelet production, it is thought that profibrotic cytokines expressed by megakaryocytes and platelets will also be increased via the action of TPO-RAs on the TPO receptor (Kuter et al. 2007). Two large studies evaluating chronic ITP patients receiving long-term TPO-RA therapy showed a low incidence of bone marrow fibrosis—1.7% in patients receiving eltrombopag for up to 5.5 years (Brynes et al. 2015) and 2% in patients receiving romiplostim for up to 5 years (Rodeghiero et al. 2013). In these large adult trials, the majority of bone marrow fibrosis was restricted to reticulin fibrosis, with rarely identified collagen fibrosis (Rodeghiero et al. 2013; Saleh et al. 2013; Brynes et al. 2015). Reticulin fibers, best seen with a reticulin stain, can be seen normally in the bone marrow of healthy individuals, although increased levels of reticulin fibrosis may be associated with various disease processes and, in fact, have been demonstrated in adult ITP patients who are treatment naïve (present in 31% of ITP patients yet to receive therapy in one study) (Rizvi et al. 2015). Collagen fibrosis, conversely, is not present in healthy bone marrow and always reflects an underlying disease process—most often a myeloproliferative disorder. These fibers are composed of type I collagen and are best seen with a trichrome stain. The one ITP patient receiving romiplostim therapy in whom collagen fibrosis was identified also had known preexisting cytogenetic abnormalities associated with myelodysplastic syndrome (Rodeghiero et al. 2013). Also of note, identification of bone marrow fibrosis in chronic ITP patients receiving eltrombopag or romiplostim did not correlate with peripheral blood count abnormalities or other unexpected morphological or quantitative bone marrow abnormalities and also appeared to be reversible or stable once TPO-RA therapy was discontinued (Rodeghiero et al. 2013; Saleh et al. 2013; Brynes et al. 2015). Although smaller studies have shown more inconclusive results, the larger body of evidence regarding accelerated bone marrow fibrosis associated with TPO-RA therapy to date demonstrates no significant concern for this risk. Therefore, experts generally do not recommend routine bone marrow monitoring in patients receiving TPO-RA therapy, but continued monitoring of peripheral blood counts and smear should occur on a routine basis; and if cytopenias or morphological abnormalities develop, a bone marrow evaluation should be obtained.

18.4.1.3 Risk of Rebound Thrombocytopenia

Rebound thrombocytopenia following discontinuation of TPO-RA therapy is a well-documented risk, and many hematologists wean rather than abruptly discontinue these agents, with continued close follow-up for at least 2–4 weeks following discontinuation of therapy. The majority of ITP patients receiving TPO-RA therapy return to pre-therapy baseline platelet levels upon discontinuation of therapy, with a small subset of patients actually achieving sustained platelet responses following discontinuation of therapy (Ghadaki et al. 2013; Bussel et al. 2015c; Biagiotti et al. 2015). Up to 10% of patients experience significant rebound thrombocytopenia, with platelet counts decreasing below pretreatment levels and remaining low for 1–3 weeks before returning to prior baseline (Kuter et al. 2008). This is likely due to the fact that endogenous TPO activity is regulated by platelet mass, which may be suppressed while platelet levels are elevated on TPO-RA therapy and cannot quickly equilibrate when therapy is abruptly discontinued. This rebound thrombocytopenia can be associated with significant risk of bleeding. Therefore, although manufacturers of both agents recommend holding the dose if the platelet count exceeds 400,000/μL, experienced providers recommend close monitoring and dose reduction, as well as initiation of low-dose ASA if platelet count exceeds 800,000/μL, to avoid the risk of rebound thrombocytopenia, which in clinical practice likely poses higher risk to the patients than a transiently elevated platelet count (Kuter et al. 2010).

18.4.1.4 Risk of Clonal Evolution

Given prior knowledge of hematopoietic precursor cell expression of c-mpl (TPO receptor), the direct action of TPO on the hematopoietic stem cells was established shortly after its purification and successful cloning in 1994 (Zeigler et al. 1994). This direct stimulation of early hematopoietic stem cells by TPO is the basis for investigating the use of TPO-RAs in refractory and, now frontline, severe aplastic anemia (SAA). However, this is also the basis for the theoretical concern about clonal evolution with the use of TPO-RAs in both SAA and myelodysplastic syndromes (MDS)/acute myelogenous leukemia (AML). Recent studies evaluating the effects of eltrombopag therapy in SAA have shown new cytogenetic abnormalities/clonal evolution in 8–18% of SAA patients treated with eltrombopag (Desmond et al. 2014; Townsley et al. 2015; Gill et al. 2017; Townsley et al. 2017), which appears consistent with the incidence of clonal evolution in historical cohorts of SAA patients treated with immunosuppressive therapy alone. This likely represents a risk associated with the disease and not eltrombopag therapy, but further investigation is needed to clarify the potential risks of clonal evolution in the treatment of SAA and MDS/AML with TPO-RAs.

18.4.2 Adverse Effects and Risks Associated with Eltrombopag

18.4.2.1 Risk of Cataract Formation

There was initial concern for increased risk of cataract formation related to eltrombopag therapy, due to preliminary findings in animal studies. However, no clinical investigation has shown an increased risk of cataracts with eltrombopag use (Bussel et al. 2009; Cheng et al. 2011). There have been cataracts reported in patients treated with both eltrombopag and romiplostim, but these patients were also exposed to significant steroid doses. There does not appear to be an increased risk of cataract in children. Some experts continue to recommend baseline ophthalmologic evaluation prior to initiation of eltrombopag therapy and annually while continuing therapy, as further clinical data accumulates.

18.4.2.2 Risk of Liver Function Abnormalities

Hepatic abnormalities have been noted with eltrombopag therapy. Elevations in serum alanine aminotransferase (ALT), aspartate aminotransferase (AST), and bilirubin occurred in 4–6% of patients receiving eltrombopag therapy (Novartis 2016). Although these hepatobiliary laboratory abnormalities are generally asymptomatic and appear to resolve with disruption or discontinuation of therapy, certain monitoring parameters and corresponding dose titration or discontinuation actions are recommended to prevent drug-induced liver injury. Large trials reporting the safety of eltrombopag therapy in ITP patients generally recommend discontinuing drug when the following parameters are met: ALT $\geq$ 5× the upper limit of normal and/or ALT $\geq$ 3× the upper limit of normal with accompanying hepatitis symptoms or rash and bilirubin $\geq$1.5× the upper limit of normal (with >35% direct fraction) (Saleh et al. 2013). Additionally, providers utilizing eltrombopag in the setting of thrombocytopenia related to chronic HCV-associated hepatitis, specifically in combination with ribavirin- and interferon-based therapies, need to be aware of the increased risk for acute hepatic decompensation in this setting (fda.gov 2017a).

18.4.2.3 Other Adverse Effects Associated with Eltrombopag

Milder side effects noted most commonly in patients receiving eltrombopag therapy include headache, nasopharyngitis, upper respiratory tract infection, and fatigue (Saleh et al. 2013). However, eltrombopag therapy is generally well tolerated.

18.4.3 Adverse Effects and Risks Associated with Romiplostim

18.4.3.1 Risk of Antibody Development

Previous experience with the first-generation recombinant TPO proteins and resultant development of cross-reactive antibodies with the use of the pegylated recombinant product generated persistent concern for the development of similar antibodies with the use of second-generation TPO-RAs as well. Eltrombopag carries no relevant risk for cross-reactive or neutralizing antibody formation though, as it is a small-molecule therapeutic and also shares no structural or epitope homology with endogenous TPO; and in clinical practice, no antibody formation has been noted. Conversely, romiplostim does carry a theoretical risk of cross-reactive antibody formation, as it acts on the same TPO receptor extra-cytoplasmic binding domain as endogenous TPO acts upon, albeit without any structural similarity to endogenous TPO. However, no cross-reactive antibody formation has occurred in 10–15 years of clinical romiplostim use. Romiplostim therapy does result in formation of neutralizing anti-romiplostim antibodies in a small subset of patients, which results in a decrease or cessation of treatment response. This phenomenon should therefore be considered and further investigated in patients previously responsive to romiplostim therapy, with subsequent loss of response (Neunert et al. 2016; Rodeghiero et al. 2013; Carpenedo et al. 2016).

18.4.3.2 Other Adverse Effects Associated with Romiplostim

The most commonly noted side effects in patients receiving romiplostim therapy are headache, fatigue, and nasopharyngitis (Rodeghiero et al. 2013), although as previously noted, romiplostim is well tolerated overall.

18.5 Use of Thrombopoietin Receptor Agonists in Immune Thrombocytopenia (ITP)

TPO-RA therapy is most extensively studied and widely utilized in the treatment of patients with ITP. Early clinical trials investigating the use of both eltrombopag and romiplostim in adults with chronic ITP resulted in an FDA indication for both agents in adult patients with chronic ITP refractory to first-line therapies (IVIG, anti-D immune globulin, and glucocorticoids) (fda.gov 2017a, b). Eltrombopag and romiplostim response rates in treatment-refractory chronic ITP patients, generally defined by achievement of platelet count ≥50,000/μL, averaged ~80% (compared to an average of 20% or less in placebo groups), also with decreased bleeding events, improved health-related quality of life scores, and no increased incidence of severe adverse effects noted in eltrombopag (Saleh et al. 2013; Bussel et al. 2009; Cheng et al. 2011; Bussel et al. 2007; Bussel et al. 2013) and romiplostim (Rodeghiero et al. 2013; Kuter et al. 2008; Kuter et al. 2010) treatment groups. Additionally, follow-up studies demonstrated maintenance of sustained treatment response and continued safety in chronic ITP patients receiving long-term eltrombopag (Saleh et al. 2013) or romiplostim (Rodeghiero et al. 2013) therapy for up to 3–5 years. Similarly, studies in pediatric ITP patients (≥1 year of age) have demonstrated the safety and efficacy of eltrombopag in this population (Bussel et al. 2013; Grainger et al. 2015), with an FDA indication for the use of eltrombopag in pediatric chronic ITP patients refractory to first-line therapies. Likewise, ongoing studies show excellent safety and efficacy profiles for romiplostim use in the treatment of pediatric ITP (Tarantino et al. 2016; Bussel et al. 2011), and this therapy is also widely utilized clinically for the treatment of childhood ITP.

In clinical practice, the role of TPO-RA therapy in ITP continues to expand significantly as further data proving the safety and efficacy of these agents is compiled. For example, TPO-RA therapy is occasionally implemented earlier in the treatment of symptomatic ITP, in an attempt to avoid splenectomy or extensive glucocorticoid exposure, prior to possible disease resolution over the first 12 months. These agents may be easily weaned during the persistent phase, as spontaneous recovery occurs. Alternatively, therapy may be continued or reinitiated as indicated, if chronic disease develops. Studies have shown that response is maintained with intermittent use (i.e., response is again achieved at similar levels when TPO-RA therapy is resumed) and extended use (Rodeghiero et al. 2013; Bussel et al. 2013) and that therapy can be discontinued with no irreversible or long-term complications once ITP resolves (Ghadaki et al. 2013). Moreover, studies show that up to 30% of ITP patients treated with TPO-RAs maintain an extended response (up to 6 months and longer) once therapy is discontinued (Ghadaki et al. 2013; Bussel et al. 2015c; Biagiotti et al. 2015), with the implication that TPO-RA therapy may be capable of inducing a sustained platelet response. More long-term follow-up data is needed to define this possibility.

The advent of TPO-RA therapies has broadened the therapeutic landscape in ITP. TPO-RAs induce reliable platelet responses in the majority of patients and are also associated with decreased bleeding events, improved health-related quality of life, and an overall favorable safety profile, including the lack of immunosuppression associated with other second-line therapies. When one TPO-RA is ineffective or not tolerated, response or tolerability could be achieved by switching to an alternate TPO-RA, with no cross-resistance noted between the two available drugs in this class.

In summary, abundant data supports consideration of treatment with TPO-RA therapies in both adults and children with chronic ITP. Treated patients often have reduced bleeding complications, fewer activity restrictions, and potentially improved quality of life (Tarantino et al. 2016; Bussel et al. 2013; Rodeghiero et al. 2013; Saleh et al. 2013; Kuter et al. 2008; Kuter et al. 2010; Bussel et al. 2009; Cheng et al. 2011; Bussel et al. 2007; Bussel et al. 2013; Grainger et al. 2015; Bussel et al. 2011). Additionally, patients may be able to avoid splenectomies or adverse effects of prolonged immunosuppression. Occasional sustained platelet responses have occurred after TPO-RA therapy is discontinued, but these agents should not be considered curative.

18.6 Use of Thrombopoietin Receptor Agonists in Severe Aplastic Anemia (SAA)

Outside of therapy for chronic ITP, eltrombopag has a clinical indication for the treatment of patients with SAA who are refractory to first-line immunosuppressive therapies and are ineligible for hematopoietic stem cell transplant (HSCT). In its original use, eltrombopag was intended to ameliorate the complications of thrombocytopenia which are associated with SAA. However, during initial trials, trilineage effects of eltrombopag were noted, with improved red blood cell (RBC) and white blood cell (WBC) parameters in addition to the improved megakaryopoiesis and platelet production which was expected (Desmond et al. 2014). As discussed previously, this is likely due to the direct action of the TPO-RAs on early hematopoietic precursors via the same mechanism as endogenous TPO (Zeigler et al. 1994), creating expansion of all hematopoietic stem cells and thereby all cell lines. This finding prompted further investigation of eltrombopag as therapy for SAA, with ongoing trials now investigating this medication as a frontline therapeutic option (in combination with immunosuppressive therapy) for SAA. Early results are promising, with a recently published trial enrolling 92 SAA patients to receive eltrombopag in combination with immunosuppressive therapy as frontline therapy (starting at either Day 1 or Day 14) showing average complete response rates of 39% at 6 months and overall response rates of 87% at 6 months, compared to complete response rates of 10% and overall response rates of 66% in historical SAA cohorts treated with immunosuppressive therapy alone (Townsley et al. 2017). Incidentally, greatest response rates were noted in the patient cohort beginning eltrombopag therapy at Day 1. In all patients receiving frontline eltrombopag, marked increases in bone marrow cellularity, $CD34^+$ stem cells, and early hematopoietic progenitors were noted. Hematopoietic progenitor stimulation does raise the concern for potential development of new cytogenetic abnormalities or clonal evolution in SAA, given that up to 1/3 of AA/SAA patients have genetic mutations typically associated with myeloid neoplasms (Yoshizato et al. 2015). However, rates of clonal evolution in this study of 92 SAA patients treated with frontline eltrombopag therapy were similar to those in historical cohorts treated with immunosuppressive therapy alone (~8%) (Townsley et al. 2017). Further investigation of TPO-RAs in the treatment of SAA is needed at this point; however, preliminary findings portend a possible paradigm shift in the management of SAA, with the introduction of eltrombopag as a frontline treatment option.

18.7 Use of Thrombopoietin Receptor Agonists in Chronic Hepatitis

A third clinical indication for the use of eltrombopag is in the treatment of chronic hepatitis C virus (HCV)-associated hepatitis. The premise of this indication is based on the frequent need for peginterferon-based therapy in patients with chronic HCV infection, which cannot be effectively completed in the setting of comorbid thrombocytopenia. Eltrombopag has proven effective in raising platelet counts in this population, leading to decreased bleeding complications and, most importantly, to successful completion of peginterferon therapy without interruptions, dose reductions, or discontinuations. This has led to an increased rate of sustained virological response during peginterferon-based antiviral therapy in this population of patients (Fried et al. 2002). As peginterferon therapy becomes less utilized in the advent of newer antiviral therapies for HCV infection, this indication for eltrombopag therapy may change. However, both eltrombopag and peginterferon therapy will likely continue to play a significant role in HCV-associated hepatitis therapy for an extended period of time, until these newer antiviral agents become more widely available and accessible throughout the world.

18.8 Off-Label Uses of Thrombopoietin Receptor Agonists, Currently Under Investigation

18.8.1 First-Line Treatment for Aplastic Anemia

Investigation of eltrombopag as first-line treatment in SAA is discussed in detail above (*Use of TPO-RAs in SAA*). Early results are promising, likely owing to generalized stimulation of early hematopoietic precursor cells by eltrombopag, ultimately resulting in multi-lineage effects.

18.8.2 Myelodysplastic Syndrome (MDS)/Acute Myelogenous Leukemia (AML)

The premise for investigation of TPO-RAs in the treatment of MDS and AML is similar to that in SAA. Thrombocytopenia is a major problem in these patients, occurring in 40–65% (Kantarjian et al. 2007) and contributing significantly to bleeding complications and morbidity/mortality in this population of patients. Eltrombopag and romiplostim are expected to ameliorate the thrombocytopenic complications associated with MDS and AML if found to be safe and effective. There are currently many ongoing trials among pediatric and adult patients with MDS/AML, mostly in advanced or refractory patients (with eltrombopag) but also in lower-risk patients (with romiplostim). Generally, treatment with both TPO-RAs has been demonstrated to be safe, although there was early concern for increased progression to AML in patients treated with romiplostim (with updated findings less clear that there is any increased risk of AML progression associated with romiplostim therapy (Kantarjian et al. 2015)).

Eltrombopag has been studied in 98 relapsed or refractory adult patients with intermediate-2- or high-risk MDS or AML, with good results. Rates of platelet and red blood cell transfusion independence were improved in the eltrombopag-treated patients vs patients receiving placebo therapy (38% vs 21% and 20% vs 6%, respectively) (Platzbecker et al. 2015). In another trial investigating the efficacy and safety of eltrombopag in intermediate-2- or high-risk MDS or AML patients, the frequency of clinically relevant thrombocytopenic events and severe bleeding was also decreased in the eltrombopag treatment group (Mittelman et al. 2016). In both of these trials, there was no increased frequency of disease progression in the eltrombopag-treated patients; and in fact, in the latter trial (Mittelman et al. 2016), there was a reduced trend of disease progression in the eltrombopag-treated arm vs placebo (42% vs 60%, respectively). Another ongoing study investigating eltrombopag therapy in adult patients with relapsed or refractory low- and intermediate-1-risk MDS has shown promising results as well, with 54% of patients receiving eltrombopag therapy having achieved a platelet response at 24 weeks, compared to 27% of patients receiving placebo therapy. Again, the incidence of AML evolution or MDS disease progression was not increased in eltrombopag-treated patients; and of note, six patients treated with eltrombopag had gone into complete remission at 24 weeks (Oliva et al. 2015).

Romiplostim therapy in MDS has been studied largely in lower-risk patients. In one year-long study in low- and intermediate-1-risk MDS patients receiving supportive care only with platelet counts ≤50,000/μL, a durable platelet response was achieved in 46% of romiplostim-treated patients. Notably, progression to AML was observed in ~5% of patients (two patients) (Kantarjian et al. 2010a). Additional smaller studies investigating the safety and efficacy of romiplostim in combination with azacitidine (Kantarjian et al. 2010b), lenalidomide (Wang et al. 2012), and decitabine (Greenberg et al. 2013) in lower-risk MDS patients all demonstrated improved thrombocytopenic events and decreased bleeding events in romiplostim-treated patients. Numbers of patients included in each study were too small to determine romiplostim effects on disease progression. At this time, further studies are needed to clarify whether romiplostim therapy in MDS or AML poses a risk for accelerated disease progression. Eltrombopag, however, appears not to be associated with risk for disease progression in MDS and AML patients (Platzbecker et al. 2015; Mittelman et al. 2016; Oliva et al. 2015). This may be due to eltrombopag's ancillary property as a divalent ion chelator—specifically as an iron chelator in this instance (Roth et al. 2012). Again, further investigations regarding potential antitumor properties of eltrombopag are yet to be completed in the clinical setting and will need further exploration before definitive associations are made.

18.8.3 Chemotherapy-Induced Thrombocytopenia

TPO-RAs have not yet been extensively studied in the setting of chemotherapy-induced or radiation-induced thrombocytopenia and/or bone marrow failure. However, small studies investigating both eltrombopag and romiplostim use among patients receiving chemotherapy for solid tumors have shown favorable results. For both TPO-RA agents, treatment resulted in decreased platelet count nadirs and fewer dose modifications and/or interruption of chemotherapy (Winer et al. 2015; Kellum et al. 2010; Parameswaran et al. 2014). Larger randomized trials are needed to determine safety and to better identify optimal treatment groups for TPO-RA therapy in chemotherapy-induced thrombocytopenia prior to recommending TPO-RA therapy in this clinical setting.

18.8.4 Thrombocytopenia Following Hematopoietic Stem Cell Transplant (HSCT)

Delayed platelet recovery following HSCT is a common problem associated with HSCT in both children and adults. No extensive investigation regarding the use of TPO-RA therapy in the setting of post-HSCT thrombocytopenia has been done. However, early and ongoing studies are promising, confirming both safety and efficacy of TPO-RAs in this setting. An ongoing phase 2 randomized controlled trial evaluating the safety and efficacy of eltrombopag in the treatment of delayed platelet recovery (≥35 days after HSCT) in adult patients undergoing HSCT demonstrated platelet response (≥50,000/μL) in 21% of eltrombopag-treated patients at 8 weeks, vs 0% of patients receiving placebo. Additionally, there was no increased morbidity/mortality or incidence of adverse effects in the group of patients receiving eltrombopag therapy (Popat et al. 2015). Similarly, two case series evaluating the use of romiplostim in delayed platelet recovery post-HSCT showed no increased adverse effects in romiplostim-treated patients and demonstrated realization of platelet response (≥50,000/μL) in all patients treated within 2–12 weeks (Calmettes et al. 2011; Poon et al. 2013). Further data is needed to determine safety and efficacy of TPO-RA approach for management of thrombocytopenia following HSCT, but early results are promising.

18.8.5 Congenital Thrombocytopenias

Very little investigation regarding the role of TPO-RAs in the setting of hereditary thrombocytopenias has been completed. However, we know that this is a rapidly expanding category of diseases given the ongoing advances in genetic diagnostic tools, with potential utility of TPO-RA therapy. Small studies have shown some benefit of eltrombopag therapy in both Wiskott-Aldrich syndrome and myosin heavy chain 9 (MYH-9)-related thrombocytopenias; but more studies are needed to delineate the safety and efficacy of TPO-RA therapy in this clinical setting.

References

Bartley TD, Bogenberger J, Hunt P, et al. Identification and cloning of a megakaryocyte growth and development factor that is a ligand for the cytokine receptor Mpl. Cell. 1994;77:1117–24.

Biagiotti C, Carrai V, Bacchiarri F, et al. Persistent remission of chronic immune thrombocytopenia after thrombopoietin mimetics discontinuation. Haematologica. Conference Publication: (var.pagings). 2015;100:124.

Brynes RK, Orazi A, Theodore D, et al. Evaluation of bone marrow reticulin in patients with chronic immune thrombocytopenia treated with eltrombopag: data from the EXTEND study. Am J Hematol. 2015;90:598–601.

Bussel JB, Cheng G, Saleh MN, et al. Eltrombopag for the treatment of chronic idiopathic thrombocytopenic purpura. N Engl J Med. 2007;357:2237–47.

Bussel JB, Provan D, Shamsi T, et al. Effect of Eltrombopag on platelet counts and bleeding during treatment of chronic idiopathic thrombocytopenic purpura: a randomised, double-blind, placebo-controlled trial. Lancet. 2009;373:641–8.

Bussel JB, Buchanan GR, Nugent DJ, et al. A randomized, double-blind study of romiplostim to determine its safety and efficacy in children with immune thrombocytopenia. Blood. 2011;118:28–36.

Bussel JB, Saleh MN, Vasey SY, et al. Repeated short-term use of eltrombopag in patients with chronic immune thrombocytopenia (ITP). Br J Haematol. 2013;160:538–46.

Bussel JB, de Miguel PG, Despotovic JM, et al. Eltrombopag for the treatment of children with persistent and chronic immune thrombocytopenia (PETIT): a randomised, multicentre, placebo-controlled study. Lancet Haematol. 2015a;2(8):e315–25.

Bussel JB, Hsieh L, Buchanan GR, et al. Long-term use of the thrombopoietin-mimetic romiplostim in children with severe chronic immune thrombocytopenia (ITP). Pediatr Blood Cancer. 2015b;62:208–13.

Bussel J, Shah KM, Brigstocke S, et al. Tapering eltrombopag in patients with chronic ITP: how successful is this and in whom does it work? Blood. 2015c;126:1054.

Calmettes C, Vigouroux S, Tabrizi R, et al. Romiplostim (AMG531, Nplate) for secondary failure of platelet recovery after allo-SCT. Bone Marrow Transplant. 2011;46:1587–9.

Carpenedo M, Cantoni S, Coccini V, et al. Response loss and development of neutralizing antibodies during long-term treatment with romiplostim in patients with immune thrombocytopenia: a case series. Eur J Haematol. 2016;97(1):101–3.

Cheng G, Saleh MN, Marcher C, et al. Eltrombopag for management of chronic immune thrombocytopenia (RAISE): a 6-month, randomised, phase 3 study. Lancet. 2011;377:393–402.
de Sauvage FJ, Hass PE, Spencer SD, et al. Stimulation of megakaryocytopoiesis and thrombopoiesis by the c-Mpl ligand. Nature. 1994;369:533–8.
Desmond R, Townsley D, Dumitriu B, et al. Eltrombopag restores trilineage hematopoiesis in refractory severe aplastic anemia that can be sustained on discontinuation of drug. Blood. 2014;123:1818–25.
Fried MW, Shiffman ML, Reddy KR, et al. Peginterferon alfa-2a plus ribavirin for chronic hepatitis C virus infection. N Engl J Med. 2002;347:975–82.
Ghadaki B, Nazi I, Kelton JG, et al. Sustained remissions of immune thrombocytopenia associated with the use of thrombopoietin receptor agonists. Transfusion. 2013;53:2807–12.
Gill H, Leung G, Lopes D, et al. The thrombopoietin mimetics eltrombopag and romiplostim in the treatment of refractory aplastic anaemia. Br J Haematol. 2017;176(6):991–4.
Grainger JD, Locatelli F, Chotsampancharoen T, et al. Eltrombopag for children with chronic immune thrombocytopenia (PETIT2): a randomised, multicentre, placebo-controlled trial. Lancet. 2015;386(10004):1649–58.
Greenberg PL, Garcia-Manero G, Moore M, et al. A randomized controlled trial of romiplostim in patients with low- or intermediate-risk myelodysplastic syndrome receiving decitabine. Leuk Lymphoma. 2013;54:321–8.
Imbach P, Crowther M. Thrombopoietin-receptor agonists for primary immune thrombocytopenia. N Engl J Med. 2011;365:734–41. (Figure 1. Copyright © 2011 Massachusetts Medical Society. Reprinted with permission.)
Kantarjian H, Giles F, List A, et al. The incidence and impact of thrombocytopenia in myelodysplastic syndromes. Cancer. 2007;109:170–1714.
Kantarjian H, Fenaux P, Sekeres MA, et al. Safety and efficacy of romiplostim in patients with lower-risk myelodysplastic syndrome and thrombocytopenia. J Clin Oncol. 2010a;28:437–44.
Kantarjian HM, Giles FJ, Greenberg PL, et al. Phase 2 study of romiplostim in patients with low- or intermediate-risk myelodysplastic syndrome receiving azacitidine therapy. Blood. 2010b;116:3163–70.
Kantarjian HM, Mufti G, Fenaux P, et al. Romiplostim in thrombocytopenic patients with low-risk or intermediate-1-risk myelodysplastic syndrome results in reduced bleeding without impacting leukemic progression: updated follow-up results from a randomized, double-blind, placebo-controlled study. ASH Annu Meet Abstr Blood. 2015;126(23).
Kato T, Ogami K, Shimada Y, et al. Purification and characterization of thrombopoietin. J Biochem (Tokyo). 1995;118:229–36.
Kellum A, Jagiello-Gruszfeld A, Bondarenko IN, et al. A randomized, double-blind, placebo-controlled, dose ranging study to assess the efficacy and safety of eltrombopag in patients receiving carboplatin/paclitaxel for advanced solid tumors. Curr Med Res Opin. 2010;26(10):2339–46.
Kuter DJ. Milestones in understanding platelet production: a historical overview. Br J Haematol. 2014;165(2):248–58.
Kuter DJ, Beeler DL, Rosenberg RD. The purification of megapoietin: a physiological regulator of megakaryocyte growth and platelet production. Proc Natl Acad Sci U S A. 1994;9(1):11104–8.
Kuter DJ, Bain B, Mufti G, et al. Bone marrow fibrosis: pathophysiology and clinical significance of increased bone marrow stromal fibres. Br J Haematol. 2007;139(3):351–62.
Kuter DJ, Bussel JB, Lyons RM, et al. Efficacy of romiplostim in patients with chronic immune thrombocytopenic purpura: a double-blind randomised controlled trial. Lancet. 2008;371:395–403.
Kuter DJ, Rummel M, Boccia R, et al. Romiplostim or standard of care in patients with immune thrombocytopenia. N Engl J Med. 2010;363(20):1889–99.
Li J, Yang C, Xia Y, et al. Thrombocytopenia caused by the development of antibodies to thrombopoietin. Blood. 2001;98:3241–8.
Lok S, Kaushansky K, Holly RD, et al. Cloning and expression of murine thrombopoietin cDNA and stimulation of platelet production in vivo. Nature. 1994;369:565–8.

Mittelman M, Platzbecker U, Afanasyev B, et al. Thrombopoietin receptor agonist eltrombopag for advanced MDS or AML and severe thrombocytopenia: 12-week, randomized, placebo-controlled, phase 2 ASPIRE study. Haematologica. 2016;101(s1):15–6.

Neunert C, Despotovic J, Haley K, et al. Thrombopoietin receptor agonist use in children: data from the pediatric ITP consortium of North America ICON2 study. Pediatr Blood Cancer. 2016;63(8):1407–13.

Novartis PROMACTA [package insert]. East Hanover, NJ: Novartis Pharmaceuticals Corporation; 2016.

Oliva EN, Santini V, Alati C, et al. Eltrombopag for the treatment of low and intermediate-1 IPSS risk myelodysplastic syndromes: interim results on efficacy, safety and quality of life of an international, multicenter prospective, randomized, trial. ASH Annu Meet Abstr Blood. 2015;91.

Parameswaran R, Lunning M, Mantha S, et al. Romiplostim for management of chemotherapy-induced thrombocytopenia. Support Care Cancer. 2014;22(5):1217–22.

Platzbecker U, Wong RS, Verma A, et al. Safety and tolerability of eltrombopag versus placebo for treatment of thrombocytopenia in patients with advanced myelodysplastic syndromes or acute myeloid leukaemia: a multicentre, randomised, placebo-controlled, double-blind, phase 1/2 trial. Lancet Haematol. 2015;2(10):e417–26.

Poon LM, Di Stasi A, Popat U, et al. Romiplostim for delayed platelet recovery and secondary thrombocytopenia following allogeneic stem cell transplantation. Am J Blood Res. 2013;3:260–4.

Popat U, Ray G, Basset R et al. Eltrombopag for post-transplant thrombocytopenia: results of phase II randomized double blind placebo controlled trial. ASH Annu Meet Abstr Blood 2015;738.

Rizvi H, Butler T, Calaminici M, et al. United Kingdom immune thrombocytopenia registry: retrospective evaluation of bone marrow fibrosis in adult patients with primary immune thrombocytopenia and correlation with clinical findings. Br J Haematol. 2015;169(4):590–4.

Rodeghiero F. Is ITP a thrombophilic disorder? Am J Hematol. 2016;91:423–36.

Rodeghiero F, Carli G. Beyond immune thrombocytopenia: the evolving role of thrombopoietin receptor agonists. Ann Hematol. 2017;96(9):1421–34. https://doi.org/10.1007/s00277-017-2953-6.

Rodeghiero F, Stasi R, Giagounidis A, et al. Long-term safety and tolerability of romiplostim in patients with primary immune thrombocytopenia: a pooled analysis of 13 clinical trials. Eur J Haematol. 2013;91:423–36.

Roth M, Will B, Simkin G, et al. Eltrombopag inhibits the proliferation of leukemia cells via reduction of intracellular iron and induction of differentiation. Blood. 2012;120:386–94.

Saleh MN, Bussel JB, Cheng G, et al. Safety and efficacy of eltrombopag for treatment of chronic immune thrombocytopenia: results of the long-term, open-label EXTEND study. Blood. 2013;121:537–45.

Tarantino MD, Bussel JB, Blanchette VS, et al. Romiplostim in children with immune thrombocytopenia: a phase 3, randomised, double-blind, placebo-controlled study. Lancet. 2016;388(10039):45–54.

Townsley D, Dumitriu B, Scheinberg P, et al. Eltrombopag added to standard immunosuppression for aplastic anemia accelerates count recovery and increases response rates. Blood. 2015;126:LBA-2.

Townsley DM, Scheinberg P, Winkler T, et al. Eltrombopag added to standard immunosuppression for aplastic anemia. N Engl J Med. 2017;376(16):1540–50.

U.S. Food and Drug Administration. Eltrombopag. Available from www.accessdata.fda.gov/scripts/cder/daf/index.cfm?event=overview.process&applno=022291. Accessed 22 May 2017a.

U.S. Food and Drug Administration. Romiplostim. Available from www.accessdata.fda.gov/scripts/cder/daf/index.cfm?event=overview.process&applno=125268. Accessed 22 May 2017b.

Wang ES, Lyons RM, Larson RA, et al. A randomized, double-blind, placebo-controlled phase 2 study evaluating the efficacy and safety of romiplostim treatment of patients with low or

intermediate-1 risk myelodysplastic syndrome receiving lenalidomide. J Hematol Oncol. 2012;5:71.
Winer ES, Safran H, Karaszewska B, et al. Eltrombopag with gemcitabine-based chemotherapy in patients with advanced solid tumors: a randomized phase I study. Cancer Med. 2015;4(1):16–26.
Yoshizato T, Dumitriu B, Hosokawa K, et al. Somatic mutations and clonal hematopoiesis in aplastic anemia. N Engl J Med. 2015;373:35–47.
Zeigler FC, de Sauvage F, Widmer HR, et al. In vitro megakaryocytopoietic and thrombopoietic activity of c-mpl ligand (TPO) on purified murine hematopoietic stem cells. Blood. 1994;84(12):4045–52.

19 Registries in Immune Thrombocytopenia: The History of the Intercontinental Cooperative ITP Study Group

Thomas Kühne

19.1 Introduction

Immune thrombocytopenia (ITP) is an acquired autoimmune-mediated thrombocytopenia, defined by a platelet count of <100 × 10^9/l based on the definitions of an international working group (Rodeghiero et al. 2009). Besides bleeding, patients are healthy, and except thrombocytopenia, all other hematological values including blood smear analysis are normal. Thrombocytopenia is the result of an increased destruction of autoantibody-coated platelets by the monocytic-phagocytic system and a certain degree of platelet production failure, because megakaryocytes in the bone marrow express the same epitopes as do platelets and are thus affected by destructive processes, which may impair development and induce apoptosis of megakaryocytes (Perera and Garrido 2017).

ITP was often referred to as Werlhof's disease according to Paul Gottlieb Werlhof, who published in 1735 a report of a female suggestive to be one of the first descriptions of ITP (Werlhof 1735). However "Morbus" Werlhof implicates a disease with a unique etiology and pathomechanism and would ask therefore for a standardized algorithm of the management. If pathophysiology could be identified by routine laboratory tests in each patient, probably patients would be treated very differently. Thus a unique approach to patients with ITP, as it is currently practiced, appears to be questionable.

Autoantibodies are not found in every patient with ITP and patients with ITP do not respond to standard therapy in the same way, suggesting that besides autoreactive antibodies, there are different mechanisms ultimately resulting in thrombocytopenia, such as cytotoxic T lymphocyte-mediated cellular toxicity (Zufferey et al.

T. Kühne, MD
Division of Oncology/Hematology, University Children's Hospital,
Postfach, Spitalstrasse 33, CH-4031 Basel, Switzerland
e-mail: thomas.kuehne@ukbb.ch

P. Imbach (ed.), *Antibody Therapy*, https://doi.org/10.1007/978-3-319-68038-5_19

2017). This mechanism has the potential to destroy platelets and to affect their development by inducing megakaryocyte maturation defects (Stasi 2012). In contrast to secondary ITP, that is defined by a known underlying disorder or trigger, primary ITP is of unknown etiology and represents a diagnosis of exclusion without any specific laboratory tests, leaving the diagnosis of primary ITP vague and imprecise. Secondary ITP is much rarer than primary ITP.

Children and adolescents of all age groups but also adults and elderly patients may exhibit age-specific clinical characteristics. The bleeding phenotype can be affected by coexisting factors other than thrombocytopenia, i.e., exogenous factors (e.g., infectious diseases, drugs), endogenous factors (e.g., age, arteriovenous malformations, gene polymorphisms influencing immune response or hemostatic reactions, and inherited disorders of hemostasis, such as von Willebrand disease or inherited platelet function disorders), comorbidities, drugs, and other factors (Kühne 2017; Michel et al. 2011; Kistanguri and McCrae 2013).

In 1996 the American Society of Hematology (ASH) published a clinical practice guideline article with a comprehensive literature review of the time between 1966 and 1994 (George et al. 1996). It was recognized that the management of children and adults with ITP is mainly based on opinion rather than on evidence-based decisions. This publication stimulated a group of pediatric hematologists to establish an international network of scientists and physicians involved in the field of ITP with the aim to promote evidence-based medicine (Imbach et al. 2002; Kühne 2013). The name of the group was Intercontinental Childhood ITP Study Group (ICIS), which was changed in 2004 to Intercontinental Cooperative ITP Study Group (ICIS), because of collaboration with adult hematology (www.itpbasel.ch). The research activities of ICIS include the planning, performing, and assessing of projects with four international registries, two of them being still open for patient registration, exchange and interpretation of data, and organization of regular meetings. This review article summarizes the activities of ICIS and reviews registries in patients with ITP (Table 19.1).

Table 19.1 Intercontinental Cooperative ITP Study Group projects[a]

Name of the project	Duration of project	Patients (N)	Investigators (N)	Institutions (N)	Countries (N)
Registry I	1997–2000	2786	228	153	41
Registry II	2002–2004	1383	96	69	42
Splenectomy Registry	Since 1998	357	80	63	27
PARC-ITP Pediatric and Adult Registry on Chron. ITP	Since 2004	3995	107	92	34

[a]As of March 31, 2017

19.2 Methods in ITP

The documentation and classification of quality of the management in medicine and the development of strict definitions of evidence-based medicine by various systems, such as the GRADE system, are important achievements. These systems use a systematic and validated approach to grading the strength of clinical practice recommendations to minimize the potential for bias, to promote evidence-based medicine, and to enhance the validity of interpretations of research results (Guyatt et al. 2008). Different methods and strategies have been developed and practiced, in order to qualify recommendations and medical decisions based on their background (opinion or evidence).

Primary ITP with its complex pathophysiology and unknown etiology represents a disturbance of the immunological balance between self and nonself. Because it is not possible to investigate the exact pathomechanisms in the daily routine, the diagnosis is associated with imprecision and vagueness. Patients with primary ITP are characterized sometimes with a change in their diagnosis to secondary ITP or to thrombocytopenia of other reasons, if an underlying cause of thrombocytopenia becomes evident. Therefore classification of ITP can be difficult and the disease may manifest an evolutionary change of diagnostic features, which may ask for adaptations in the management. The clinician caring for patients with ITP must always consider the adequacy of the diagnosis and be ready to initiate new diagnostic procedures, if new insights arise, such as changes in physical signs and symptoms, new laboratory results, therapy refractoriness, and other unexpected clinical occurrences. Constant adaptations of the clinical management are typical for autoimmune disorders. Practice guidelines and recommendations exhibit a certain degree of rigidity in following such an evolution and do not replace best physical judgments, making physicians' experience and networking important prerequisites to manage children and adults with ITP. General algorithms for the management of patients with ITP must be therefore interpreted carefully, particularly in patients with chronic ITP. The management of patients with ITP is characterized by a rather individualized concept, which can be further influenced by patients' preferences, making the measurement and interpretation of health-related quality of life important (Haverman et al. 2017).

Evidence-based medicine qualifies research according to strict rules. For example, the revised ASH 2011 evidence-based practice guideline used the GRADE system, which categorizes the quality of the contributing evidence and the strength that the evidence brings to the recommendations (Neunert et al. 2011). The system consists of numbers indicating the strength of a recommendation and letters indicating the quality of the underlying evidence, e.g., randomized controlled trials, observational studies, or case series. Additionally, the process of achieving a recommendation must include a declaration of all individuals' potential and existing conflicts of interests, which may influence such recommendations.

Registries are widely used in medicine and represent ideal scientific tools for the study of rare diseases with the opportunity to collect multicenter data of a large number of patients from all continents within short time period (Gliklich et al. 2014). Registry data may be the basis to elaborate scientific questions and to prepare clinical trials, particularly to investigate inclusion and exclusion criteria of patients, to evaluate the relevance of scientific objectives and the feasibility of clinical research. The design and infrastructure of the registry depend upon the requirements and research plans of the research groups, the epidemiology of the disease to be investigated, and the availability and duration of funding (Gliklich et al. 2014).

There are attractive features and advantages of registries that include an immediate access to research, interim analyses, and a structure that allows flexibility with adaptations and modifications when new scientific questions arise during data analyses or new knowledge occurs from the scientific community. Additionally a registry permits "learning effects" during data acquisition, resulting in consecutive changes of registry questions and structures. The database is often accessible by the Internet and allows fast reporting and structured screening of entered data by the system but also by the central office as part of a quality program to avoid erroneous data.

There are also limitations of registries. Despite its flexibility, registries are under control of scientific groups and regular authorities, and thus changes of their structure could be associated with high work load and need adaptations by their users. There are both population-based national and international registries and case-based registries. The former type presumes a controlled and thus costly endeavor to include a preferably complete number of patients representing the population of a given geographical area. Often, such registries are designed for other purposes than the study of a specific disease or for the study of a disease group, such as public health and cancer registries. Exact case definitions are often missing in such registries. Case-based registries depend often on voluntary registration by physicians participating in a network. They are often designed for the study of a specific disease and benefit from its flexibility by changes of its structure, should new data and knowledge of the disease occur. There are also economic problems particularly for investigator-driven case-based registries. Remuneration of participating investigators and institutions and financial aspects of the development and maintenance of the database and its structures must be considered for budgets. Databases of registries depend on sophisticated software applications and need specialists in informatics. International multicenter data may contain multilevel biases based on country-, region-, and institution-specific characteristics which may affect quality. However, quality can be controlled by the structure of the registry, by continuous modifications of Internet access software, by the knowledge of participating institutions and investigators, and by quality control measures, such as regular interim analyses and on-site monitoring procedures. Quality control can be expensive and must be considered in preparing budgets. Case-based registries collect data of consecutive patients by voluntary reporting of investigators. This must be considered when assessing results.

19.3 History and Development of ICIS

In 1997 ICIS was founded and started immediately with the activation of registries. Based on the lack of clinical data in ITP and the fact that many, if not most clinical decisions in children with ITP were based on expert opinion (George et al. 1996), the objectives of ICIS included the establishment of a well-functioning and accessible international network of scientists and clinicians involved in the field of thrombocytopenia and ITP, the prospective collection of clinical and laboratory data from children with ITP by registries, and regular publications and organization of meetings to exchange experience and scientific achievements. In 2004 ICIS decided to change its structure to a group of pediatric and adult hematologists, because ITP—although different in some aspects—shares many common characteristics throughout age groups, including the rarity, the challenges to perform research, and clinical features. Furthermore the extension of the group will benefit from an increased strength of more experts in the field. The ICIS registries represent ideal tools to learn more about demographics of patients, the natural history of ITP, and management issues.

Since 2003, ICIS performs international expert meetings every third year in Switzerland and published them in peer-reviewed scientific journals (Imbach et al. 2003; Kühne and Imbach 2006, 2010, 2013, 2016). These meetings are opportunities for experts to exchange knowledge and to discuss further projects. ICIS investigators can share their research results and get most actual information in these meetings. The most recent meeting took place in 2015 in central Switzerland with the topic "immunomodulation and management in ITP and other autoimmune disorders." For the first time, experts not only from hematology and basic sciences but also from other disciplines with autoimmune disorders, such as dermatology, rheumatology, pneumology, immunology, neurology, and gastroenterology, were invited to give a lecture and write a manuscript on the topic "immunomodulation." The meeting was an exciting and successful scientific exchange of many experts (Kühne and Imbach 2016). ICIS is currently preparing its sixth expert meeting, which will be held in Arosa, Switzerland, in 2018 with the topic "to treat or not to treat." Another stimulating scientific event can be expected.

19.4 ICIS Registry I (1997–2000)

Registry I was the first initiative by ICIS with the aim to collect data of children with ITP from all continents within short time period and to learn more about the natural history of pediatric ITP in different countries. It was designed to register data at the time of first presentation, with follow-up data 6 and 12 months later. The management and outcome was assessed with a main focus on watchful waiting, corticosteroids, and intravenous high-dose immunoglobulins (IVIG). Findings of several analyses included:

(1) Clinical characterization of children of different age groups.
(2) The percentage of children with chronic ITP at 6 and 12 months (at that time chronic ITP was defined with 6 months' duration of thrombocytopenia, and thrombocytopenia was defined with a platelet count of <150 × 10^9/l): 31% had chronic ITP without a difference between boys and girls.
(3) A low frequency of severe and life-threatening bleeding despite a very low platelet count of less than 20 × 10^9/l at presentation. Intracranial hemorrhage was reported in 2 of 1496 children with data available at 6 months after the initial presentation.
(4) Predictive factors for chronic ITP included a higher platelet count at diagnosis and older age.
(5) The outcome of children at 6 months after initial presentation did not depend on whether they received drug treatment or were managed without drugs (Kühne et al. 2001).

Another analysis revealed age-specific characteristics of ITP, including 203 infants who exhibited a lower incidence of chronic ITP (Kühne et al. 2003). It has been shown that boys are more frequently affected with ITP during infancy. The reason for this observation remains unclear. Interestingly it has been shown that among older adults men are again more frequently seen than women (Moulis et al. 2014). An important observation was that 25% of children recovered from their ITP, who were observed during 6 and 12 months after the diagnosis of ITP (Imbach et al. 2006). The maintained potential of remission during 1 year resulted in a discussion at an ICIS expert meeting and finally leads to a change of the definition of chronic ITP to be of rather 12 than of the earlier used 6-month duration of thrombocytopenia (Rodeghiero et al. 2009; Imbach et al. 2006; Ruggeri et al. 2006). In a matched pair analysis and calculated odds ratios of ICIS Registry I data, the influence of the initial treatment on the course of ITP was investigated. Assuming that a platelet count of <50 × 10^9/l is of more clinical relevance, the matched pair analysis was repeated with a platelet count of <50 × 10^9/l as an alternate definition for chronic ITP and compared with patients with a platelet count of ≥50 × 10^9/l (Tamminga et al. 2009). Based on this analysis, a subgroup of children who were treated with IVIG exhibited a smaller risk of chronic ITP compared with children not receiving IVIG; it is however not clear which clinical and laboratory factors define such a subgroup (Tamminga et al. 2009).

19.5 ICIS Registry II (2002–2004)

The observation that a majority of children with newly diagnosed ITP has often no, mild, or moderate bleeding in spite of a low platelet count stimulated ICIS to design a cohort study with the aim to test the hypothesis, that major hemorrhage in children with newly diagnosed ITP is uncommon (Neunert et al. 2008). Major hemorrhage was defined broadly with Intracranial or other overt internal or mucous membrane bleeding, which results in anemia or which requires local treatment to stop hemorrhage. Physical examination included bleeding assessment by using the bleeding scale of Bolton-Maggs and Moon (1997) and Bolton-Maggs (2003). Between June 2001 and December 2004, 1106 children were enrolled by 74 investigators and observed during 2 years at initial presentation, during the first 4 weeks, at 6, 12, and 24 months. Severe, moderate, and no or mild hemorrhage was found in 3, 20, and 77%, respectively (Neunert et al. 2008). These numbers were almost identical with those found by Bolton-Maggs in her national survey in the United Kingdom (Bolton-Maggs and Moon 1997). New bleeding and admission because of bleeding complications during the 2-year observational time were rare (Neunert et al. 2013), which was confirmed by others (Rosthøj et al. 2012; Neunert et al. 2014). However, it is important to be reminded that bleeding and its severity in ITP are difficult to be studied, because of the lack of standardized case definitions, the difficulties in assessing and reporting bleeding with bleeding scores, and the omission of reporting bleeding outcomes in many clinical studies, registries, and administrative databases (Arnold 2015). Prognostic factors for the individual outcome and for chronic ITP can now be estimated with ICIS Registry I and II data and with other sources, based on several factors, such as insidious onset of bleeding symptoms, mild bleeding at initial presentation, a higher platelet count at presentation, age more than 10 years, and no preceding infectious disorders (Zeller et al. 2005; Glanz et al. 2008; Revel-Vilk et al. 2013; Heitink-Pollé et al. 2014; Chotsampancharoen et al. 2017).

19.6 Pediatric and Adult Registry on Chronic ITP (PARC-ITP) (Since 2004)

In 2004, ICIS decided to collaborate with adult hematologists, and therefore, a new global network of investigators involved in basic and clinical science was initiated. The Pediatric and Adult Registry on Chronic ITP (PARC-ITP) was activated with the aim to learn more about common and different clinical and laboratory aspects of ITP in children and adults, to expand our knowledge in the natural history of ITP and its management, and to gather data which may enable the design of future trials. The registry has the potential to add modules to the central database. Thus, amendment 1 was added in 2005, which is a DNA bank available for genetic projects in ITP, and amendment 2 was added in 2008 with the expansion of more clinical questions including personal and family history of bleeding and thrombotic diseases, comorbidities of patients, co-medications, and safety surveillance of drug treatment. Data are registered by Internet access (https://www.parc-itp.net/parc-itp/) with data administration at the ICIS office in Basel, Switzerland. In 2011 an interim analysis with data of 1784 children and 340 adults with newly diagnosed ITP unexpectedly revealed that there have been more common clinical and laboratory findings of children and adults at the time of first presentation, including the bleeding phenotype and the occurrence of no or mild bleeding, as well as the severity of thrombocytopenia at first presentation and the likelihood to be treated for bleeding (Kühne et al. 2011). A second interim analysis is currently undertaken and was published at the ASH annual meeting in 2016 in preliminary form (Kühne and Schifferli 2016). The patient population consisted of 3360 children and 420 adults with newly diagnosed ITP. Follow-up data at 6, 12, and 24 months after the diagnosis of ITP were available in 67, 49, and 31% of children and in 77, 64, and 47% of adults, respectively. Of children and adults with a platelet count of $<100 \times 10^9/l$ at 6 months, 36 and 28% achieved again a remission at 12 months, suggesting that the potential of recovery, which is observed in children, can also be observed in adult patients. Patients with persistent and chronic ITP at 6, 12, and 24 months after the diagnosis of ITP received drug treatment for their ITP in similar frequency in 58, 46, and 47% of children and in 58, 52, and 40% of adults, respectively. The PARC-ITP Registry will continue to accept new patient data and perform analyses.

19.7 The Splenectomy Registry (Since 1998)

Splenectomy is a successful therapy with the potential to cure ITP (Kaznelson 1916; Kojouri et al. 2004; Aslam et al. 2017). The procedure is not frequently undertaken in children with chronic ITP, because of the potential of improvement of or even recovery from ITP and of complications of splenectomy including life-threatening infections caused by encapsulated bacteria and thromboembolic complications. A further disadvantage of the procedure includes the burden of life after splenectomy, such as preparing for traveling, reacting when fever occurs, and taking regular medical controls. Additionally, vaccinations must be performed prior to surgery and afterwards, as well as antibiotic prophylaxis. The timing and the management of the splenectomy is not standardized. The Splenectomy Registry was opened in the early ICIS time of 1998 and contains data of 357 children from 80 investigators of 27 countries as of February 2017. The aim of the registry is to learn more about clinical and laboratory characteristics of children who are planned for splenectomy and to study their management and their outcome. An interim analysis of 134 children confirmed that splenectomy is also successful in pediatric patients with a stable course during 5 years (Kühne et al. 2007). Half of the children were openly splenectomized and half were splenectomized by laparoscopical technology. More than 86% of patients responded with a platelet count of $>150 \times 10^9/l$ within 90 days after the procedure, and another 9% had a partial response. One year later, 80% of the complete responders maintained their platelet count, and most of them remained stable during the following 3–4 years. In seven children a sepsis without fatal outcome was observed. The analysis revealed several aspects of management including presurgical vaccination and postsplenectomy antibiotic prophylaxis, time point, and indication of splenectomy, which did not follow current recommendations and guidelines and may be basis for further discussions and attempts for consensus. There is still a significant lack of clinical data and the indication and timing of splenectomy remains individually based and controversial (Schifferli and Kühne 2013).

19.8 Outlook

Clinical research in children and adults with ITP faces several problems: difficulties and high costs in recruiting patients because of the rarity of the disease, the heterogeneous pathomechanisms, which are usually unidentified by routine laboratory, the diagnostic difficulties with missing laboratory tests to prove ITP, resulting in a high degree of heterogeneity of study subjects, and the imprecision of treatment endpoints (e.g., platelet count, bleeding, quality of life, reduction of concomitant therapies, and patient preferences). Therefore, clinical research and daily practice differ significantly. These problems may be at least in part resolved by registries and represent their major advantages: cost-effectiveness, reflection of "real life" of patients and physicians, ideal tools for the study of rare diseases, international research with registration of a large number of patients from different origins, and assessing results, which may serve as a basis for clinical trials. Registries may reveal information serving as new ideas and focusing on unexpected areas of research. In most countries registries are feasible with minimal administrative investment. Internet, software developments, biostatistics, and database technologies underlie fast-changing processes, and their application and knowledge are the basis for successful registries.

In summary the performance of registries represents a success story of ICIS since 20 years in the attempt to fill the gaps and increase knowledge of ITP in children and adults by establishing an international network, bringing physicians and scientists together to exchange their ideas, and coordinating research with a careful use of resources.

Acknowledgments The author thanks the numerous ICIS investigators and their patients for providing their data and for their ongoing support. Many thanks go to Paul Imbach for his invitation to write this article and for his help. I thank Caroline Martin Asal, Verena Stahel, and Monika Imbach of the ICIS office in Basel, Switzerland, for their patience and help and all members of the ICIS Board for their continuous support of our group.

References

Arnold DM. Bleeding complications in immune thrombocytopenia. Hematol Am Soc Hematol Educ Program. 2015;2015:237–42.

Aslam R, et al. The spleen dictates platelet destruction, anti-platelet antibody production, and lymphocyte distribution patterns in a murine model of immune thrombocytopenia. Exp Hematol. 2017. https://doi.org/10.1016/j.exphem.2016.07.004.

Bolton-Maggs P. Severe bleeding in idiopathic thrombocytopenic purpura. J Pediatr Hematol Oncol. 2003;25(Suppl 1):S47–51.

Bolton-Maggs PH, Moon I. Assessment of UK practice for management of acute childhood idiopathic thrombocytopenic purpura against published guidelines. Lancet. 1997;350:620–3.

Chotsampancharoen T, et al. Predictive factors for resolution of childhood immune thrombocytopenia: experience from a single tertiary center in Thailand. Pediatr Blood Cancer. 2017;64:128–34.

George JN, et al. Idiopathic thrombocytopenic purpura: a practice guideline developed by explicit methods for the American Society of Hematology. Blood. 1996;88:3–40.

Glanz J, et al. A population-based, multisite cohort study of the predictors of chronic idiopathic thrombocytopenic purpura in children. Pediatrics. 2008;121:e506–12.

Gliklich R, et al., editors. Registries for evaluating patient outcomes: a user's guide. Third edition. Two volumes. (Prepared by the outcome DEcIDE Center [Outcome Sciences, Inc., a Quintiles company] under contract no. 290 2005 00351 TO7.) AHRQ Publication No. 13(14)-EHC111. Rockville, MD: Agency for Healthcare Research and Quality; 2014. http://www.effectivehealthcare.ahrq.gov/registries-guide-3.cfm

Guyatt GH, et al. Grades of recommendation for antithrombotic agents: American College of Chest Physicians Evidence-Based Clinical Practice Guidelines (8th edition). Chest. 2008;133(6 Suppl):123S–31S.

Haverman L, et al. Paediatric health-related quality of life: what is it and why should we measure it? Arch Dis Child. 2017. https://doi.org/10.1136/archdischild-2015-310068.

Heitink-Pollé KMJ, et al. Clinical and laboratory predictors of chronic immune thrombocytopenia in children: a systematic review and meta-analysis. Blood. 2014;124:3295–307.

Imbach P, et al. Historical aspects and present knowledge of idiopathic thrombocytopenic purpura. Br J Haematol. 2002;119:894–900.

Imbach P, et al., Guest editors. Intercontinental childhood ITP Study Group (ICIS): state-of-the-art expert meeting on ITP, September 23–25, 2003 – Buergenstock, Switzerland. J Pediatr Hematol Oncol. 2003;25(Suppl 1):1–84.

Imbach P, et al. Childhood ITP: 12 months follow-up data from the prospective registry I of the Intercontinental Childhood ITP Study Group (ICIS). Pediatr Blood Cancer. 2006;46:351–6.

Kaznelson P. Verschwinden der hämorrhagischen Diathese bei einem Falle von essentieller Thrombopenie (Frank) nach Milzexstirpation. Wien Klin Wochenschr. 1916;29:1451–4.

Kistanguri G, McCrae KR. Immune thrombocytopenia. Hematol/Oncol Clin N Am. 2013;27:495–520.

Kojouri K, et al. Splenectomy for adult patients with idiopathic thrombocytopenic purpura: a systematic review to assess long-term platelet count responses, prediction of response, and surgical complications. Blood. 2004;104:2623–34.

Kühne T. Update on the Intercontinental Cooperative ITP Study Group (ICIS) and on the pediatric and adult registry on chronic ITP (PARC ITP). Pediatr Blood Cancer. 2013;60(Suppl 1):S15–8.

Kühne T. Diagnosis and management of immune thrombocytopenia in childhood. Hamostaseologie. 2017;37:36–44.

Kühne T, Imbach P, Guest editors. 2nd Intercontinental Childhood ITP Study Group (ICIS) expert meeting on "critical issues and future research of ITP", September 16–18, 2006, Yverdon, Switzerland. Special issue 2006. Pediatr Blood Cancer. 2006;47:649–745.

Kühne T, Imbach P, Guest editors. 3rd Intercontinental cooperative ITP Study Group (ICIS) expert meeting on consensus and development of strategies in ITP. Basel, Switzerland, September 3–5, 2009. Ann Hematol. 2010;89(Suppl 1):1–109.

Kühne T, Imbach P, Guest editors. 4th Intercontinental cooperative ITP Study Group (ICIS) expert meeting on "changes in ITP of children and adults", Montreux, Switzerland, September 13–15, 2012. Semin Hematol. 2013;50(Suppl 1):S1–S126.

Kühne T, Imbach P, Guest editors. 5th Intercontinental cooperative ITP Study Group (ICIS) expert meeting on "immunomodulation and management in ITP and other autoimmune disorders", Flüeli-Ranft, Switzerland, September 24–26, 2015. Semin Hematol. 2016;53(Suppl 1):S1–S72.

Kühne T, Schifferli A. On behalf of the Intercontinental Cooperative ITP Study Group (ICIS). A comparative prospective observational study of children and adults with immune thrombocytopenia: 2-year follow-up. 58th ASH annual meeting. Abstract. Blood. 2016;128(22):3741.

Kühne T, et al. Newly diagnosed idiopathic thrombocytopenic purpura in childhood: an observational study. Lancet. 2001;358:2122–5.

Kühne T, et al. A prospective comparative study of 2540 infants and children with newly diagnosed idiopathic thrombocytopenic purpura (ITP) from the Intercontinental Childhood ITP Study Group. J Pediatr. 2003;143:605–8.

Kühne T, et al. Splenectomy in children with idiopathic thrombocytopenic purpura: a prospective study of 134 children from the Intercontinental Childhood ITP Study Group. Pediatr Blood Cancer. 2007;49:829–34.

Kühne T, et al. Newly diagnosed immune thrombocytopenia in children and adults: a comparative prospective observational registry of the Intercontinental Cooperative Immune Thrombocytopenia Study Group. Haematologica. 2011;96:1831–7.

Michel M, et al. Characteristics and outcome of immune thrombocytopenia in elderly: results from a single center case-controlled study. Am J Hematol. 2011;86:980–4.

Moulis G, et al. Epidemiology of incident immune thrombocytopenia: a nationwide population-based study in France. Blood. 2014;124:3308–15.

Neunert CE, et al. Severe hemorrhage in children with newly diagnosed immune thrombocytopenic purpura. Blood. 2008;112:4003–8.

Neunert C, et al. The American Society of Hematology 2011 evidence-based practice guideline for immune thrombocytopenia. Blood. 2011;117:4190–207.

Neunert CE, et al. Bleeding manifestations and management of children with persistent and chronic immune thrombocytopenia: data from the Intercontinental Cooperative ITP Study Group (ICIS). Blood. 2013;121:4457–62.

Neunert C, et al. Severe bleeding events in adults and children with primary immune thrombocytopenia: a systematic review. J Thromb Haemost. 2014;13:457–64.

Perera M, Garrido T. Advances in the pathophysiology of primary immune thrombocytopenia. Hematology. 2017;22:41–53.

Revel-Vilk S, et al. Age and duration of bleeding symptoms at diagnosis best predict resolution of childhood immune thrombocytopenia at 3, 6, and 12 months. J Pediatr. 2013;163:1335–9.

Rodeghiero F, et al. Standardization of terminology, definitions and outcome criteria in immune thrombocytopenic purpura (ITP) of adults and children. Report from an international working group. Blood. 2009;113:2386–93.

Rosthøj S, et al. Duration and morbidity of chronic immune thrombocytopenic purpura in children: five-year follow-up of a Nordic cohort. Acta Paediatr. 2012;101:761–6.

Ruggeri M, et al. Heterogeneity of terminology and clinical definitions in adult idiopathic thrombocytopenic purpura: a critical appraisal from literature analysis. Pediatr Blood Cancer. 2006;47:653–6.

Schifferli A, Kühne T. Chronic immune thrombocytopenia in children: who needs splenectomy? Semin Hematol. 2013;50(Suppl 1):S58–62.

Stasi R. Immune thrombocytopenia: pathophysiologic and clinical update. Semin Thromb Hemost. 2012;38:454–62.

Tamminga R, et al. Possible lower rate of chronic ITP after IVIG for acute childhood ITP an analysis from registry I of the Intercontinental Cooperative ITP Study Group (ICIS). Br J Haematol. 2009;146:180–4.

Werlhof PG. De Variolis et Anthracibus. Hannover; 1735.

Zeller B, et al. Childhood idiopathic thrombocytopenic purpura in the Nordic countries: epidemiology and predictors of chronic disease. Acta Paediatr. 2005;94:178–84.

Zufferey A, et al. Pathogenesis and therapeutic mechanisms in immune thrombocytopenia (ITP). J Clin Med. 2017;6(2):1–21.

Part IV

Translation from Polyclonal to Monoclonal Antibody Treatment

Therapeutic Monoclonal Antibodies as Immunomodulators and Anti-Cancer Agents: Development, Evidence of Efficacy, Mechanisms of Actions, Adverse Effects

20

Tim Niehues

Abbreviations

Abs	Antibodies
ACR	American College of Rheumatology
ADAs	Anti-drug antibodies
ADCC	Antibody-dependent cellular cytotoxicity
ADCP	Antibody dependent cellular phagocytosis
AEs	Adverse events
AML	Acute myeloid leukemia)
APC	Antigen-presenting cell
BRM	Biological response modifiers
CDC	Complement Dependent Cytotoxicity
CDCC	Complement Dependent Cell mediated Cytotoxicity
CDCP	Complement Dependent Cell mediated Phagocytosis
CDRs	Complementarity determining regions
CMC	Complement dependent cytotoxicity
CSA	Ciclosporine A
DAMP	Damage-associated molecular pattern

Declaration COI: Tim Niehues is receiving honoraria from Up2date.com as a reviewer and author.

T. Niehues
Zentrum für Kinder- und Jugendmedizin, HELIOS KLINIKUM Krefeld,
Lutherplatz 40, 47805 Krefeld, Germany

Akad. Lehrkrankenhaus, RWTH Aachen, Aachen, Germany
e-mail: tim.niehues@helios-gesundheit.de

P. Imbach (ed.), *Antibody Therapy*, https://doi.org/10.1007/978-3-319-68038-5_20

EGFR (synonyms erbb1, HER1)	Epithelial growth factor receptors
ESR	Erythrocyte sedimentation rate
EULAR	European League against Rheumatism
Fab	Variable region of antibody, antigen-binding fragment
FAEs	Fatal adverse events
Fc	Constant region of antibody, crystalizable fragment
FcR	Fc receptors
FcRn	Neonatal FC receptor
FDA	Food and Drug Administration (USA)
GD2	Glykolipiddisialoganglioside
GMCSF	Granulocyte macrophage colony stimulating factor
HAMAs	Human anti-mouse antibodies
HAT	Medium containing hypoxanthine, aminopterin, thymidine
HER-2	Human epidermal growth factor receptor 2
IBD	Inflammatory bowel disease
Ig	Immunoglobulin
irAEs	Immune related adverse events
ITP	Idiopathic thrombocytopenic purpura
IVIG	Intravenous immunoglobulins
JAK	Janus Kinase
JC virus	John Cunningham virus
JiA	Juvenile idiopathic arthritis
mAbs	Monoclonal antibodies
MAC	Membrane attack complex
MS	Multiple sclerosis
MTX	Methotrexate
NSAIDS	Non-steroidal and anti-inflammatory drugs
PAMP	Pathogen-associated molecular pattern
PDGFR	Platelet-derived growth factor receptor
PEG	Polyethylene glycol
PJP	Pneumocystis jiroveci pneumonia
PIGF	Placental growth factor
PML	Progressive multifocal leukoencephalopathy
PRRs	Pathogen recognition receptors
RA	Rheumatoid arthritis
RANK	Receptor activator of nuclear factor kappaB
RANKL	Receptor activator of NFκb ligand
SIRs	Standard infusion reactions
sJIA	Systemic onset JIA
SLE	Systemic lupus erythematosus
SYK	Spleen tyrosine kinases
TAA	Tumor associated antigens
TCR	T-cell receptor
TDM	Therapeutic drug monitoring
TNF	Tumor necrosis factor
Tregs	T-regulatory cells
VEGF	Vascular endothelial growth factor

20.1 Introduction

Immunotherapy has been a long wish among immunologists. In the late 19th century, the first proof of immunotherapy was probably the successful treatment of diphtheria by Emil von Behring, using serum (Behring and Kitasato 1890). In 1952, Ogden Bruton showed that patients devoid of immunoglobulins (X-linked agammaglobulinemia) can successfully be treated with plasma containing polyclonal antibodies (Bruton et al. 1952). In 1981, Paul Imbach and colleagues demonstrated that polyclonal antibody preparations can be used to treat immune-mediated disease (idiopathic thrombocytopenic purpura (ITP)) (Imbach et al. 1981).

In 1948 Astrid Fagraeus had published the first detailed chemical structure of antibodies (Fagraeus 1948). In the early 1970s Milstein and colleagues used transformed B-cells (myelomas) and myeloma fusion partners to generate hybrid cells (so-called hybridomas) that produced large amounts of different antibodies. Georges Köhler joined Milstein in 1973, immunized mice with sheep red blood-cells and then fused the lymphocytes from their spleen with myelomas. These hybridomas produced specific antibodies to sheep red blood-cells with a single type of specific antibody termed monoclonal antibodies (mAbs) (Köhler and Milstein 1975). Milstein and Köhler received the Nobel Prize in 1984 but never patented their findings. In 2014, the top ten therapeutic mAbs sold for annual global sales of more than 72 billion dollars (https://www.thebalance.com/top-biologic-drugs-2663233). In 2020, it is estimated that 70 monoclonal antibody products will be on the market with worldwide sales of nearly 125 billion dollars (Ecker et al. 2015).

20.2 Definitions

Monoclonal antibodies (*mAbs*) resemble human physiological molecules with high molecular complexity and belong to the group of biologics. There are different terms for *mAbs* used as therapeutic agents: Biological response modifiers (BRM), biologics, biologicals, therapeutic antibodies, biologic agents, biopharmaceuticals, etc.

Biologics describe any agent that is made by a biological process. According to FDA definitions biologics are medical products made from living sources (human, animal, microorganisms), e.g. vaccines, blood products, allergenic extracts, gene therapies, cellular therapies, etc.

Difference of Biologics to conventional drugs: Conventional drugs consist of chemical substances with known structures. Biologics are complex mixtures that are not easily identified or characterized. They tend to be heat-sensitive and susceptible to microbial contamination.

Biosimilars are copies of biologics (see Table 20.1). According to WHO a biosimilar is a biotherapeutic product which is similar in terms of quality, safety, and efficacy to an already licensed reference biotherapeutic product. It has the same primary amino acid sequence as the reference product and has undergone rigorous analytic and clinical testing in comparison with its reference product (Anonymous 2009; Chingcuanco et al. 2016; Kay 2016). Based on sufficient biosimilarity and interchangeability, biosimilars have been successfully used in patients (e.g., TNFα inhibitors, Etanercept, Adalimumab, Infliximab, and Rituximab).

Table 20.1 Targets for therapeutic morbs on hematopoietic cells other than lymphocytes, licensed by FDA (last updated in 03/2017)

Target system	Target molecule	Antibody	Brand name	Type of antibody/protein	Route	Indication (FDA)
Granulocytes (adhesion molecules)						
	Alpha-4 integrin	**Natalizumab**	Tysabri	Humanized IgG4κ	i.v.	Relapsing forms of MS, Crohn's disease
	Integrin $\alpha_4\beta_7$ (LPAM-1, lymphocyte Peyer's patch adhesion molecule 1)	**Vedolizumab**	Entyvio	Humanized	i.v.	Ulcerative colitis
Platelets						
	GPIIb/IIIa	**Abciximab**	ReoPro	Chimeric/human monoclonal antibody; Fab portion	i.v.	Cardiac ischemia

Comments/Meta-analyses (emphasis on Cochrane library, last 10 years):

MS: In relapsing remitting multiple sclerosis Interferons, Natalizumab, Alemtuzumab, Daclizumab, and other drugs were examined. Alemtuzumab, Natalizumab, and Fingolimod were the best choices of preventing clinical relapse in a 24-month follow-up. For prevention of disability only Natalizumab showed a beneficial effect (Tramacere, Cochrane Database Syst Rev. 2015 Sep 18;(9):CD011381)

IBD: Controlled randomized trials on moderate to severe Crohn's disease or ulcerative colitis were examined regarding mucosal healing as an endpoint (observation periods of 6–12 weeks for induction, 32–54 weeks for maintenance). Anti-TNF was more effective than placebo for maintaining mucosal healing in Crohn's disease. In ulcerative colitis Adalimumab was inferior to Infliximab. Both Infliximab and Adalimumab were similar in Crohn's disease. (Cholapraneh, Elementary pharmacology and therapeutics 2017;45:1291–1302)

Table 20.2 Targets for therapeutic mabs licensed by FDA (last updated in 03/2017) on lymphocytes, T-cells and antigen-presenting cells (APC), B cells and soluble targets (B cell specific cytokines)

Target system	Target molecule	Antibody	Brand name	Type of antibody/protein	Route	Indication (FDA)
Lymphocyte subpopulation						
	CD52	**Alemtuzumab**	Campath, Lemtrada	Humanized IgG1κ, recombinant	i.v.	Chronic B-lymphocyte Leukemia (B-CLL)
T-lymphocytes						
	IL2RA	**Basiliximab**	Simulect	Chimeric IgG1κ, recombinant	i.v.	Prophylaxis of acute organ rejection in adults
	IL2R	**Daclizumab**	Zinbryta	Humanized	s.c.	Multiple sclerosis
	IL-2R	**Denileukin diftitox**	ONTAK	Recombinant fusion protein expressing amino acid residues of diphtheria toxin fragment A & B, followed by the sequence for IL-2	i.v.	Recurrent CD25 positive, cutaneous T-cell lymphoma
	CD3/CD19	**Blinatumomab**	Blincyto	Mouse, bispecific	i.v.	Precursor B-cell acute lymphoblastic leukemia

(continued)

Table 20.2 (continued)

Target system	Target molecule	Antibody	Brand name	Type of antibody/protein	Route	Indication (FDA)
T-lymphocyte/APC (synapse)						
	B7-1 (CD80), B7-2 (CD86)	**Abatacept**	Orencia	CTLA4-Human IgG1 Fusion protein	s.c.	Rheumatoid Arthritis, Juvenile Rheumatoid Arthritis
	CD80, CD86	**Belatacept**	Nulojix	CTLA fused to the Fc portion of human IgG1	i.v.	Prophylaxis of organ rejection after kidney transplant
	CTLA-4	**Ipilimumab**	Yervoy	Chimeric IgG1κ, recombinant monoclonal antibody	i.v.	Melanoma that is metastatic or unresectable
	PD-1	**Nivolumab**	Opdivo	Fully human	i.v.	Metastatic melanoma, Metastatic squamous non-small cell lung carcinoma
	PD-1	**Pembrolizumab**	Keytruda	Humanized	i.v.	Metastatic melanoma
	PD-L1	**Atezolizumab**	Tecentriq	Humanized	i.v.	Urothelial carcinoma
	PD-L1	**Durvalumab**	Imfinzi	Fully human	i.v.	Urothelial carcinoma
	PD-L1	**Avelumab**	Bavencio	Fully human	i.v.	Metastatic Merkel cell carcinoma
Comments/Meta-analyses (emphasis on Cochrane library, last 10 years):						
Metastatic melanoma: Various immunotherapy agents alone or in combination with chemotherapy have been used (checkpoint inhibitors: Ipilimumab, Pembrolizumab, Nivolumab). No systematic Cochrane reviews available						
Metastatic non-small cell lung carcinoma: Nivolumab, pembrolizumab have been used as some of the tumors overexpress PDL1.ipilimumab as inhibitor of CTLA4. No systematic Cochrane reviews available						
Urothelial carcinoma: Atezolizumab has been used in metastatic disease. No systematic Cochrane reviews available						
B cells and B cell specific cytokines						
	BLyS (BAFF)	**Belimumab**	Benlysta	Human monoclonal antibody IgG1-lambda	i.v.	Systematic lupus erythematosus (SLE)
	CD20	**Ocrelizumab**	Ocrevus	Humanized	i.v.	Systemic lupus erythematosus (SLE), Multiple sclerosis (MS)
	CD20	**Rituximab**	Rituxan	Chimeric IgG1κ, recombinant	i.v.	Rheumatoid arthritis; B-cell non-Hodgkin's lymphoma
Comments/Meta-analyses (emphasis on Cochrane library, last 10 years):						
SLE: Belimumab showed a significant benefit compared to standard-of-care treatment in patients with primary cutaneous and musculoskeletal manifestations of SLE (Navarra SV, Lancet 2011;377:721; Furie, Arthritis and Rheumatism 2011;63:3918). Atacicept, a fusion protein blocking BLYS and APRIL showed no difference to placebo at a standard dose (Isenberg, Annals of rheumatic diseases 2015;74:2006)						

Table 20.3 Therapeutic mabs and fusion proteins against tumor necrosis factor (TNF), licensed by FDA (last update 03/2017)

Target molecule	Antibody	Brand name	Type of antibody/protein	Route	Indication (FDA)
TNF	**Adalimumab**	Humira	Human IgG1κ, recombinant	s.c.	Rheumatoid arthritis; juvenile idiopathic arthritis; psoriatic arthritis; ankylosing spondylitis; Crohn's disease; plaque psoriasis
TNF	**Certolizumab pegol**	Cimzia	Humanized, recombinant Fab' fragment conjugated to polyethylene glycol	s.c.	Crohn's disease
TNFα and TNFβ	**Etanercept**	Enbrel	TNFR-IgG1 Fc fusion protein	s.c.	Rheumatoid arthritis; juvenile idiopathic arthritis; psoriatic arthritis; ankylosing spondylitis; Crohn's disease; plaque psoriasis
TNF alpha	**Infliximab**	Remicade	Chimeric IgG1k, recombinant monoclonal antibody	i.v.	Rheumatoid arthritis (in combination with methotrexate); Ankylosing spondylitis; Psoriatic arthritis; Plaque psoriasis; Crohn's disease; Ulcerative colitis; Pediatric ulcerative colitis
TNF	**Infliximab-dyyb**	Inflectra	Chimeric, biosimilar	i.v.	Crohn's disease, Ulcerative colitis, Ankylosing spondylitis, Psoriatic arthritis, Plaque psoriasis
TNF	**Golimumab**	Simponi Aria	Fully human	i.v.	Rheumatoid arthritis

(continued)

Table 20.3 (continued)

Target molecule	Antibody	Brand name	Type of antibody/protein	Route	Indication (FDA)
TNF	**Golimumab**	Simponi	Human IgG1κ, recombinant	s.c.	Rheumatoid arthritis; Psoriatic arthritis; Ankylosing spondylitis
TNF	**Adalimumab-atto**	Amjevita	Fully human, biosimilar	s.c.	Rheumatoid arthritis
TNF	**Infliximab-abda**	Renflexis	Chimeric, biosimilar	i.v.	Crohn's disease, Ulcerative colitis, Rheumatoid arthritis, Ankylosing spondylitis, Psoriatic arthritis, Plaque psoriasis

Comments/Meta-analyses (emphasis on Cochrane library, last 10 years):

Rheumatoid arthritis RA: Abatacept, Adalimumab, Etanercept, Infliximab, and Rituximab were associated with significant improvement in the ACR 50 rate. Anakinra was less effective than all the other biologics. (Singh CMAJ, Canadian Medical Association Journal 2009;181:787). Patients were more likely to withdraw from the trials if they were on biologics. There is no evidence that any one of the TNF inhibitors has greater efficacy than the others (Medical Letters drugs therapy 2010:52(1338):38)

Ankylosing spondylitis: TNF inhibitors increase the chance of achieving partial remission and slight improvement of spinal inflammation as measured by MRI. (Maxwell, Cochrane Database Syst Rev. 2015 Apr 18;(4):CD005468). In the biologics group more patients dropped out of the studies because of side-effects. Compared to placebo, improvement with TNF blockers was rated between 25 and 40%. Partial remission was reached in 10–44%. TNFα blockers were shown to improve disease activity and functional capacity in a clinically meaningful manner (Callhoff et al. Annals of Rheumatic Diseases 2015;74:1241)

JIA Polyarthritis: The majority of trials show a flawed trial design (so-called withdrawal design). The only properly designed double blind randomized placebo controlled trial did not show a significant effect regarding efficacy of Infliximab (Ruperto, Arthritis and Rheumatism 2007;56:3098)

Pediatric psoriasis: There is a single randomized controlled trial (industry sponsored and observation of 12 weeks) Sanclemente, Cochrane Skin Group 2015 DOI: 10.1002/14651858.CD010017.pub2)

Table 20.4 Therapeutic mabs and fusion proteins against Interleukin 1 (IL 1) and Interleukin 6 (IL 6), licensed by FDA (last update 03/2017)

Target system	Target molecule	Antibody	Brand name	Type of antibody/protein	Route	Indication (FDA)
Interleukin 1						
	Interleukin-1 type I receptor (IL-1RI)	**Anakinra**	Kineret	Recombinant, nonglycosylated form of the human interleukin-1 receptor antagonist (IL-1Ra)	s.c.	Moderately to severely active rheumatoid arthritis, in patients 18 years of age or older who have failed 1 or more disease modifying antirheumatic drugs
	IL1B	**Canakinumab**	Ilaris	Human anti-human-IL-1β IgG1 monoclonal antibody	s.c.	Treatment of CAPS, including Familial Cold Autoinflammatory Syndrome (FCAS), and Muckle-Wells Syndrome (MWS), in adults and children 4 years of age and older
	IL-1 beta (IL-1β)	**Rilonacept**	Arcalyst	Dimeric fusion protein; ligand-binding domains of IL-1 receptor (IL-1R) & IL-1 receptor accessory protein (IL-1RAcP) linked to human IgG1	s.c.	Cryopyrin-associated periodic fever syndromes (CAPS), including Muckle-Wells syndrome (MWS) and familial cold autoinflammatory syndrome (FCAS) in children 12 years and older
Interleukin 6						
	IL6	**Siltuximab**	Sylvant	Chimeric	i.v.	Multicentric Castleman's disease
	IL6R	**Tocilizumab**	Actemra	Humanized	i.v., s.c.	Rheumatoid arthritis, Polyarticular juvenile idiopathic arthritis, Systemic juvenile idiopathic arthritis

Comments/Meta-analyses (emphasis on Cochrane library, last 10 years):

RA: The Il1-blocking Anakinra was less effective than all the other biologics. (Singh, Canadian Medical Association Journal 2009;181:787)

Crohn's disease: A Tocilizumab trial has been stopped as a number of bowel perforations were observed that might have been obscured by the fact that CRP levels cannot be judged in antiIL6R treatment because CRP levels depend on IL6

Castleman's disease: Is due to an excessive release of pro-inflammatory cytokines and excess proliferation of B-and T-cells. Targeting IL6 may be a promising approach to treat HHV8 negative multicentric Castleman's disease

Table 20.5 Therapeutic mabs against IgE, Interleukin 4 (IL4) and Interleukin 5 (IL5), licensed by FDA (last update 03/2017)

Target system	Target molecule	Antibody	Brand name	Type of antibody/ protein	Route	Indication (FDA)
IgE						
	IgE	**Omalizumab**	Xolair	Humanized IgG1κ, recombinant	i.v.	Moderate to severe IgE-mediated, persistent asthma (US) or severe asthma (EU), in adults and children over 12 years old, inadequately controlled by inhaled corticosteroid treatment
Interleukin 4						
	IL4RA	**Dupilumab**	Dupixent	Fully human	s.c.	Atopic dermatitis
Interleukin 5						
	IL5	**Mepolizumab**	Nucala	Humanized IgG1κ monoclonal antibody	s.c.	Severe eosinophilic asthma in patients aged 12 years or older
	IL5	**Reslizumab**	Cinqair	Humanized	i.v	Severe asthma

Comments/Meta-analyses (emphasis on Cochrane library, last 10 years):

Asthma: Omalizumab was effective in reducing asthma exacerbations and hospitalizations as an adjunctive therapy to inhaled steroids and during steroid tapering phases of clinical trials. It remains to be tested prospectively whether the addition of omalizumab has a prednisolone-sparing effect and whether there is a threshold level of baseline serum IgE for optimum efficacy of omalizumab. Given the high cost of the drug, identification of biomarkers predictive of response is of major importance for future research. (Normansell, The Cochrane Library: 13 January 2014; DOI: 10.1002/14651858.CD003559.pub4)

Severe eosinophilic asthma: There is a single study on Mepolizumab in participants with severe eosinophilic asthma: improvement in health-related quality of life scores and reduction of asthma exacerbations. There are no studies reporting results from children. (Powell, Cochrane Database of Systematic Reviews 2015, Issue 7. Art. No.: CD010834. DOI: 10.1002/14651858.CD010834.pub2))

Table 20.6 Therapeutic mabs against Interleukin 17 (IL 17), Interleukin 12 (IL 12), and Interleukin 23 (IL 23), licensed by FDA (last update 03/2017)

Target system	Target molecule	Antibody	Brand name	Type of antibody/ protein	Route	Indication (FDA)
Interleukin 17						
	IL17A	**Ixekizumab**	Taltz	Humanized	s.c.	Plaque psoriasis
	IL17A	**Secukinumab**	Cosentyx	Human immunoglobulin G1k (IgG1k) subclass monoclonal antibody	s.c.	Moderate to severe plaque psoriasis; ankylosing spondylitis; psoriatic arthritis
	IL17RA	**Brodalumab**	Siliq	Chimeric	s.c	Plaque psoriasis
Interleukin 12, Interleukin 23						
	IL12	**Ustekinumab**	Stelara	Human IgG1k monoclonal antibody	s.c	Adult patients (18 years or older) with moderate to severe plaque psoriasis who are candidates for phototherapy or systemic therapy

Comments/Meta-analyses (emphasis on Cochrane library, last 10 years):

Severe Crohn's disease: Ustekinumab was not significantly better than placebo in moderate to severe Crohn's disease (Rogler, Digestive diseases 2017;35:5–12)

Psoriasis: Biologics are highly effective for the treatment of moderate to severe psoriasis, and anti-IL-17 drugs have the same, or even greater, efficacy than anti-tumor necrosis factor (TNF) and anti-IL-12/23 drugs. (de Carvalho, Drugs R D. 2017 Mar; 17(1): 29–51)

Table 20.7 Targets on vessels and bone as well as soluble targets (complement) for therapeutic mabs and fusion proteins, licensed by FDA (last update 03/2017)

Target system	Target molecule	Antibody	Brand name	Type of antibody/protein	Route	Indication (FDA)
Complement						
	Complement component 5	**Eculizumab**	Soliris	Humanized	i.v.	Paroxysmal nocturnal hemoglobinuria
Vessels: Vascular and placental growth factors and receptors						
	VEGF, PIGF	**Aflibercept**	Eylea	Fusion protein: IgG Fc, and ligand binding domains of VEGFR-1, VEGFR-2	Intravitreal injection	Wet age-related macular edema; Macular edema following central retinal vein occlusion
	VEGF	**Bevacizumab**	Avastin	Humanized monoclonal antibody	i.v.	Metastatic colorectal cancer; unresectable, locally advanced, recurrent or metastatic non-small cell lung cancer
	VEGFR1	**Ranibizumab**	Lucentis	Humanized IgG1κ Fab fragment	Intravitreal injection	Neovascular (wet) age-related macular degeneration
	VEGFR2	**Ramucirumab**	Cyramza	Fully human	i.v.	Gastric cancer
	VEGF, PIGR	**Ziv-aflibercept**	Zaltrap	Fusion protein: IgG Fc, and ligand binding domains of VEGFR-1 and VEGFR-2	i.v.	Metastatic colorectal cancer
Bone: osteoclast activation						
	RANKL	**Denosumab**	Prolia, Xgeva	Human IgG2 monoclonal antibody	Subcutaneous	Xgeva: Prevention of skeletal-related events in patients with bone metastases from solid tumors; Prolia: treatment of postmenopausal osteoporosis; treatment of men receiving androgen deprivation

Comments/Meta-analyses (emphasis on Cochrane library, last 10 years):

*Metastatic colorectal cancer***:** Bevacizumab has varying success

Metastatic non-small cell lung carcinoma: Addition of Bevacizumab to Carboplatin and Paclitaxel may increase overall survival and progression-free survival in some patients (Sandler, NEJM 2006;355:2542)

Gastric cancer: Ramucirumab has been used in cases of advanced gastric cancer. It is unclear how effective it is

Table 20.8 Tumor associated antigenes (TAA) and growth factor receptors as targets for therapeutic mabs, licensed by FDA (last update 03/2017)

Target molecule	Antibody	Brand name	Type of antibody/protein	Route	Indication (FDA)
HER2	**Ado-trastuzumab emtansine**	Kadcyla	Humanized IgG1κ mAb	i.v.	HER-2 positive metastatic breast cancer
EGFR	**Cetuximab**	Erbitux	Chimeric monoclonal antibody	i.v.	Metastatic colorectal cancer, head and neck cancer
GD2	**Dinutuximab**	Unituxin	Chimeric	i.v.	Pediatric high-risk neuroblastoma
EGFR	**Panitumumab**	Vectibix	Recombinant human IgG2κ monoclonal antibody	i.v.	Treatment of EGFR-expressing, metastatic colorectal carcinoma with disease progression on or following fluoropyrimidine-, oxaliplatin-, and irinotecan- containing chemotherapy regimens
HER2	**Pertuzumab**	Perjeta	Humanized IgG1κ monoclonal antibody, glycosylated	i.v.	HER2 overexpressing breast cancer, in combination with trastuzumab and docetaxel
PDGFRA	**Olaratumab**	Lartruvo	Fully human	i.v.	Soft tissue sarcoma
HER2	**Trastuzumab**	Herceptin	Humanized receptor antagonist	i.v.	HER2 overexpressing breast cancer
EGFR	**Necitumumab**	Portrazza	Fully human	i.v.	Metastatic squamous non-small cell lung carcinoma

Comments/Meta-analyses (emphasis on Cochrane library, last 10 years):

Breast cancer: Trastuzumab has improved 5-year disease-free survival in tumors overexpressing the receptor HER2 significantly

Neuroblastoma: Dinutuximab and addition of cytokines GMCSF, IL2 and Isotretinoin improves outcome (Yu, NEJM 2010)

Metastatic colorectal cancer: Cetuximab and Panitumumab have varying success

Soft-tissue sarcoma including gastrointestinal tumors: Studies have focused on inoperable metastatic and/or recurrent disease using Olaratumab either with Doxorubicin or without

Table 20.9 Targets on hematopoietic malignant cells, licensed by FDA (last update 03/2017)

Target system	Target molecule	Antibody	Brand name	Type of antibody/protein	Route	Indication (FDA)
	CD38	**Daratumumab**	Darzalex	Fully human	i.v.	Multiple myeloma
	SLAMF7	**Elotuzumab**	Empliciti	Humanized	i.v.	Multiple myeloma
	CD19	**Blinatumomab**	Blincyto	Mouse, bispecific	i.v.	Precursor B-cell acute lymphoblastic leukemia
	CD30	**Brentuximab vedotin**	Adcetris	Chimeric IgG1k monoclonal antibody conjugated to a microtubule disrupting agent MMAE by a protease-cleavable linker	i.v.	Hodgkin's lymphoma, Systemic anaplastic large cell lymphoma
	CD20	**Ibritumomab tiuxetan**	Zevalin	Murine IgG1κ monoclonal antibody, conjugated to a chelator (tiuxetan) for labeling with Indium-111 or Yttrium-90	i.v.	Non-Hodgkins Lymphoma (CD20 positive, low-grade or follicular) which is relapsed or refractory to rituximab, in combination with rituximab
	CD20	**Tositumomab**	Bexxar	Murine, monoclonal; covalently bound to Iodine-131		Non-Hodgkins Lymphoma (CD20 positive, follicular) which is refractory to rituximab and relapsed following chemotherapy
	CD20	**Obinutuzumab**	Gazyva	Humanized IgG1 monoclonal antibody	i.v.	Chronic Lymphocytic Leukemia in combination with chemotherapy in treatment-naïve patients
	CD20	**Ofatumumab**	Arzerra	Human IgG1κ monoclonal antibody, recombinant	i.v.	Chronic lymphocytic leukemia resistant to fludarabine and alemtuzumab

Comments/Meta-analyses (emphasis on Cochrane library, last 10 years):

Lymphoma B-cell chronic lymphocytic leukemia, Non-Hodgkins Lymphoma, Hodgkins Lymphoma and Anaplastic large-cell lymphoma: Rituximab has been used for B-cell Non-Hodgkins Lymphoma and is included in current chemotherapy standard chemotherapy protocols as it has been shown to be effective (Chop-R). Brentuximab has been used in Hodgkin lymphoma but is not part of the standard chemotherapy protocols

Chronic Lymphocytic Leukemia (CLL): Obinutuzumab and Ofatumumab, Alemtuzumab have been used but are not part of the standard protocols. Rituximab plus chemotherapy is more effective than chemotherapy alone. (Bauer, Cochrane Library 2012, DOI: 10.1002/14651858.CD008079.pub2)

Multiple Myeloma High-dose chemotherapy with autologous hematopoietic stem cell transplantation has become the treatment of choice in patients under 65 years of age. In relapses Elotuzumab and Daratumumab have been tried

Table 20.10 Targets for therapeutic mabs on microorganisms, liver cells, and drugs licensed by FDA (lcs update 3/2017)

Target system	Target molecule	Antibody	Brand name	Type of antibody/ protein	Route	Indication (FDA)
Microorganisms						
	F protein of RSV	**Palivizumab**	Synagis	Humanized IgG1κ	Intramuscular	Prevention of serious lower respiratory tract disease caused by respiratory syncytial virus (RSV) in pediatric patients at high risk of RSV disease
	Protective antigen of Bacillus anthracis	**Raxibacumab**	Raxibacumab	Human IgG1-lambda mAB	i.v.	Inhalational anthrax
	Protective antigen of the Anthrax toxin	**Obiltoxaximab**	Anthem	Chimeric	i.v.	Inhalational anthrax
	Clostridium difficile toxin B	**Bezlotoxumab**	Zinplava	Fully human	i.v.	Prevent recurrence of Clostridium difficile infection
Liver cells/LDL-receptors						
	PCSK9	**Evolocumab**	Repatha	Fully human	s.c.	Heterozygous familial hypercholesterolemia; Refractory hypercholesterolemia
	PCSK9	**Alirocumab**	Praluent	Fully human	s.c.	Heterozygous familial hypercholesterolemia; Refractory hypercholesterolemia
Drugs						
	Dabigatran	**Idarucizumab**	Praxbind	Humanized Fab	i.v.	Emergency reversal of anticoagulant dabigatran

Kinase inhibitors are relative simple chemical compounds, having Janus (JAK) and Spleen tyrosine kinases (SYK) as targets. Kinase inhibitors may result in similar effects as they may target the same pathway as a monoclonal antibody. Unlike biologics they are not proteins and hence not biologics. They may have similar effects on immune-mediated diseases as many mAbs, as some of them inhibit the downstream signaling of proinflammatory cytokines (Patterson et al. 2014; Wu et al. 2015). In this article I focus on mAbs, biosimilars, and engineered proteins (e.g., fusion proteins, bispecific antibodies) that have entered clinical practice.

20.3 Terminology

The USAN (United States Adopted Names) Council has proposed guidelines for the naming of mAbs (https://www.ama-assn.org/about/monoclonal-antibodies). Starting from the end of the name all monoclonal antibodies end with the suffix –mab (Fig. 20.1) (Ballow 2005). Any monoclonal antibody name is composed of combining key elements

1. Prefix
2. Infix, representing the target or disease and/or indicating the source
3. Stem used as suffix

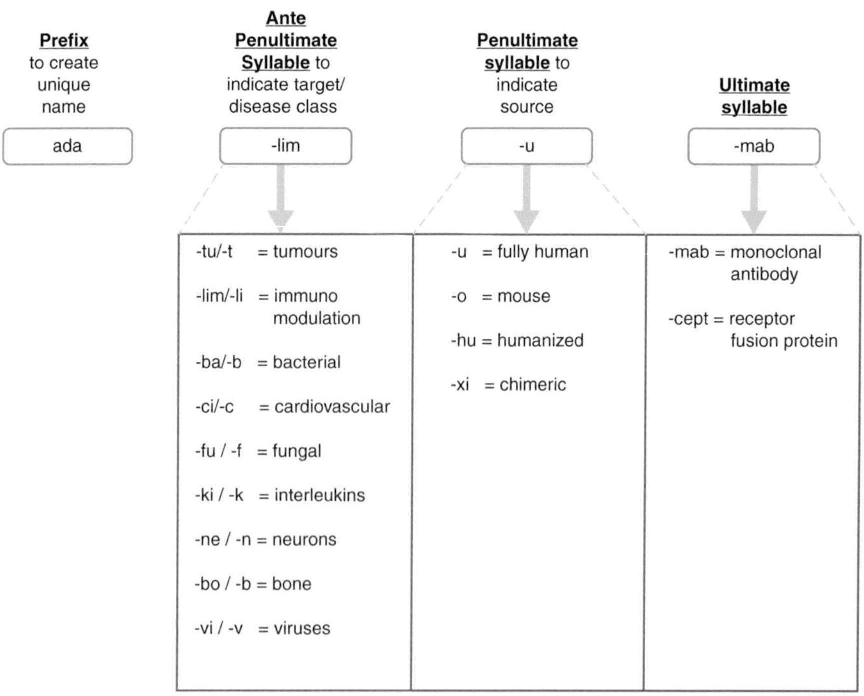

Fig. 20.1 Nomenclature INN (International non-priority names) for biologicals and biotechnology substances. Adapted from www.ama-assu.org/about monoclonal-antibodies

Prefixes are used to create a unique name, a distinct compatible syllable as the starting prefix. The choice of inflix is determined by the available information regarding clinical indications and antibody action. The target disease inflix has been truncated with a single letter when the source inflix begins with a vowel. Examples for target/disease class inflixes are shown in Fig. 20.1.

Recently, it has become quite difficult to capture the mAbs vowel in a single syllable, so terminology is changing (Parren et al. 2017).

20.4 Antibody Structure and Engineering

The basis for development of therapeutic antibodies is the precise knowledge of the normal IgG antibody structure and activity, which is schematically outlined in Fig. 20.2a. IgG can be engineered to a higher specificity, longer half-life, and better bio-availability (summarized in Fig. 20.2b) The function of antibodies is dependent on their binding affinity and target specificity. Instability or aggregation hotspots in the antibodies CDRs can be removed, the hinge can be stabilized and glycosylation inhibited (e.g., aglycosylated IgG4). In the variable region (Fab), affinity can be altered and may allow targeting antigens even more selectively.

The Fc region of any antibody interacts with immune cells carrying Fc receptors (FcR) (e.g., macrophages). By engineering glycosylation status antibody dependent cellular cytotoxicity can be altered. The half-life of the antibody can be engineered by altering binding of the Fc part of the mAb to the neonatal FC receptor (FcRn) (e.g., on endothelial cells). MAbs can be associated with highly cytotoxic drugs, cytokines, toxins, etc.

Bispecific antibodies with a simultaneous blockade of two or more targets may be even more promising than inhibition of a single target (e.g., the bispecific antibody Blinatumomab).

20.5 Production Technology

MAbs are typically made by fusing myeloma cells with mouse spleen cells that have been previously immunized with the desired antigen and future target. Myeloma cells have lost the ability to grow in standard media. This can be exploited by supplementing standard culture media with so-called HAT medium containing hypoxanthine, aminopterin, and thymidine and thus selectively grow hybridomas. Single cell clones are grown on microtiter wells and the antibodies secreted by different clones are assayed for their ability to bind antigen. The most productive and stable clones are selected for future use. Injected into mice, these hybridomas can produce antibody-rich fluid (ascites), containing large amounts of monoclonal antibody. In 1986, the first murine monoclonal antibody Muromonab (CD3 specific) was used clinically. Initial therapeutic antibodies were composed of all mouse protein which were highly immunogenic leading to human anti-mouse antibodies (HAMAs) and toxicities.

Moreover, mAbs are heterogeneous as they contain aggregates, degradation products, glycosylation variants, oxidized side chains, as well as amino and carboxyl

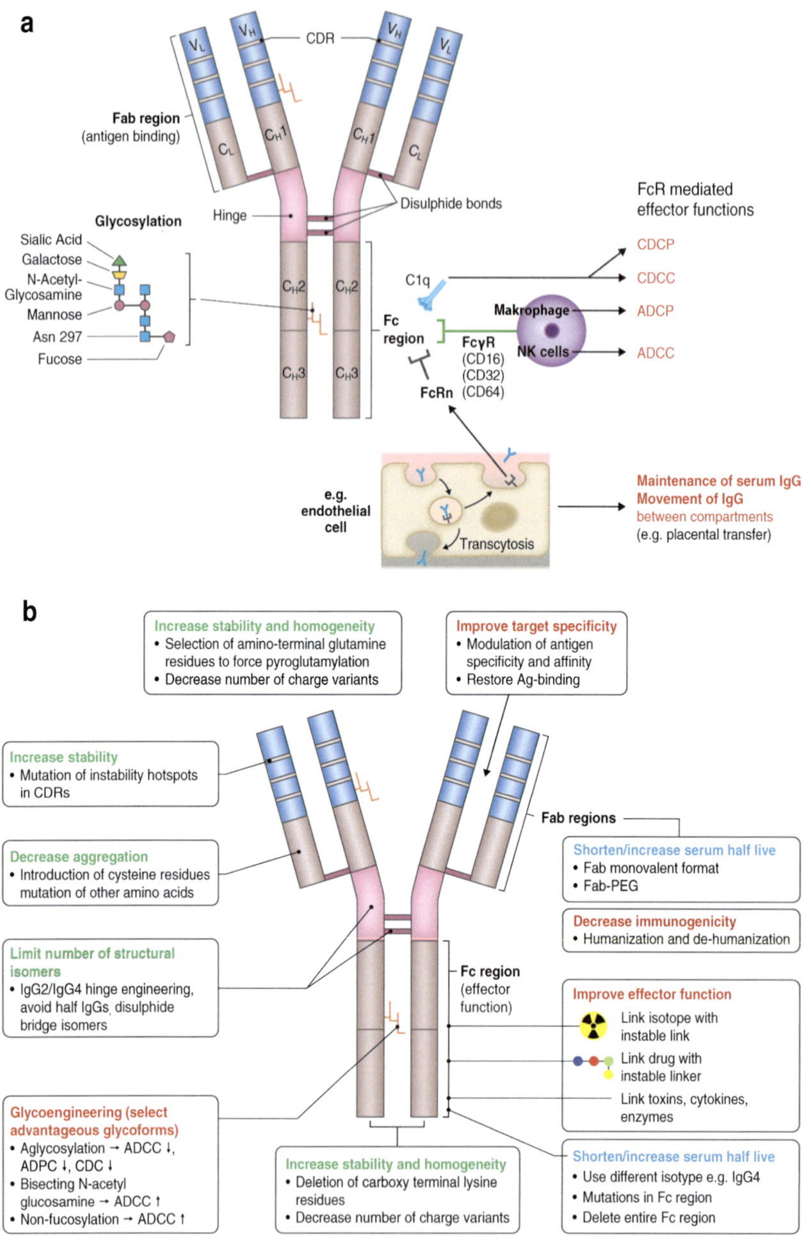

Improvement/modulation of pharmaceutical progerties is depicted in green; Improvement of antibody function in red and Modulation of pharmacokinetics/pharmacodynamics in blue

amino acid additions. All of these can have consequences for product potency, bio-availability, and immunogenicity. Moreover, mAbs do not experience the post-translational modification that physiological abs get from mammalian cells (e.g., glycosylation).

In 1984, antibody chimerization had been described by Morrison et al. (1984). Chimeric antibodies had been created by combining murine monoclonal antibody variable regions with the constant region of a human antibody. In 1986, antibody humanization was described by Jones et al. (1986). Humanized mAbs were developed which incorporated only the hypervariable or complementarity determining regions (CDRs) of the murine monoclonal antibody to the remaining portions of the human IgG molecule. Such a humanized antibody then had less than 10% of their murine constituent.

In the early 1990s Phage display technology, single B-cell cultures, and usage of transgenic mice allowed for fully humanized and then fully human antibodies (Beck et al. 2010).

20.6 Pharmacokinetics

From polyclonal IgG preparations it is known that IgG has a half-life of 3–4 weeks. The half-life will be influenced by lysosomal degradation that can be prevented by binding to a scavenger receptor, the neonatal FC receptor (FcRn), e.g. expressed in endothelial cells. The bio-distribution of mAbs was studied by using radio-labelled mAbs and measuring their distribution by positron emission tomography PET: mAbs are cleared gradually from the circulation by liver, spleen, and kidneys and specifically accumulate at the target site. MAbs even are located to the human brain, which originally was thought to be a sanctuary (Oosting et al. 2015).

Fig. 20.2 (**a**) Normal IgG 1 structure and its interaction at the Fc region with complement and effector cells via different Fc receptors (e.g. Fc γ receptor, Fc receptor n) (**b**) Engineering of IgG1. Adapted from Beck et al. (2010), Chan and Carter (2010), and Weiner (2015). Illustration: Oliver Hippmann, Schwarzenbruck. ADCC = antibody dependent cellular cytoxicity; ADCP = antibody dependent cellular phagocytosis; Asn = Asparagine at position 297; CD16 = FcγR on NK cells, mast cells, basophils, DC; CD32, CD64 = FcγR on Makrophage, neutrophils, eosinophils, DC; CDC = complement dependent cytotoxicity; ;CDCC = complement dependent cell mediated cytotoxicity; CDCP = complement dependent cell mediated phagocytosis; CDR = complementarity determining region; C_{L1-3} = constant region light chain 1–3; C_{H1-3} = constant region heavy chain 1–3; Fab = fragment antigen binding; Fc = fragment crystallizable; FcR = Fc receptor; FcRn = neonatal Fc receptor; MAC = membrane attack complex; PEG = polyethylen glycol; V_L = variable region light chain; V_H = variable region heavy chain

20.6.1 Factors Influencing Pharmacokinetics

Pharmacokinetics is influenced by significant inter-patient variability (Oude Munnink et al. 2016). It is influenced by demographic variables (body weight, body surface area, gender). Most mAbs are dosed based on body weight or body surface area to equalize monoclonal antibody exposure between patients. As circulating plasma volume is not linearly correlated with body weight, it has been suggested to use fixed dosing instead of weight or surface adapted dosing to reduce variability in exposure. For the monoclonal antibody Panitumumab, Rituximab, Bevacizumab, and Infliximab clearance in females was 23–39% lower and distribution volume 14–22% smaller compared to males. In other studies, this effect was not shown, so dosing of mAbs is still gender-independent and bodyweight/surface dependent.

There is no specific clearance and subsequent degradation. Pharmacokinetics is dependent on disease activity. After having entered the interstitial space and specific binding to the target antigen has taken place, the antigen immune complex is prone to FcR mediated phagocytosis by immune cells and clearance. Target-mediated degradation is dependent on target antigen availability which is likely to be higher in active or non-controlled disease, e.g. in patients with active inflammatory bowel disease or RA, e.g. high levels of TNFα are associated with an increased clearance of Infliximab. Interestingly, in the Atlas Study Infliximab and Adalimumab concentration in tissue biopsies correlated with serum concentrations of the TNFα antibodies. The better the correlation was between serum and tissue antibody concentrations, the more likely patients were in endoscopic remission of their inflammatory bowel disease. High tissue levels of TNFα appear to act as a sink for monoclonal anti TNFα antibodies (Yarur et al. 2016). Similarly, a high tumor load in lymphoma patients is associated with low Rituximab serum concentrations (Golay et al. 2013).

Immunogenicity may limit bioavailability and function of therapeutic mAbs. The less human the therapeutic antibody is, the more likely is the generation of anti-drug antibodies (ADAs). In a study with Infliximab in inflammatory bowel disease ADAs were found in a third of the patients and were associated with high Infliximab clearance (Dotan et al. 2014).

Drugs coadministered with mAbs may delay the clearance of mAbs, e.g. intravenous immunoglobulins (IVIG), which may saturate Fc receptors on endothelial cells/macrophages/monocytes/tissue macrophages. Co-administration of Methotrexate with anti-TNF antibodies like Infliximab and Adalimumab seems to be advantageous because Methotrexate may significantly lower ADAs induction. Lastly, the route of administration is influencing drug levels as subcutaneous administration only appears to have 50–80% bioavailability.

20.6.2 Therapeutic Drug Monitoring TDM

As a consequence, it appears to be logical to do therapeutic drug monitoring in patients treated with mAbs, which is routinely applied in conventional drugs like antibiotics, anti-epileptics, immunosuppressive drugs, etc. The rationale of TDM is to correlate serum concentration and response in order to document interpatient variation in pharmacokinetics, to define the therapeutic window and to allow for flexibility in dosing. Subtherapeutic monoclonal antibody concentrations may result in disease progression which in turn means increased target antigen expression calling for a higher dosage of therapeutic monoclonal antibody in patients with active disease. This vicious cycle may be associated with lowered response and prospective randomized clinical trials have been initiated to explore whether systematic TDM may have a place in treatment algorithms of inflammatory and malignant diseases treated with mAbs.

20.6.2.1 TDM in Immune Mediated Diseases

Antibody trough levels have been estimated for Adalimumab, Infliximab in rheumatologic and inflammatory bowel diseases in several studies. For Adalimumab trough level cut-offs have been 5–8 mg/l in Rheumatoid Arthritis (RA), 0.3–8.1 mg/l in Inflammatory Bowel Disease (IBD). For Infliximab, the cut-off-level has been 1–2.5 mg/l in RA and 0.5–6.2 mg/l in IBD.

20.6.2.2 TDM In Oncology Diseases

Only a few studies have been done to determine trough levels of mAbs and clinical response. For Rituximab the cut-off for trough levels was as variable as 0.3-8.1 mg/l in B-cell lymphoma. In malignant disease the amount of monoclonal antibody necessary to control the tumor might be quite variable. In most of the studies convincing exposure—response relationships provide encouraging evidence for the further exploration of therapeutic drug monitoring TDM.

20.7 Targets

20.7.1 Targets in Immune Mediated Diseases

Targets of mAbs used in the treatment of immune mediated diseases are shown in Fig. 20.3. The inflammation starts with recognition of any antigen (be it antigen, tumor antigen, and allergen) by cells of the innate immune system and amplification of antigen recognition signals by specialized receptors (PRRs: pathogen recognition receptors, e.g. TOLL-like receptors). PRRs are activated by ligands that have a damage-associated molecular pattern DAMP or have a pathogen-associated molecular pattern PAMP (e.g., DNA, RNA from damaged cells or lipopolysaccharides LPS on microorganisms). PRRs are expressed on tissue macrophages and other efficient professional antigen-presenting cells. After decades of research, the events of the initial pathological immune activation are still unclear in many diseases. If setting and exact nature of autoantigens would be known it may be possible to intervene earlier in the disease process by antigen-specific regulation (e.g., by vaccinations). As of now, targets of biologics are mainly downstream of the induction at the stage of perpetuation of chronic inflammation or tissue/organ destruction as depicted in Fig. 20.3.

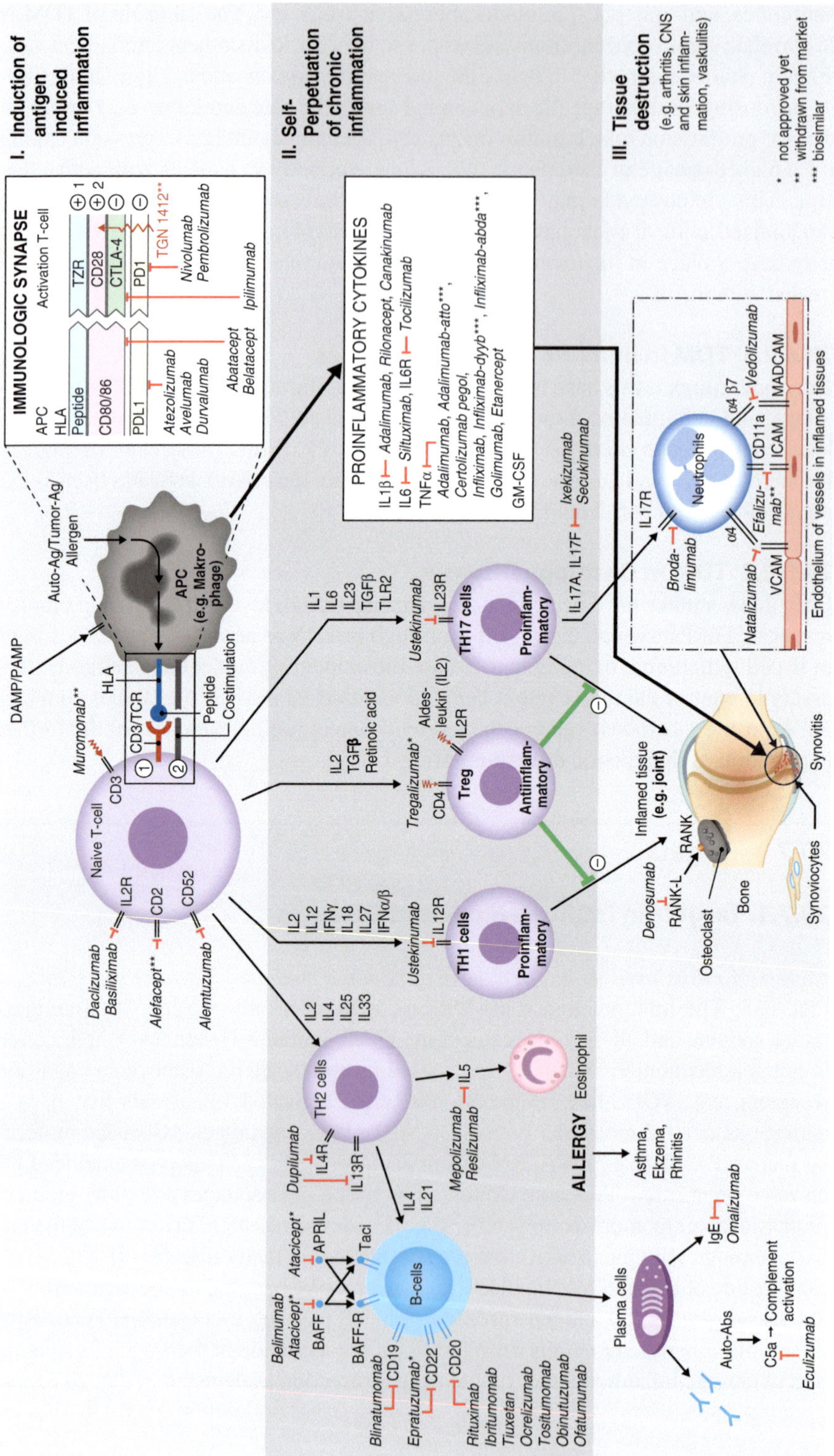
I. Induction of antigen induced inflammation
II. Self-Perpetuation of chronic inflammation
III. Tissue destruction
(e.g. arthritis, CNS and skin inflammation, vaskulitis)
* not approved yet
** withdrawn from market
*** biosimilar
IMMUNOLOGIC SYNAPSE
APC
HLA
Peptide
CD80/86
PDL1
Activation T-cell
TZR
CD28
CTLA-4
PD1
TGN 1412**
Atezolizumab
Avelumab
Durvalumab
Abatacept
Belatacept
Ipilimumab
Nivolumab
Pembrolizumab
PROINFLAMMATORY CYTOKINES
IL1β ⊣ Adalimumab, Rilonacept, Canakinumab
IL6 ⊣ Siltuximab, IL6R ⊣ Tocilizumab
TNFα ⊣
Adalimumab, Adalimumab-atto***,
Certolizumab pegol,
Infliximab, Infliximab-dyyb***, Infliximab-abda***,
Golimumab, Etanercept
GM-CSF
DAMP/PAMP
Auto-Ag/Tumor-Ag/Allergen
APC (e.g. Makrophage)
HLA
Peptide
Costimulation
CD3/TCR
Muromonab**
CD3
Naive T-cell
IL2R
CD2
CD52
Daclizumab
Basiliximab
Alefacept**
Alemtuzumab
IL2
IL12
IFNγ
IL18
IL27
IFNα/β
IL2
TGFβ
Retinoic acid
IL1
IL6
IL23
TGFβ
TLR2
Ustekinumab
IL12R
TH1 cells
Proinflammatory
Tregalizumab*
CD4
Treg
Antiinflammatory
Aldesleukin (IL2)
IL2R
Ustekinumab
IL23R
TH17 cells
Proinflammatory
IL17A, IL17F ⊣ Ixekizumab Secukinumab
IL17R
Brodalimumab
Neutrophils
α4
Efalizumab**
CD11a
α4 β7
Vedolizumab
Natalizumab
VCAM
ICAM
MADCAM
Endothelium of vessels in inflamed tissues
Inflamed tissue (e.g. joint)
Denosumab
RANK-L
RANK
Osteoclast
Bone
Synoviocytes
Synovitis
IL2
IL4
IL25
IL33
TH2 cells
Dupilumab
IL4R
IL13R
Mepolizumab
Reslizumab
IL5
Eosinophil
ALLERGY
Asthma, Ekzema, Rhinitis
IL4
IL21
Belimumab
Atacicept*
BAFF
Atacicept*
APRIL
BAFF-R
Taci
B-cells
CD19
CD22
CD20
Blinatumomab
Epratuzumab*
Rituximab
Ibritumomab
Tiuxetan
Ocrelizumab
Tositumomab
Obinutuzumab
Ofatumumab
Plasma cells
IgE
Omalizumab
Auto-Abs
C5a → Complement activation
Eculizumab

20.7.2 Targets in Oncology

Targets in cancer immunotherapy are shown in Fig. 20.4.

20.7.2.1 Targeting of Tumor Associated Antigens (TAA)

Tumor associated antigens (TAA) represent soluble factors and receptors that are overexpressed in tumors and are optimal blocking targets to avoid cancer cell proliferation, e.g. Epithelial growth factor receptors (EGFR (synonyms erbb1, HER1)), Vascular endothelial growth factor (VEGF), Placental growth factors (PLGF1 and PLGF2), Platelet-derived growth factor receptor (PDGFR), Glykolipiddisialoganglioside (GD2), Receptor activator of NFκb ligand (RANKL) as well as antigens on cells of the hematopoietic lineage etc.

20.7.2.2 Enhancement of Tumor Immunity

The anticancer immune response or inflammation is complex and compartmentalized in blood, lymph nodes, and tumors. Its success depends on priming and activation of anticancer T-cells, the rate of migration of anticancer T-cells from the lymph node to the blood and the rate of T-cell infiltration into the tumor as well as the rate of T-cell efflux from tumors to blood (Chen and Mellman 2017). The so-called checkpoint inhibitors target T-cell activation within the immunological synapse (PD1, PD ligand 1, CTLA4). These checkpoint inhibitors prevent effector T-cells (that fight cancer successfully) from getting exhausted and hyperexhausted (Figs. 20.3 and 20.4). An effective amplifier of the immune system is the use of bispecific antibodies like Blinatumomab, an anti-CD3/anti-CD19 bispecific antibody which simultaneously binds tumor antigen (CD19) and recruits T-cells (CD3). Similar approaches are thought of in neuroblastoma and osteosarcoma (Majzner et al. 2017).

20.8 Mechanism of Action

There are five non-overlapping mechanisms described. Clearly some therapeutic mAbs use multiple mechanisms to reach their effect. Five mechanisms are described (Chen and Mellman 2017).

1. Ligand blockade

   Full length IgG therapeutic antibodies, antibody fragments (e.g., Certolizumab) or receptor fusion proteins (Etanercept) prevent the ligand from engaging with their cognate receptors.
2. Receptor blockade

   Antibodies can be directed directly to their cognate receptors and thus inhibit receptor activation. Examples are Tocilizumab, Natalizumab, Vedolizumab, and Abatacept.

Fig. 20.3 Targets of monoclonal antibodies, fusion proteins and biosimilars in different disease stages of immune-mediated diseases. Adapted from Burmester et al. (2014), Davis and Ballas (2017), and Her and Kavanaugh (2016). Illustration: Oliver Hippmann, Schwarzenbruck

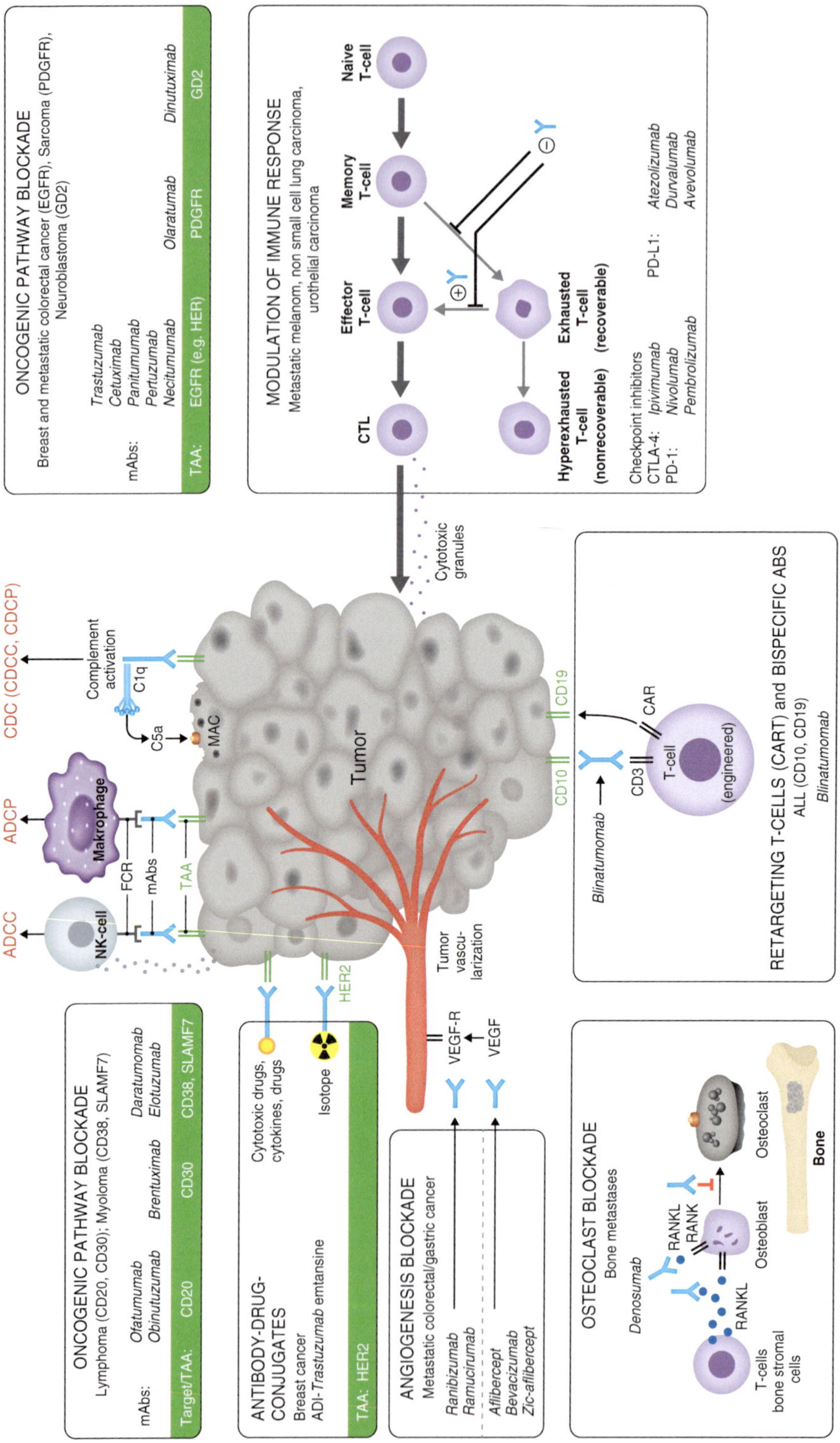
ONCOGENIC PATHWAY BLOCKADE
Breast and metastatic colorectal cancer (EGFR), Sarcoma (PDGFR), Neuroblastoma (GD2)
mAbs: Trastuzumab Cetuximab Panitumumab Pertuzumab Necitumumab
Olaratumab
Dinutuximab
TAA: EGFR (e.g. HER) PDGFR GD2
MODULATION OF IMMUNE RESPONSE
Metastatic melanom, non small cell lung carcinoma, urothelial carcinoma
Naive T-cell
Memory T-cell
Effector T-cell
CTL
Exhausted T-cell (recoverable)
Hyperexhausted T-cell (nonrecoverable)
Checkpoint inhibitors
CTLA-4: Ipivimumab
PD-1: Nivolumab Pembrolizumab
PD-L1: Atezolizumab Durvalumab Avevolumab
Cytotoxic granules
ADCC
ADCP
CDC (CDCC, CDCP)
NK-cell
Makrophage
FCR
mAbs
TAA
Complement activation
C1q
C5a
MAC
Tumor
Tumor vascu-larization
HER2
CD10
CD19
Blinatumomab
CD3
CAR
T-cell (engineered)
RETARGETING T-CELLS (CART) and BISPECIFIC ABS
ALL (CD10, CD19)
Blinatumomab
ONCOGENIC PATHWAY BLOCKADE
Lymphoma (CD20, CD30); Myoloma (CD38, SLAMF7)
mAbs: Ofatumumab Obinutuzumab
Brentuximab
Daratumomab Elotuzumab
Target/TAA: CD20 CD30 CD38, SLAMF7
ANTIBODY-DRUG-CONJUGATES
Breast cancer
ADI-Trastuzumab emtansine
Cytotoxic drugs, cytokines, drugs
Isotope
TAA: HER2
VEGF-R
VEGF
ANGIOGENESIS BLOCKADE
Metastatic colorectal/gastric cancer
Ranibizumab Ramucirumab
Aflibercept Bevacizumab Zic-aflibercept
OSTEOCLAST BLOCKADE
Bone metastases
Denosumab
RANKL
RANK
T-cells bone stromal cells
Osteoblast
Osteoclast
Bone

3. Receptor downregulation
   Instead of blocking the receptor binding of the antibody might lead to a downregulation of receptors and to their internalization. Examples are Omalizumab, Otelixizumab, Teplizumab, and Epratuzumab.
4. Binding to the cell surface receptor may result in depletion of all or a majority of receptor carrying cells. Depletion of cells will be achieved by complement mediated cytotoxicity (CMC) and/or antibody-dependent monocyte/macrophage mediated phagocytosis ADCP (antibody dependent cellular phagocytosis) antibody-dependent cellular cytotoxicity (ADCC) (e.g., by NK-cells) (Fig. 20.2a). Examples are Rituximab, Ofatumumab, Ocrelizumab, Alemtuzumab, Muromonab, and Epratuzumab.
5. Signaling induction
   Instead of blocking the receptor therapeutic antibodies may activate signals after binding to the receptor. Examples are mAbs binding to the T-cell receptor TCR/CD3, e.g. Teplizumab and Muromonab.

20.9 Indications and Efficacy

FDA-approved indications related to each agent are listed in Table 20.1.

Biologics (mAbs and fusion proteins) have been used in very different diseases and disease subtypes. Biologics are used off label in many indications, which cannot be covered in this chapter. There is strong evidence that they will benefit patients in some situations which cannot easily be studied in clinical trials (e.g., Alemtuzumab (anti CD52) CAMPATH in stem cell transplantation used for conditioning). In the following I will focus on main indication areas for biologics in the treatment of immune mediated diseases and cancer. Cochrane and other meta-analyses of the main indications (RA, Psoriasis, IBD, MS (Multiple Sclerosis)) were reviewed.

The quality of meta-analyses can differ substantially. The type of funding sources, author conflicts of interest, and author networks compromise study quality and risk of bias as impressively shown for psoriasis (Gomez-Garcia et al. 2017;

Fig. 20.4 Targets in antibody-based cancer immunotherapy. Adapted from Hendricks et al. (2017), Her and Cavanaugh (2016), Martin-Liberal et al. (2017), Weiner (2015), Batlevi et al. (2016), and Sukshari et al. (2017) Chen (2017) Illustration: Oliver Hippmann, Schwarzenbruck. ALL = acute lymphoblastic leukemia, CART = chimeric antigen receptor T-cells, CTL = cytotoxic T-cell, CDCC = complement dependent cellular cytotoxicity, CDCP = complement dependent cell mediated phagocytosis, MAC = membrane complex, TAA = tumor associated antigen, EGFR = epithelial growth factor receptor, PDGFR = platelet derived growth factor receptor, GD2 = glucolipidsialoganglyosid, PD1 = programmed cell death 1PD-L1 = programmed cell death ligand 1, CTLA4 = cytotoxic T-lymphocyte associated protein 4, ADCC = antibody dependent cell mediated cytotoxicity ADCP = antibody dependent cell mediated phagocytosis, VEGFR = vascular endothelial growth factor receptor, VEGF = vascular endothelial growth factor, HER2 = human epidermal growth factor receptor 2, RANK = receptor activator of nuclear factor kB, RANKL = receptor activated of nf kB ligand

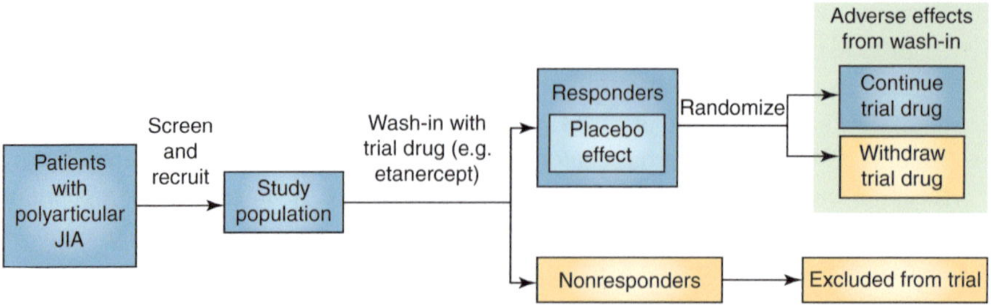

Fig. 20.5 Example of flawed trial design. The so-called withdrawal trial design is used in the majority of controlled trials in polyarticular JIA. Flaws include false-high response rates by inclusion of the placebo response and exclusion of non-responders as well as carry-over of adverse events in both study (continued drug) and control (withdrawal drug) groups. Adapted from Niehues (2015)

Sanz-Cabanillas et al. 2017). There clearly is an urgent need for investigator-initiated trials which are independent are properly developed consensus treatment protocols. The majority of trials in all indication areas of therapeutic mAbs are industry-initiated and industry-sponsored. A large body of data on therapeutic mAbs derives from industry-sponsored registries with a high degree of bias. Patient registries are commonly used as a convenient shortcut to answer questions regarding efficacy and safety of mAbs/fusion proteins to avoid expensive and laborious trials. Registries have repeatedly shown to provide data of low and non-reliable quality (Anderson 1994; Windeler 2014).

Trial design has been flawed in trials regarding industry-initiated clinical trials on mAbs. A striking example are the many trials on mAbs in Pediatric Rheumatology: With very few exceptions the so-called withdrawal trial design was used. The trial design results in falsely high responder rates and lower rates of AEs in the study drug and measures whether a drug can be withdrawn but not whether a drug is efficacious (Niehues 2015) (Fig. 20.5). Any clinician is interested whether a drug prescribed is effective and less so whether this drug can be withdrawn. Needless to say that the drug wouldn't be prescribed in the first place if it were not effective.

20.9.1 Immune Mediated Diseases

20.9.1.1 Rheumatoid Arthritis (RA)

In all of diseases below (RA, JIA, Uveitis, MS, IBD, etc.) information from trials is of limited value because of the short observation periods in trials (max. 2 years) for diseases that last for 30–40 years. Especially regarding safety data longer observation periods are key.

RA is characterized by acute and chronic inflammation in the synovium which is associated with a destruction of joint tissues.

Early use of DMARDS (disease modifying antirheumatic drugs, e.g. Methotrexate MTX) is key to the success of RA treatment (Burmester and Pope 2017; Moreland 2016). According to ACR and EULAR recommendations (ACR American College of Rheumatology, EULAR European League against Rheumatism) initial treatment does not consist of TNFα inhibitors but one DMARD or combination of two DMARDs, non-steroidal and anti-inflammatory drugs (NSAIDS) and/or glucocorticoids (systemic and/or intra-articular). Only if there is no remission after 3–6 months of treatment, a TNF inhibitor can be added. Meta-analyses showed that addition of a biological to a conventional DMARD is more effective than a conventional DMARD alone (Nam et al. 2017). In adults with RA who are naive to Methotrexate biologics (Abatacept, Adalimumab, Etanercept, Golimumab, Infliximab, Rituximab) in combination with MTX probably improve signs and symptoms of RA while the use of TNF biologics alone does not make a difference regarding signs and symptoms of RA or chances of RA remission (Singh et al. 2017).

20.9.1.2 Juvenile Idiopathic Arthritis (JIA)

Juvenile idiopathic arthritis usually has a much less severe disease course as compared to RA and can be subdivided into Oligoarthritis and Polyarthritis (involving more than five joints). Notably, there are no clinical trials on the use of biologics in the most common subtype of JIA (persistent oligoarthritis). It is quite worrying that a large proportion of children with JIA oligoarthritis are treated with biologics without any evidence from properly conducted clinical trials (Davies et al. 2017). In most JIA subtypes MTX has been shown to be effective repeatedly in investigator-initiated trials. If Methotrexate fails, clinicians feel that TNF inhibitors are efficient drugs, however, the evidence for the overall efficacy of biologicals in JIA remains unclear as the trial design has been exclusively an inadequate industry-initiated withdrawal design trial (see above, Fig. 20.5) (Niehues 2015).

In JIA with systemic onset (SJIA) (Stills disease) two randomized placebo-controlled trials claimed efficacy for Tocilizumab and Canakinumab which were industry-initiated and limited by their very short observation periods of their double-blind phases (12 weeks, 29 days) (De Benedetti et al. 2012; Ruperto et al. 2012).

20.9.1.3 Uveitis

Adalimumab can be considered as second-line immunomodulatory agent. In patients with JIA associated uveitis and ongoing ocular inflammation despite systemic and local glucocorticoid therapy Adalimumab has been shown to be effective in an investigator-initiated trial (Ramanan et al. 2017).

Data on non-JIA associated inflammatory uveitis and biologicals are lacking. In Behçet's disease and its ocular manifestations Infliximab and Adalimumab can be considered as first-line treatment. Infliximab and Adalimumab are considered as potential second-line immunomodulatory agents for Posterior Uveitis, Panuveitis, severe Uveitis associated with seronegative spondylarthropathy, Scleritis. In contrast, Etanercept has been linked to the induction of De novo-Uveitis.

20.9.1.4 Systemic Lupus Erythematosus (SLE)

SLE is characterized by high titers of antinuclear antibodies, in particular anti-double-stranded DNA antibodies which are thought to play a role in SLE pathogenesis. Therefore, B-cells and antibody-producing plasma cells have been thought to be an important target for biologics in the disease, but the results of some well-designed controlled trials (e.g., rituximab) were disappointing (Merrill et al. 2010; Rovin et al. 2012).

20.9.1.5 Psoriasis

Psoriasis is a chronic inflammatory skin disease (Feldman 2017). Limited plaque psoriasis responds to topical corticosteroids and emollients, or alternatively Vitamin D analogs or topical retinoids. Severe psoriasis requires phototherapy or systemic therapy with MTX, cyclosporine (CSA), or biologics (anti-TNF agents, anti-IL12/IL23, anti-IL17) (see Tables 20.1 and 20.2). The British dermatologists recommend offering biologics to patients who require systemic therapy, if MTX and CSA have failed, are not tolerated or contraindicated, and psoriasis is extensive or particularly severe at localized sites (Smith et al. 2017). Biologics can be considered earlier and after MTX has failed, if there is psoriatic arthritis.

20.9.1.6 Multiple Sclerosis (MS)

MS is an immune mediated inflammatory demyelinating disease of the central nervous system that is a leading cause of disability in young adults. Biologics (cytokines: Interferon β1a¸mAbs: Natalizumab, Daclizumab, Alemtuzumab) play an important role in the treatment of patients with relapsing remitting multiple sclerosis. The initial choice depends on disease activity and patient values and preferences (Olek 2017). For prevention of disability only Natalizumab shows a beneficial effect. Natalizumab is recommended for patients with more active disease and patients who value effectiveness above safety and convenience. Daclizumab, a humanized monoclonal antibody binding the alpha chain of the high affinity IL2 receptor and Alemtuzumab depleting CD52 positive cells (T-cells, B-cells) have both been shown to reduce disability progression compared to placebo, however, their clinical utility is likely to be limited by severe adverse events (cytokine storm, serious infections, autoimmune disorders). Rituximab and Ocrelizumab (licensed in 2017) targeting CD20 appear to be effective but long-term data from trials are lacking.

20.9.1.7 Inflammatory Bowel Disease

In mild or moderately active Crohn's disease immunomodulators or biologics are not necessary. In patients who are refractory to treatment with first-line agents like glucocorticoids, 5-aminosalycilate therapy and antibiotics Azathioprine, Methotrexate, and/or mAbs are used (TNF/Integrin inhibitors) (see Table 20.1).

In a recent systematic review on induction and maintenance of mucosal healing in moderate to severe Crohn's disease or ulcerative colitis (trial observation periods of 6–12 weeks for induction, 32–54 weeks for maintenance trials) anti-TNF treatment was more effective than placebo for maintaining mucosal healing in Crohn's disease. In ulcerative colitis, anti-TNFs and anti-integrin therapy with Vedolizumab were more effective than placebo and Adalimumab was inferior to Infliximab. Both Infliximab and Adalimumab were similar in Crohn's disease (Cholapranee et al. 2017).

20.10 Adverse Events (AEs)

Target-related and unrelated AEs for biologics are listed in Table 20.2. In general terms, pharmacodynamically large quantities (hundreds of milligrams per milliliter) have to be administered to achieve target saturation and the half-life of IgG is usually quite long at around 3–4 weeks. Adverse events may occur late and span over a longer time-span than in conventional chemical compound drugs.

AEs tend to be underreported. A striking example is the TENDER trial in sJIA. Although published in a top-ranking journal, fatal adverse events in the study drug group are not mentioned in the abstract (De Benedetti et al. 2012):

Six patients of 112 included discontinued treatment (increase in liver enzymes, macrophage activation syndrome). Three patients died during treatment from pneumothorax at week 50, a traffic accident in week 90 and a streptococcal sepsis at week 104. Three more patients in the treatment group died after being withdrawn from the study, two died from pulmonary hypertension after 6 months while one more patient died from probable macrophage activation syndrome 13 months after withdrawing from the study.

Long-term pharmacosurveillance is key in the safety of these many new compounds. Pharmacosurveillance within the biological drug class is almost exclusively done in industry-financed patient registries. Patient registries have multiple flaws and are not the adequate tool to monitor long-term side-effects of mAbs (see above).

Mechanistically, AEs can be classified into the categories immune stimulation, immunodeficiency alteration of homeostasis, off target activity (Boyman et al. 2014; Davis and Ballas 2017).

20.10.1 Immune Stimulation

Standard infusion reactions (SIRs) occur but they usually remain moderate (Boyman et al. 2014). Therapeutic mAbs resemble physiological antibodies and are highly complex molecules. They are not identical to the human proteins and thus are recognized by the hosts' immune system leading to hypersensitivity reactions (Picard and Galvao 2017). Immediate hypersensitivity reactions are the result of degranulation of mast cells, may be more severe, and can progress to life-threatening condition within minutes. Immediate hypersensitivity reactions usually do not occur after the first infusion and are triggered by subsequent infusions similar to IgE mediated reactions. Apart from neutralizing the biologic agent anti-drug antibodies can cause clinical hypersensitivity reactions.

Antibodies to a target can lead to activation of the receptor-bearing cell (e.g., T-cell). This has been documented for Muromonab leading to a cytokine storm and severe hypotension and multi-organ failure, etc. The most drastic example of a cytokine storm and uncontrolled immunostimulation occurred when an anti-CD28 activating monoclonal antibody TGNIH2 was infused resulting in a cytokine storm and multiorgan dysfunction (Suntharalingam et al. 2006) which received world-wide press coverage.

20.10.2 Immunodeficiency, Infections and Cancer

Efficient targeting of an important molecule in immunophysiology may lead to a clinical phenotype resembling an inborn Primary Immunodeficiency. Similarly, autoimmune diseases in which endogenous monoclonal autoantibodies are produced against cytokines (e.g., IL17) lead to the clinical phenotype of chronic mucocutaneous candidiasis that is indistinguishable from inherited primary immunodeficiency (caused by mutations in genes responsible for development of TH17 cells: STAT1 gain of function). Therefore, most of the infections occurring in patients treated with exogenous mAbs against well-known immune system targets show characteristic infectious disease profiles, e.g. tuberculosis reactivation upon anti-TNF treatment (Fig. 20.6).

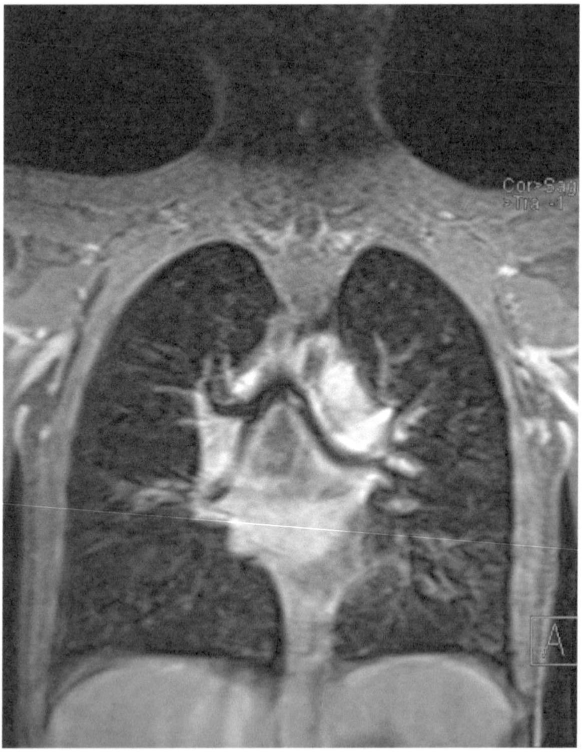

Fig. 20.6 Tuberculosis reactivation after 7 months of adalimumab treatment in a 16-year-old boy with Crohn's disease. MRI shows interstitial changes, enlarged lymph nodes, infracarinal tuberculoma with colliquative necrosis

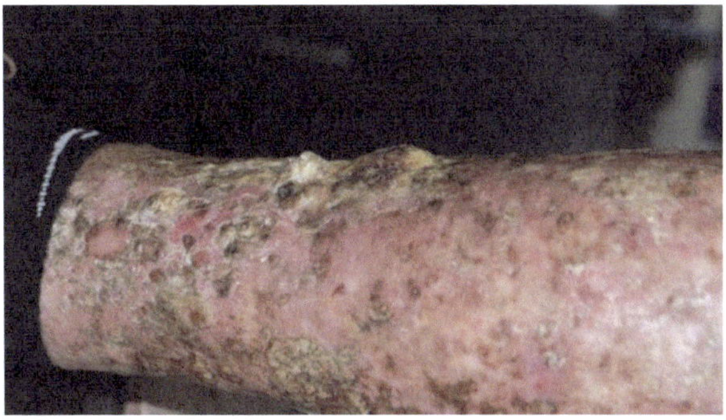

Fig. 20.7 Multiple squamous cell carcinomas on lower limb apparent after commencing ustekinumab as treatment of moderate to severe plaque type psoriasis. Also note pre–existing actinic damage and evidence of chronic venous stasis. Adapted from Young and Czarnecki (2012)

Moreover, it is known that in primary immunodeficiencies immunosurveillance is hampered and thus cancers may arise (e.g., squamous cell carcinoma arising upon anti-IL-12/23 treatment, Fig. 20.7). Major indications for biologic treatments (mAbs, biosimilars, and fusion proteins) are immune mediated diseases and cancer. Both immune-mediated diseases and/or cancer cause a disease-related immunodeficiency. The use of immune-modulating agents and biologics amplifies this immunodeficiency in patients. The combination of both, a conventional immunosuppressive drug and a biological drug in the same patient significantly increases the risk of infection and/or cancer. So outside of controlled trials it is difficult to clearly allocate severe side-effects to biologics only.

20.10.3 Alteration of Homeostasis and Inflammatory Diseases

Some of the targets blocked by therapeutic mAbs may be important in maintaining peripheral tolerance, e.g. cytokines important for both pro-inflammatory and anti-inflammatory functions. Accordingly blocking TNF may lead to an array of autoimmune diseases, e.g. Uveitis (Fig. 20.8) vasculitis, demyelinating CNS disease (Figs. 20.9 and 20.10), IL17 blockade (Secukinumab) may lead to Crohn's disease. A large array of autoimmune diseases, so-called immune-related adverse events (IrAEs) have resulted from blocking molecules important for T-cell activation (checkpoint inhibitors), some of them fatal.

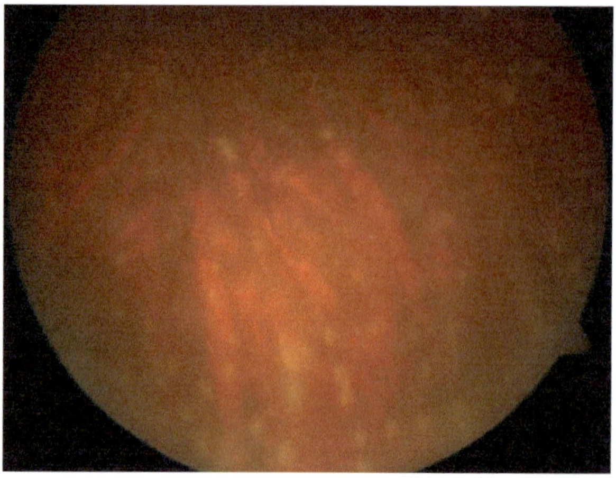

Fig. 20.8 Induction of uveitis by etanercept. Funduscopy of left eye showing snow-balls in the inferior vitreous cavity (Fonollosa A, Artaraz J, Les I, Martinez-Berriotxoa A, Izquierdo JP, Lopez AS, Gardeazaba J, Berasategui B, Martinez-Alday N: Sarcoid intermediate uveitis following etanercept treatment: a case report and review of the literature. *Ocul Immunol Inflamm* 2012,20(1):44–48)

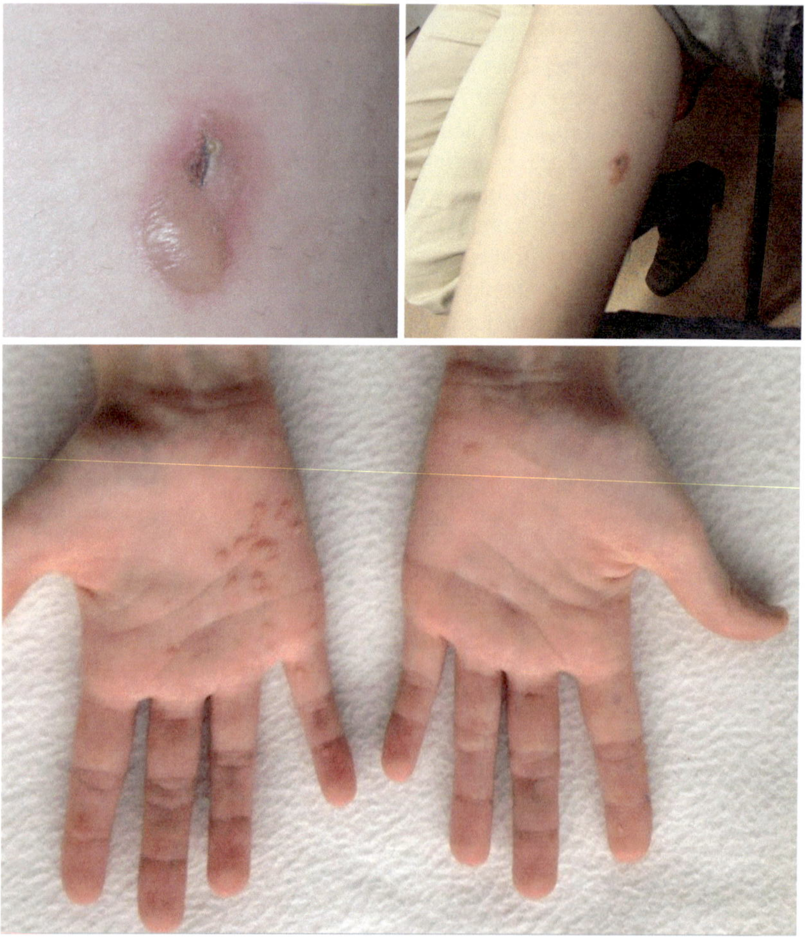

Fig. 20.9 Cutaneous AEs of TNF blocking agents: Verrucae vulgares after 3 months treatment with adalimumab in a 13-year-old girl with polyarticular JIA (*lower panel*); vasculitis on right calf of 13-year-old girl treated with etanercept for polyarticular JIA (*upper panel*)

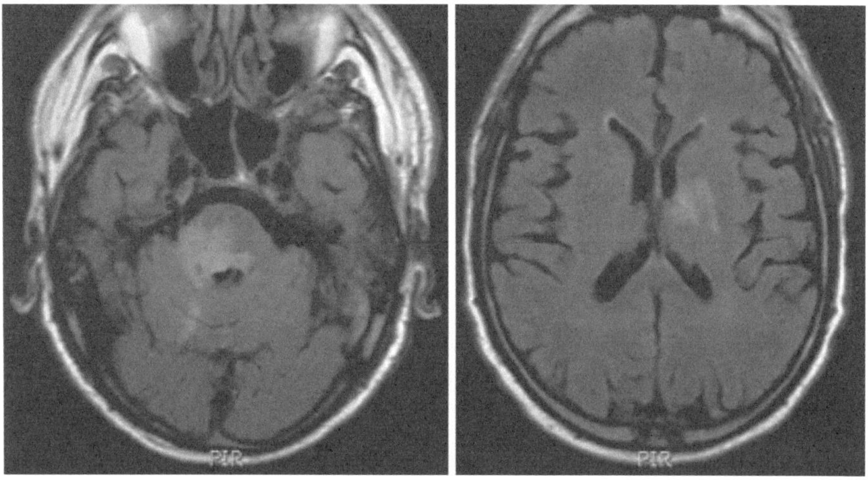

Fig. 20.10 Demyelinating CNS disease 57-year-old man with RA managed with infliximab, methotrexate, and low-dose prednisone presented with 5 days of progressive encephalopathy. Brain MRI with and without contrast. Fluid-attenuated inversion recovery sequences demonstrate T2 hyperintense lesions in the pons, right middle cerebellar, bilateral basal ganglia, left frontal and parietal lobes (not shown). The patient had started infliximab 4 months prior to presentation. The patient's neurologic examination and the brain MRI lesions progressed over several days, and he was treated with high-dose steroids for a presumed autoimmune demyelinating syndrome. The patient died from septic shock. There was pathologic proof of a demyelinating process following TNF antagonism: Brain histopathology demonstrated an acute demyelinating process. Adapted from Bradshaw et al. (2016)

20.10.4 Off-Target Activity (e.g. Progressive Multifocal Leukoencephalopathy PML)

As antibodies are highly specific for their target it appears unlikely that off-target activity occurs. However, regarding severity and localization some unexpected clinical findings have been made upon administration of biologics (e.g., CNS side-effects: PML in Integrin inhibitors, TNF inhibitor side-effects in the skin).

20.11 Summary

Immunotherapy with antibodies has moved from the use of polyclonal IgG plasma derived mixtures to engineered, monoclonal abs. Precise understanding of the protein-chemistry of antibodies, and modern production technologies allow us to generate designer abs, that almost resemble human abs. They target specifically molecules that appear central to pathophysiological processes. While this has been a significant medical progress, caution is strongly advised:

1. These new drugs need to be as rigorously tested for efficacy and safety as conventional drugs within properly designed, randomized, and placebo-controlled clinical trials and followed up in independent registries long-term. Notably in many biologics this has not yet been done. Just because these drugs are highly complex and very precise in targeting it doesn't mean they are effective and safe.
2. Nihil nocere is a prime duty for every ethically aware clinician. MAbs, biosimilars, and fusion proteins have repeatedly caused severe AEs and death, which to some degree appears to be underreported. In light of their potential harm and currently very high cost for our health systems a strictly evidence-based approach for using biologics is needed.

Acknowledgement Without the careful and skillful help of Andrea Groth the preparation of this manuscript would not have been possible. I thank Kathrin Siepermann, Gregor Dückers, and Antje Ballauff for discussing interesting cases of treatment with biologics within our team at the HELIOS Children's Hospital in Krefeld, Germany. I thank Ina Bruins for her additional help in manuscript preparation.

Table 20.11 Target-and target system associated adverse events of therapeutic monoclonal antibodies, biosimilars and fusion proteins (licensed by FDA, some taken from market, some in development): Hematopoietic cells (granulocytes, platelets)

Target system	Target molecule	Antibody	Brand name	Physiology/pathophysiology (Fig. 3)
Granulocytes (adhesion molecules)				
	Alpha-4 integrin	**Natalizumab**	Tysabri	A first step in migration of inflammatory cells (especially leukocytes) to the inflamed tissue is their adherence to endothelial cells in vessels. The endothelial cells express selectins and integrins. Adhesion molecules are expressed both on the endothelial side and the surface of inflammation cells (neutrophil granulocytes). Inability of neutrophil granulocytes to adhere to endothelial cells or blood vessels in inborn adhesion defects leads to very severe necrotic infections with a lack of pus and extremely high leukocyte numbers in blood. Neutrophil granulocytes that adhere to endothelial cells express Beta integrins (CD18, LFA1 lymphocyte function associated antigen) on the cell surface of neutrophil granulocytes. These integrins bind to adhesion molecule receptors on activated endothelial cells (ICAM1, ICAM2, MadCAM-1). Natalizumab binds to the α4 subunit found in α4β1 (VLA-4) and α4β7 integrins which are ligands for VCAM 1 and MADCAM 1 adhesion molecules.
	Alpha-4 integrin	**Vedolizumab**	Entyvio	
	CD11a	**Efalizumab**	Raptiva	
Adverse Events (AEs): Blocking the ingress of neutrophils into inflamed tissue sites may lead to *immunodeficiency and severe infections*: localized herpes zoster reactivation, pneumonia, urinary tract infections. *PML progressive multifocal leukoencephalopathy* results from reactivation of the JC virus (John Cunningham) and has been fatal in many cases. Inhibition of entry of CD4 cells to the CNS as well as a mobilization of stem cells that might harbor the JC virus are hypothesized to be responsible for this very severe side-effect. Natalizumab as well as Efalizumab had been withdrawn from the market but in need of effective drugs for multiple sclerosis Natalizumab was reintroduced in 2006. The risk for JC virus reactivation depends on the length of treatment and prior use of immunosuppressants. Because of the PML risk Natalizumab should not be combined with other immunosuppressants.				
Platelets				
	GPIIb/IIIa	**Abciximab**	ReoPro	GPIIb/IIIa is expressed on activated platelets
Adverse Events (AEs) *Excessive or abnormal bleeding* sometimes associated with thrombocytopenia. *Hypersensitivity* reaction including anaphylaxis				

Table 20.12 Target-and target system associated adverse events of therapeutic monoclonal antibodies, biosimilars, and fusion proteins (licensed by FDA, some taken from market, some in development): Lymphocytes, T-Lymphocytes, T-Lymphocyte/APC (synapse)

Target system	Target molecule	Antibody	Brand name	Physiology/pathophysiology) (Fig. 4)
Lymphocyte subpopulation				
	CD52	**Alemtuzumab**	Campath, Lemtrada	CD52: cell surface protein of unknown function, found on neutrophils, monocytes, macrophages, lymphocytes including T, B, and NK cells
Adverse events (AEs):				
It may induce *severe lymphopenia*, sometimes for more than 10 years. Phenotype similar to severe combined immunodeficiency. *Severe systemic viral, fungal, bacterial, and protozoal infections* have been described as well as *TB reactivation*. Viruses (VZV, HSV, CMV, EBV) fungi (Candida, aspergillus, cryptococcus, mucor). Due to altered hematopoiesis *ITP hemolytic anemia neutropenia* and *pancytopenia* have been observed. Live vaccines should not be used. Emergence of *autoimmune thyroid disease* and immune thrombocytopenia with a case of *fatal intracranial hemorrhage* has been documented.				
T-lymphocytes				
	IL2RA	**Basiliximab**	Simulect	IL-2, the most important cytokine for T-cell proliferation and activation, binds to the IL2 receptor. The IL2 receptor is composed of the alpha chain and a common gamma chain which is a shared receptor for other cytokines. Recombinant human IL2 (Aldesleukin) which may be useful in the activation of tumor specific lymphocytes (metastatic renal cell carcinoma, metastatic melanoma)
	IL2R	**Daclizumab**	Zinbryta (Zanaprax until 2009)	
		Denileukin diftitox	ONTAK	
	CD3	**Blinatumomab**	Blincyto	CD3: classical lineage specific marker for T-cells. By stimulating CD3, Teplizumab is supposed to induce IL10-producing CD4 cells and CD8 positive T-regulatory cells (Tregs)
		Muromonab	Orthoclone OKT3	
		Teplizumab	N. N.	
	CD2	**Alefacept**	Amevive	CD2: Expressed on T cell, B cells, and NK cells.
Adverse Events (AEs):				
By activating the IL2 receptor T-cells may be overtly stimulated leading to post *administration anaphylaxis and a so-called cytokine storm, which may be fatal. Hypotension, angina pectoris, arrhythmia, tachycardia, dyspnea, pulmonary edema, thrombocytopenia, thrombosis* all have been described. Basiliximab is used in transplant patients thus underlying diseases or coadministered drugs may also be responsible for AEs. *Infections* observed with IL2 blocking agents have been respiratory tract infections, herpes simplex, and herpes zoster skin infections. Daclizumab was taken from the market in 2009 and later reintroduced for MS patients. Muromonab (Orthoclone OKT3) was the first licensed therapeutic monoclonal antibody and used in renal and liver transplantation but was withdrawn from the market in 2010. It was effective in preventing graft rejection but caused *frequent systemic infections* as well as *cytokine storm*. Teplizumab is not expected to have the same adverse events as muromonab because it is engineered not to bind to FcR The LFA3 IgG1 FC fusion protein (LFA3 is the ligand for CD2), alefacept was used in psoriasis but withdrawn from the market in 2011.				

T-lymphocyte/APC (synapse)				
	B7-1 (CD80), B7-2 (CD86)	**Abatacept**	Orencia	As the crucial initial step of T-cell activation, the immunological synapse is formed between antigen-presenting cell (APC) and T-cell. Within the synapse there are many targets for the use of biologics (Figure 3). Following ligand receptor pairs can be inhibited by mabs: CD28/CTLA4 and CD80/CD86, PD1 and PD-L1/PD-L2 (CD274)CD27 and CD70, CD40 ligand and CD40, CD137, OX40, LAG3, TIM3 may be future targets.
	CD80, CD86	**Belatacept**	Nulojix	
	CTLA-4	**Ipilimumab**	Yervoy	
	PD-1	**Nivolumab**	Opdivo	
		Pembrolizumab	Keytruda	
	PD-L1	**Atezolizumab**	Tecentriq	
		Durvalumab	Imfinzi	
		Avelumab	Bavencio	
Adverse Events (AEs):				
Immune checkpoint inhibitors have a unique and broad profile of adverse events (*immune related adverse events irAEs*), expected to occur in about 10–20% of cases. Temporary immunosuppression with other immunosuppressive drugs may be necessary (e.g., with corticosteroids). (Postow, Journal of clinical oncology 2015;33:1974). *Fatal Adverse Events (FAEs)* are significantly increased with ipilimumab. (Zhu, Exp Opin Drug Saf 2017; Zhang, Eur J Cancer 2017). Frequently a *reticular macropapular erythematous rash on extremities or trunk* has been reported as well as *Stevens Johnson Syndrome* and *Toxic epidermal necrolysis*. Diarrhea results of *colitis* and occurs approximately 6 weeks into treatment as a result of altered homeostasis. *Endocrinopathies* effecting hypopituitary, adrenal, and thyroid glands occur. *Opportunistic infections* result from treating the irAEs. *Autoimmune encephalitis* due to NMDA receptor antibodies has been described.				

Table 20.13 Target-and target system associated adverse events of therapeutic monoclonal antibodies, biosimilars and fusion proteins (licensed by FDA, some taken from market, some in development): B-cells and B-cell specific cytokines

Target molecule	Antibody	Brand name	Physiology/pathophysiology (Fig. 3)
BLyS (BAFF)	**Belimumab**	Benlysta	B-cell activating factors are BAFF (B-cell activating factor, synonym: BLYS and APRIL (a proliferation inducing ligand), and share the ability to bind to TACI (= Transmembrane activator and CAML interactor) expressed on mature B-cells, plasma cells, and activated T-cells and BCMA (also known as B-cell maturation antigen) expressed on B-cells and plasma cells. BAFF can also interact with BAFF receptor Monoclonal antibodies can interact with B-cell differentiation by binding to BAFF and APRIL (Atacicept = fusion protein of human IgG FC protein and TACI); Belimumab or Tabalumab, block BAFF
CD20	**Ocrelizumab**	Ocrevus	CD20 is not expressed on pro B-cells or antibody-producing plasma cells, an exclusive marker for mature B-cells and expressed on more than 95% of B-cells in blood and lymphoid organs
	Rituximab	Rituxan	
	Tositumomab	Bexxar	
CD22	**Epratuzumab**	Lyphocide (planned name)	CD22 is a member of the lectin-like immunoglobulin superfamily and expressed to a higher extent in naïve versus memory B-cells. It is part of the CD19/CD21/CD22/BCR (B-cell receptor complex)

Adverse Events (AEs):

Belimumab seems to have a less broad adverse event profile than the B-cell depleting antibodies. However, in clinical trials cases of *opportunistic infections* with acinetobacterand CMV were seen. The general experience is still limited, *fatal infections* have been described.

Rituximab has been widely used, a lot of side-effects have been reported, many of them occur in conjunction with chemotherapy/steroids for Lymphoma. Regarding infections one would expect the clinical phenotype of a primary antibody or B-cell deficiency (like in Bruton's agammaglobulinemia). Accordingly, *bacterial infections* like *osteomyelitis*, *otitis*, *conjunctivitis*, *cellulitis* all have been observed. Accordingly, *PJP (Pneumocystis jirovecii pneumonia) with poor outcome* (30% fatal) (Martin-Garrido, Chest 2013) and *PML* have been observed. A recent study found an increased incidence of *AML (acute myeloid leukemia)* after Rituximab treatment for B-cell lymphomas. (Tao, British Journal of Hematology 2017).

Epratuzumab is used in SLE systemic lupus erythematosus and leads to a moderate peripheral B-cell reduction (approximately 30%) and inhibition of B-cell proliferation.

Table 20.14 Target-and target system associated adverse events of therapeutic monoclonal antibodies, biosimilars, and fusion proteins (licensed by FDA, some taken from market, some in development): TNF

Target molecule	Antibody	Brand name	Physiology/pathophysiology (Fig. 3)
TNF	**Adalimumab**	Humira	Cytokines are small proteins (5–20 kilodalton) that are important in cell signaling. They are part of a complex network regulating humoral and cell-based immune responses. TNF is involved in cytokine and chemokine inducing apoptosis, endothelial cell activation, induction of adhesion molecules and growth of new blood vessels as well as regulation of fibroblasts, synoviocytes, and osteoclasts.
TNF	**Certolizumab pegol**	Cimzia	
TNFα and TNFβ	**Etanercept**	Enbrel	
TNF	**Infliximab**	Remicade	
TNF	**Infliximab-dyyb**	Inflectra	
TNF	**Golimumab**	Simponi Aria	
TNF	**Golimumab**	Simponi	
TNF	**Adalimumab-atto**	Amjevita	
TNF	**Infliximab-abda**	Renflexis	

Adverse Events (AEs):

The most characteristic side-effect is reactivation of *latent tuberculosis* (see Fig. 7). Higher incidence of *pneumonia* and *sepsis* as well as *serious bacterial* (particularly intracellular) and *viral infections*. *Opportunistic infections* such as *histoplasmosis*, *PJP*, *candida,* and *aspergillus* have been described, in many of the reported cases concomitant immunosuppressive medication was present

Immunologically mediated side-effects include *fatal infusion reactions*, *reactivation of hepatitis B* and *cytopenias*. Outside of the immune system *cardiac arrhythmias* and *bowel obstruction* have been described: Caution has to be used in patients with *Congestive Heart Failure*. A whole array of autoimmune diseases or immune mediated diseases associated with TNFα blocking therapy have been described: cutaneous side effects such as *psoriasis*, *cutaneous lupus*, *necrotizing vasculitis*, *induction of anti double-stranded DNA antibodies*, *dermatomyositis*, *polymyositis, antiphospholipid antibody syndrome*, *exacerbations of IBD* have been described. *Uveitis* has been repeatedly induced by Etanercept (see Fig. 6), in 2007 Ramos Casals had already described 234 cases of autoimmune diseases induced by TNF target therapies (Ramos Casals, Medicine 2007;86:242)

It is controversial to what extent anti-TNF treatment is associated with the induction of *lymphomas* (*Hodgkins*, *Cutaneous T-cell Lymphoma*). Rare but almost uniformly fatal is *hepatosplenic* γδ *T-cell-lymphoma* in IBD patients. There is an increased risk of *melanoma* and *non-melanoma skin cancers*. Regular skin cancer screening is advised. In many meta-analyses there has been no significant increase in the occurrence of lymphomas. It is difficult to discriminate between the effects of the underlying disease, concomitant medication and induction by TNF antagonists

CNS leukoencephalopathy and *cerebral edema* have been described with Etanercept treatment (Deutsches Ärzteblatt 2015;40:b1357). *Demyelinating acute disseminated encephalomyelitis* (Fig. 10) has been described as well as *peripheral neuropathies* (Guillain Barré syndrome), multifocal motor neuropathy, chronic inflammatory demyelinating polyradiculoneuropathy. TNF inhibitors should not be given in first degree relatives of patients with Multiple Sclerosis

Table 20.15 Target-and target system associated adverse events of therapeutic monoclonal antibodies, biosimilars, and fusion proteins (licensed by FDA, some taken from market, some in development): Interleukin 1 and Interleukin 6

w

Target system	Target molecule	Antibody	Brand name	Physiology/pathophysiology
Interleukin 1				
	Interleukin-1 type I receptor (IL-1RI)	**Anakinra**	Kineret	IL1 has pleiotropic effects: It initiates inflammation and fever, as one of the most important effects. IL1α and β are important for infection immunity. Uncontrolled release of Interleukin1β leads to severe tissue damage and systemic inflammation (deafness and blindness due to optical and acoustic nerve inflammation, treatment-resistant fever, joint destruction, etc). IL1 receptor antagonist (IL-1RA) is a soluble, naturally occurring antagonist which was the model for the development of the synthetic IL-1RA Anakinra.
	IL1B	**Canakinumab**	Ilaris	
	IL-1 beta (IL-1β)	**Rilonacept**	Arcalyst	
Adverse Events (AEs):				
Bacterial and viral infections (with a higher rate in Canakinumab due to its long half-life) opportunistic infections appear not to be significantly increased. The FDA has not approved Canakinumab for the treatment of gout because of increased incidents of *severe infections particularly in the elderly population*. (Dinarello, Nature reviews Rheumatology 2016;12:). *Fatal myocarditis* has been described in a child with systemic onset juvenile idiopathic arthritis on treatment with Anakinra. (Zeft, Pediatric Rheumatology 2012;10:8). Immune mediated side-effects of all IL1 antagonists include *pneumonitis*, *colitis*, *hepatitis*, *endocrinopathies*, *nephritis*, *dermatitis*, *encephalitis*, *psoriasis,* and *vitiligo*. In some cases *neutropenia* occurs				

Interleukin 6				
	IL6	**Siltuximab**	Sylvant	IL6 is a pro-inflammatory cytokine and binds to the IL6 receptor composed of 2 functional chains IL6 receptor α and a common signal transducing chain (GP130). IL6 receptor α is expressed only on a few cell types (mainly hepatocytes, leukocytes). However IL6 is also able to activate GP130 expressing cells which are abundant. IL6 induces the acute phase proteins in the liver (e.g., C-reactive protein), is part of inducing fever and leukocytosis, induces hematopoiesis and angiogenesis at inflammation sites. Increased IL6 in chronic inflammation induces anemia through induction of hepcidin from hepatocytes, activates T- and B-lymphocytes, plasma cells and induces the differentiation of T-helper 17 lymphocytes (among other cytokines IL1β, TGFβ, IL21, IL23). It induces ACTH, cortisol, and prolactin and inhibits the secretion of TSH and growth hormones (in chronic inflammation: growth retarding). IL6 increases insulin resistance and is associated with the development of a type-2 diabetes mellitus. It induces the cytokine RANKL and may induce osteoporosis. Il-6 mediated fibroblast proliferation may result in joint destruction.
	IL6R	**Tocilizumab**	Actemra	

Adverse Events (AEs):

Blocking of IL6 may have quite drastic adverse events with a relatively high number of deaths in trials. Blocking IL6 effectively means that there will be no c-reactive protein and ESR elevation, which normally can be used as lab tests to detect inflammation. *Severe infections* have been reported: *Pneumonia*, *urinary tract infection*, *gastroenteritis*, *diverticulitis*, *bacterial arthritis,* and *sepsis*. Infections include *opportunistic infections* with *aspergillus*, *candida,* and *pneumocystis species*. Therapy should not be started in patients with active infections of any kind. Live viral vaccines should not be given. The risk of acquiring a serious infection is > 10% on Tocilizumab trials. *Macrophage activation syndrome is common and fatal in some cases*. Other fatalities in Tocilizumab trials have been due to *bacterial sepsis*, *Pneumothorax*, *Pulmonary hypertension*, *vasculitis,* and *heart failure* (reviewed in Machado 2017). Infections with *hepatitis B or C* may severely reactivate. *Neutropenia* (< 1000 neutrophils/μL) occurs in some patients

In patients with systemic onset juvenile idiopathic arthritis (sJIA) one *anaphylactic reaction* was observed as well as a *gastrointestinal hemorrhage* from diffuse acute or chronic *colon ulceration*. Liver enzyme and LDL cholesterol elevation was observed

Regarding immune mediated adverse events the occurrence of *psoriasis* or the worsening of a pre-existing psoriasis has been reported (Deutsches Ärzteblatt 111:14, April 2014 b25)

Table 20.16 Target-and target system associated adverse events of therapeutic monoclonal antibodies, biosimilars, and fusion proteins (licensed by FDA, some taken from market, some in development): Interleukin 4 and Interleukin 5

Target system	Target molecule	Antibody	Brand name	Physiology/pathophysiology (Fig. 3)
Interleukin 4				
	IL4RA	**Dupilumab**	Dupixent	IL4 is the signature cytokine for TH2 cells.TH2 cells stimulate antibody production by B-cells and augment eosinophil responses. TH2 cells produce IL4, IL5, IL10, IL13. Th2 cells carry IL4 receptors and the cytokines IL5 and IL13 are key to IgE production. Increased activation of TH2 cells is characteristic of allergic diseases.
Adverse Events (AEs):				
Dupilumab has been approved by the FDA just recently, there is very limited experience on the safety of this drug. No serious adverse events were reported in the trial on persistent asthma with elevated eosinophil levels (Wenzel, NEJM 2013;368:2455)				
Interleukin 5				
	IL5	**Mepolizumab**	Nucala	
		Reslizumab	Cinqair	
Adverse Events (AEs):				
Reactions at the site of injection have been reported more often than in placebo mepolizumab)				
For reslizumab *oropharyngeal pain* has been the most common adverse effect. The experience with these drugs is still very limited				

Table 20.17 Target-and target system associated adverse events of therapeutic monoclonal antibodies, biosimilars, and fusion proteins (licensed by FDA, some taken from market, some in development), Interleukin 17, Interleukin 12 and Interleukin 23, GM-CSF

Target system	Target molecule	Antibody	Brand name	Physiology/pathophysiology
Interleukin 17				
	IL17A	**Ixekizumab**	Taltz	IL17 has a central role in the defense against extracellular bacteria and fungi. IL17 is the signature cytokine for TH17 cells, which respond to IL6 and TGFβ and IL23, IL17. IL17 is a highly inflammatory cytokine acting on immune cells, epithelial cells, and fibroblasts. IL17A and IL17F are specifically upregulated in inflammatory conditions leading to recruitment and activation of neutrophils, lymphocytes, and macrophages and tissue damage, including the expression of matrix metalloproteinases. TH17 cells are thought to be the main culprit in the initiation and progression of chronic inflammatory disease (Review Burmester, Nature Reviews Rheumatology 2014; 10:77–87). Effector functions of TH17 cells also appear to be osteoclastogenesis and bone erosion
	IL17A	**Secukinumab**	Cosentyx	
	IL17RA	**Brodalumab**	Siliq	
Adverse Events (AEs): *Severe infections with extracellular bacteria and fungi* and worsening symptoms in patients with *Crohn's disease* (a reduced control of candida in the gut microbiome could be a reason). For Brodalumab reports of *increased suicidal ideation* were unexpectedly observed, which may be due to an increase of IL17 concentration in the periphery when IL17 receptor is blocked. (Dinarello, Nature Reviews rheumatology 2016;12)				
Interleukin 12, Interleukin 23				
	IL12, IL23	**Ustekinumab**	Stelara	IL12 and IL23 are members of a cytokine family that regulate early-phase immune responses towards activation of TH1 and TH17 cells. IL12 and IL23 play a key role in the psoriatic plaque and mediate inflammation. IL12 and IL23 share a peptide chain (P40) that is targeted by Ustekinumab. Pure IL23 inhibitors (anti P19) Tildrakizumab and Guselkumab are being tested.
GMCSF/GMCSF-R				
	GMCSF-R common β chain	**Mavrilimumab**	N. N.	GMCSF is involved in the generation, survival and activation of cells from the myeloid compartment. It regulates the function of neutrophils, eosinophils, and macrophages within the proinflammatory network. It acts through the GMCSF receptor α heterodimer of an alpha chain for specific binding and a common β-chain shared with IL3 and IL5 receptors
Adverse Events (AEs): *Disseminated infection* caused by *mycobacteria*, *salmonella,* and *BCG* was an expected finding (Molinelli, Current drug safety 2016;11:35). Common AEs are *respiratory tract infections*, *diverticulitis*, *cellulitis*, *pneumonia*, *appendicitis*, *sepsis*, *osteomyelitis*, *cholecystitis*, *gastroenteritis*, *bronchitis,* and *urinary tract infections*. *Non-melanoma skin cancer* has been described (Figure 8) (Ehrmann, Inflammatory bowel disease 2012;18:e199; Young, Australian journal of dermatology 2012;53:57–60.) In the latter report *multiple squamous cell carcinomas* developed 2–5 months after starting Ustekinumab. A single case of *posterior leukoencephalopathy syndrome* is reported (Gratton, Acta dermatologica 2011;147:1197) *Pulmonary alveolar proteinosis* can be caused by endogenous autoantibodies against GMCSF, so this may be a safety concern with mavrilimumab				

Table 20.18 Target-and target system associated adverse events of therapeutic monoclonal antibodies, biosimilars, and fusion proteins (licensed by FDA, some taken from market, some in development): complement, vessels and vascular growth, bone (osteoclast differentiation)

Target system	Target molecule	Antibody	Brand name	Physiology/pathophysiology
Complement				
	Complement component 5	**Eculizumab**	Soliris	The complement protein cascade is key to the recognition and killing of encapsulated bacteria and clearance of immune complexes from blood. Dysregulation of complement activation, e.g. unregulated production of C5A may result in hemolytic-uremic syndrome (HUS)
Adverse Events (AEs)				
Expectedly, a blockade of C5 will mimic inherited complement deficiency. Inherited deficiencies of complement are associated with *susceptibility to infections with Neisseria species*. Neisseria meningitidis is a significant risk, upon eculizumab treatment. Encapsulated bacteria of concern are *Streptococcus pneumoniae*, *haemophilus*, *gonococci* (Gleesing, Pediatric infectious disease journal 2012;31:543)				
Vessels Vascular growth				
	VEGF, PIGF	**Aflibercept**	Eylea	VEGF, PIGF1 and 2 are key to angiogenesis, which is a key feature of new inflammation, macular edema, or tumor spread and tumor growth
	VEGF	**Bevacizumab**	Avastin	
	VEGFR1	**Ranibizumab**	Lucentis	
	VEGFR2	**Ramucirumab**	Cyramza	
	VEGF, PIGR	**Ziv-aflibercept**	Zaltrap	
Adverse Events (AEs):				
Problems with *wound dehiscence* can lead to the development of *gastrointestinal perforation* sometimes associated with *intraabdominal abscess* *Bleeding* can be serious. *Intracranial hemorrhage* has been reported (Nishimura, World Journal of Gastroenterology 2011;17:4440). *Fatal Hemoptysis* has occurred quite frequently in patients with lung cancer. *Hypertensive crisis*, *nephrotic syndrome*, *congestive heart failure* are listed in the FDA warnings. Aflibercept and Ranibizumab are administered intravitreally into the eye and major safety concerns include *endophthalmitis*, *retinal detachment*, *increased intraocular pressure*. *Arterial thrombotic events* such as *strokes* or *myocardial infarctions* have been observed. In Ziv-aflibercept *perforation*, *gastrointestinal hemorrhage* and *reversible posterior leukoencephalopathy* have been described, notably in combination with 5-FU and irinotecan based chemotherapy.				

Bone				
	RANKL	**Denosumab**	Prolia, Xgeva	Tumor cells interact with bone matrix and provoke osteoclast activation and bone destruction. Osteoclasts are activated by receptor activator of NFκb ligand (RANKL). RANKL binds to receptor activator of nuclear factor kappaB (RANK). RANK (CD265) is found on pre-osteoclasts. Bone homeostasis relies on constant and continuous balance between bone breakdown by osteoclasts and bone synthesis by osteoblasts. The absence of RANKL-RANK signaling prevents to some extent bone resorption/destruction. Breast and prostate cancer as well as some hematological conditions like multiple myeloma metastasize to the bone

Adverse Events (AEs)

Denosumab is *contraindicated in hypocalcemia*. Both calcium and vitamin D supplementation need to be completed before start of Denosumab therapy. As RANKL is also expressed on some T-cells immune mediated side effects may occur, a slightly increased number of *serious infections (mainly bacterial)* have been observed (Watts, Osteoporosis international 2012;23:327)

Table 20.19 Target-and target system associated adverse events of therapeutic monoclonal antibodies: Epithelial growth factor receptors and other tumor associated antigens (TAA)

Target molecule	Antibody	Brand name	Physiology/pathophysiology
HER2	**Ado-trastuzumab emtansine**	Kadcyla	The epithelial growth factor receptor EGFR acts as a point of integration for signals arising from g-protein-coupled receptors and cytokine receptors and is also activated by neurotransmitters, lymphokines, and stress inducers. The epithelial growth factor receptor signaling is key to the growth and development of human carcinomas. (Review Chiavenna SM, Journal of Biomedical Science 2017. 24:15)
EGFR	**Cetuximab**	Erbitux	
GD2	**Dinutuximab**	Unituxin	Glykolipiddisialoganglioside (GD2) belongs to the glycosphingolipid class and is overexpressed on the cell surface of neuroblastomas. GD2 was also found to be expressed in melanomas, small-cell lung cancer and bone and soft-tissue sarcomas
EGFR	**Panitumumab**	Vectibix	
HER2	**Pertuzumab**	Perjeta	
PDGFRA	**Olaratumab**	Lartruvo	Platelet-derived growth factor receptor α PDGFRα is a tyrosine kinase receptor expressed on hematopoietic cells and cells of mesenchymal origin in central nervous system, gonads, lung, intestines, skin, and skeleton. It has been aberrantly expressed in several human cancers and its signaling can contribute to the maintenance of the tumor microenvironment
HER2	**Trastuzumab**	Herceptin	
EGFR	**Necitumumab**	Portrazza	

Adverse Events (AEs):

A main concern with blockage of human epidermal growth factor receptor 2 (HER-2) has been *ventricular dysfunction* and *congestive heart failure*. *Severe cardiac side effects* were seen in Nezitumumab (*cardiopulmonary arrest* and/or *sudden death* in combination with Gemcitabine and Cisplatin). *Hypomagnesemia* occurred in 83% and may aggravate cardiac problems. As the drugs are usually used in combination with chemotherapy typical side effects like *anemia*, *leukopenia*, *diarrhea*, *infections*, *hypothyroidism*, *metabolic changes*, *pathological fractures*, *bone necrosis*, *convulsions*, *skin infections,* and *kidney failure* among others are listed in the drug sheet. The use of mAbs against EGFRs in solid tumors is associated with an *increased risk of FAEs* (Li, PlosOne 2013)

Infusion reactions can occur and are as common as 3%. With Cetuximab they can be fatal. Cetuximab is associated with pulmonary and dermatological toxicity, infections. An *acneiform* rash appears to be typical of Cetuximab and Panitumumab. *Dermatologic toxicities* may be complicated by infection including *sepsis* as well as *abscesses* requiring incisions and drainage

Dinutuximab can cause *severe pain* by irritating nerve cells as well as *nerve damage* and *life-threatening infusion reactions*. Common other side-effects are *pyrexia*, *capillary leak syndrome*, *hypotension*, *infections,* and *sepsis*

Olaratumab: Hematological problems like *neutropenia* in more than 50% of patients and *lymphopenia*. These will be aggravated with combining the drug with chemotherapy

Table 20.20 Target-and target system associated adverse events of therapeutic monoclonal antibodies, biosimilars, and fusion proteins (licensed by FDA, some taken from market, some in development): Surface markers on hematopoietic malignancies

Target system	Target molecule	Antibody	Brand name	Physiology/pathophysiology
	CD38	**Daratumumab**	Darzalex	CD38: Transmembrane protein, ubiquitously expressed with intra- and extracellular function, regulates intracellular Calcium. Disease marker for Lymphomas/Myelomas. Loss of CD38 function is associated with immunodeficiency, metabolic/behavioral alterations (Malavasi, Physiol. Rev 2008)
	CD319 (SLAMF7)	**Elotuzumab**	Empliciti	CD319: marker of normal plasma cells
	CD19	**Blinatumomab**	Blincyto	Present physiologically on immature B-cells in the bone marrow, mature B-cells and on some plasma cells as well as on many leukemia/lymphoma cells. Overexpression of CD19 has been linked with development of autoimmunity.
	CD30	**Brentuximab vedotin (TNF receptor SF8)**	Adcentris	CD30: expressed by activated T- and B-cells and belongs to the tumor necrosis factor receptor family. It is classically expressed on Hodgkin lymphoma Reed-Sternberg cells.
	CD20	**Ibritumomab tiuxetan**	Zevalin	See above, Table 20.13
	CD20	**Tositumomab**	Bexxar	
	CD20	**Obinutuzumab**	Gazyva	
	CD20	**Ofatumumab**	Arzerra	
	CD33	**Gemtuzumab Ozogamicin**	Mylotarg	CD33 is widely expressed on bone marrow cells, precursor cells of the myeloid and lineage and expressed in many acute myeloid leukemias (AML)

Adverse Events (AEs):

All monoclonal abs in this group: Will be used in combination before or after chemotherapy so that a clean allocation of drug-specific side-effects is difficult

Blinatumomab: *a cytokine release syndrome* can occur and may be life-threatening. *Neurological toxicities* which may be severe and life-threatening as well as fatal have been observed (FDA product information)

Blinatumomab: Infusion reactions, interference with blood compatibility testing

Brentuximab: Cases with *PML* have been reported (Jalan P, Clinical neurologic neurology and neurosurgery 2012;114:1335)

Gemtuzumab/Ozogamicin caused *bone marrow suppression* with *severe neutropenia*, *severe bacterial and fungal infections*. It is unclear whether it is effective against AML and was withdrawn from the market in 2010

Table 20.21 Target-and target system associated adverse events of therapeutic monoclonal antibodies, biosimilars, and fusion proteins (licensed by FDA, some taken from market, some in development): Microorganisms, liver cells

Target system	Target molecule	Antibody	Brand name
Microorganisms			
	F protein of RSV	**Palivizumab**	Synagis
	Protective antigen of Bacillus anthracis	**Raxibacumab**	Raxibacumab
	Protective antigen of the Anthrax toxin	**Obiltoxaximab**	Anthem
	Clostridium difficile toxin B	**Bezlotoxumab**	Zinplava
Adverse Events (AEs): Palivizumab: There have been rare cases of *anaphylaxis* and *hypersensitivity* reactions as well as *severe thrombocytopenia* Raxibakumab: Only mild to moderate *infusion reactions* were observed in normal human volunteers similar to Palivizumab Obiltoxaximab: *Hypersensitivity* and *anaphylaxis* have been observed. Bezlotoxumab: *Heart failure* was reported more commonly in patients with a history of congestive heart failure. *Hypersensitivity*, *anaphylaxis*			
Liver cells/LDL-receptors			
	PCSK9	**Evolocumab**	Repatha
	PCSK9	**Alirocumab**	Praluent
Adverse Events (AEs):			
There have been no drug specific side effects reported so far in the initial clinical trials. However, both drugs were licensed in 2015 and large-scale experience is lacking			
Drugs			
	Dabigatran	**Idarucizumab**	Praxbind
Adverse Events (AEs): Hypersensitivity reactions and anaphylaxis may occur as in most of the other monoclonal antibodies			

RSV respiratory syncytial virus

PCSK9 Proprotein convertase subtilisin/Kexin type 9 binds to the receptor für LDL (low density lipoprotein) particles

References

Anderson C. Measuring what works in health care. Science. 1994;263(1080):1082.

Anonymous. WHO Expert committee on biological standardization guidelines on evaluation of similar biotherapeutic products. In: WHO technical report series no. 977. Geneva; 2009.

Anonymous Monoclonal Antibodies. In: Association AM (ed) USAN Naming Guidelines for monoclonal antibodies; https://www.ama-assn.org/about/monoclonal-antibodies

Ballow M. ximab this and -zumab that! Has the magic bullet arrived in the new millennium of medicine and science? J Allergy Clin Immunol. 2005;116:738–43.

Batlevi CL, Matsuki E, Brentjens RJ, et al. Novel immunotherapies in lymphoid malignancies. Nat Rev Clin Oncol. 2016;13:25–40.

Beck A, Wurch T, Bailly C, et al. Strategies and challenges for the next generation of therapeutic antibodies. Nat Rev Immunol. 2010;10:345–52.

Behring E, Kitasato S. Ueber das Zustandekommen der Diphtherie-Immunität und der Tetanus-Immunität bei Thieren. Dtsch Med Wochenschr. 1890;16:1113–4.

Boyman O, Comte D, Spertini F. Adverse reactions to biologic agents and their medical management. Nat Rev Rheumatol. 2014;10:612–27.

Bradshaw MJ, Mobley BC, Zwerner JP, et al. Autopsy-proven demyelination associated with infliximab treatment. Neurol Neuroimmunol Neuroinflamm. 2016;3:e205.

Bruton OC, Apt L, Gitlin D, et al. Absence of serum gamma globulins. AMA Am J Dis Child. 1952;84:632–6.

Burmester GR, Pope JE. Novel treatment strategies in rheumatoid arthritis. Lancet. 2017;389:2338–48.

Burmester GR, Feist E, Dorner T. Emerging cell and cytokine targets in rheumatoid arthritis. Nat Rev Rheumatol. 2014;10:77–88.

Chan AC, Carter PJ. Therapeutic antibodies for autoimmunity and inflammation. Nat Rev Immunol. 2010;10:301–16.

Chen DS, Mellman I. Elements of cancer immunity and the cancer-immune set point. Nature. 2017;541:321–30.

Chingcuanco F, Segal JB, Kim SC, et al. Bioequivalence of biosimilar tumor necrosis factor-alpha inhibitors compared with their reference biologics: a systematic review. Ann Intern Med. 2016;165:565–74.

Cholapranee A, Hazlewood GS, Kaplan GG, et al. Systematic review with meta-analysis: comparative efficacy of biologics for induction and maintenance of mucosal healing in Crohn's disease and ulcerative colitis controlled trials. Aliment Pharmacol Ther. 2017;45:1291–302.

Davies R, Gaynor D, Hyrich KL, et al. Efficacy of biologic therapy across individual juvenile idiopathic arthritis subtypes: a systematic review. Semin Arthritis Rheum. 2017;46:584–93.

Davis BP, Ballas ZK. Biologic response modifiers: indications, implications, and insights. J Allergy Clin Immunol. 2017;139:1445–56.

De Benedetti F, Brunner HI, Ruperto N, et al. Randomized trial of tocilizumab in systemic juvenile idiopathic arthritis. N Engl J Med. 2012;367:2385–95.

Dotan I, Ron Y, Yanai H, et al. Patient factors that increase infliximab clearance and shorten half-life in inflammatory bowel disease: a population pharmacokinetic study. Inflamm Bowel Dis. 2014;20:2247–59.

Ecker DM, Jones SD, Levine HL. The therapeutic monoclonal antibody market. MAbs. 2015;7:9–14.

Eisenberg R. Immune compromise associated with biologics. In: Stiehm ER, Sullivan KE, editors. Stiehm's immune deficiencies. London: Elsevier; 2014. p. 889–904.

Fagraeus A. The plasma cellular reaction and its relation to the formation of antibodies in vitro. J Immunol. 1948;58:1–13.

Feldman SR. Epidemiology, clinical manifestations, and diagnosis of psoriasis. In: Dellavalle R, editor; 2017.

Fonollosa A, Artaraz J, Les I, et al. Sarcoid intermediate uveitis following etanercept treatment: a case report and review of the literature. Ocul Immunol Inflamm. 2012;20:44–8.

Golay J, Semenzato G, Rambaldi A, et al. Lessons for the clinic from rituximab pharmacokinetics and pharmacodynamics. MAbs. 2013;5:826–37.

Gomez-Garcia F, Ruano J, Aguilar-Luque M, et al. Systematic reviews and meta-analyses on psoriasis: role of funding sources, conflict of interest and bibliometric indices as predictors of methodological quality. Br J Dermatol. 2017;176:1633–44.

Hendriks D, Choi G, De Bruyn M, et al. Antibody-based cancer therapy: successful agents and novel approaches. Int Rev Cell Mol Biol. 2017;331:289–383.

Her M, Kavanaugh A. Alterations in immune function with biologic therapies for autoimmune disease. J Allergy Clin Immunol. 2016;137:19–27.

Imbach P, Barandun S, D'apuzzo V, et al. High-dose intravenous gammaglobulin for idiopathic thrombocytopenic purpura in childhood. Lancet. 1981;1:1228–31.

Jones PT, Dear PH, Foote J, et al. Replacing the complementarity-determining regions in a human antibody with those from a mouse. Nature. 1986;321:522–5.

Kay J. Editorial: biosimilars: new or Deja Vu? Arthritis Rheumatol. 2016;68:1049–52.

Kohler G, Milstein C. Continuous cultures of fused cells secreting antibody of predefined specificity. Nature. 1975;256:495–7.

London NJ, Garg SJ, Moorthy RS, et al. Drug-induced uveitis. J Ophtha Inflamm Infect. 2013;3:43.

Majzner RG, Simon JS, Grosso JF, et al. Assessment of programmed death-ligand 1 expression and tumor-associated immune cells in pediatric cancer tissues. Cancer. 2017.

Martin-Liberal J, Ochoa De Olza M, Hierro C, et al. The expanding role of immunotherapy. Cancer Treat Rev. 2017;54:74–86.

Merrill JT, Neuwelt CM, Wallace DJ, et al. Efficacy and safety of rituximab in moderately-to-severely active systemic lupus erythematosus: the randomized, double-blind, phase II/III systemic lupus erythematosus evaluation of rituximab trial. Arthritis Rheum. 2010;62:222–33.

Molinelli E, Campanati A, Ganzetti G, et al. Biologic therapy in immune mediated inflammatory disease: basic science and clinical concepts. Curr Drug Saf. 2016;11:35–43.

Moreland LW. General principles of management of rheumatoid arthritis in adults. In: O'Dell JR, editor. uptodate; 2016.

Morrison SL, Johnson MJ, Herzenberg LA, et al. Chimeric human antibody molecules: mouse antigen-binding domains with human constant region domains. Proc Natl Acad Sci U S A. 1984;81:6851–5.

Nam JL, Takase-Minegishi K, Ramiro S, et al. Efficacy of biological disease-modifying antirheumatic drugs: a systematic literature review informing the 2016 update of the EULAR recommendations for the management of rheumatoid arthritis. Ann Rheum Dis. 2017;76:1113–36.

Niehues T. Optimizing treatment in paediatric rheumatology--lessons from oncology. Nat Rev Rheumatol. 2015;11:493–9.

Olek MJ. Disease-modifying treatment of relapsing-remitting multiple sclerosis in adults. In: González-Scarano F, editor; 2017.

Oosting SF, Brouwers AH, Van Es SC, et al. 89Zr-bevacizumab PET visualizes heterogeneous tracer accumulation in tumor lesions of renal cell carcinoma patients and differential effects of antiangiogenic treatment. J Nucl Med Off Publ Soc Nucl Med. 2015;56:63–9.

Oude Munnink TH, Henstra MJ, Segerink LI, et al. Therapeutic drug monitoring of monoclonal antibodies in inflammatory and malignant disease: translating TNF-alpha experience to oncology. Clin Pharmacol Ther. 2016;99:419–31.

Parren P, Carter PJ, Pluckthun A. Changes to international nonproprietary names for antibody therapeutics 2017 and beyond: of mice, men and more. mAbs. 2017:1–9.

Patterson H, Nibbs R, Mcinnes I, et al. Protein kinase inhibitors in the treatment of inflammatory and autoimmune diseases. Clin Exp Immunol. 2014;176:1–10.

Picard M, Galvao VR. current knowledge and management of hypersensitivity reactions to monoclonal antibodies. J Allergy Clin Immunol Pract. 2017;5:600–9.

Ramanan AV, Dick AD, Jones AP, et al. Adalimumab plus Methotrexate for Uveitis in Juvenile Idiopathic Arthritis. N Engl J Med. 2017;376:1637–46.
Rovin BH, Furie R, Latinis K, et al. Efficacy and safety of rituximab in patients with active proliferative lupus nephritis: the Lupus Nephritis Assessment with Rituximab study. Arthritis Rheum. 2012;64:1215–26.
Ruperto N, Brunner HI, Quartier P, et al. Two randomized trials of canakinumab in systemic juvenile idiopathic arthritis. N Engl J Med. 2012;367:2396–406.
Sanz-Cabanillas JL, Ruano J, Gomez-Garcia F, et al. Author-paper affiliation network architecture influences the methodological quality of systematic reviews and meta-analyses of psoriasis. PLoS One. 2017;12:e0175419.
Shoushtari AN, Wolchok J, Hellman M. Principles of cancer immunotherapy. In: Atkins MB, editor; 2017.
Singh JA, Hossain A, Mudano AS, et al. Biologics or tofacitinib for people with rheumatoid arthritis naive to methotrexate: a systematic review and network meta-analysis. Cochrane Database Syst Rev. 2017;5:CD012657.
Smith CH, Jabbar-Lopez ZK, Yiu ZZ, et al. British Association of Dermatologists guidelines for biologic therapy for psoriasis 2017. Br J Dermatol. 2017.
Suntharalingam G, Perry MR, Ward S, et al. Cytokine storm in a phase 1 trial of the anti-CD28 monoclonal antibody TGN1412. N Engl J Med. 2006;355:1018–28.
Weiner GJ. Building better monoclonal antibody-based therapeutics. Nat Rev Cancer. 2015;15:361–70.
Windeler J. No new Insights. Dtsch Arztebl Int. 2014;111:646.
Wu P, Nielsen TE, Clausen MH. FDA-approved small-molecule kinase inhibitors. Trends Pharmacol Sci. 2015;36:422–39.
Yarur AJ, Jain A, Sussman DA, et al. The association of tissue anti-TNF drug levels with serological and endoscopic disease activity in inflammatory bowel disease: the ATLAS study. Gut. 2016;65:249–55.
Young L, Czarnecki D. The rapid onset of multiple squamous cell carcinomas in two patients commenced on ustekinumab as treatment of psoriasis. Australas J Dermatol. 2012;53:57–60.

Monoclonal Anti-CD20 (B-Cell) Antibody and Autoimmune Diseases

21

Bertrand Godeau

Abbreviations

AAV	ANCA-associated vasculitis
AchR	Acetylcholine receptor
AIDs	Autoimmune diseases
AIN	Autoimmune neutropenia
ANCA	Antineutrophil cytoplasmic antibody
APL	Antiphospholipid
APS	Antiphospholipid syndrome
BAFF	B-cell activating factor
CAD	Cold-agglutinin disease
CAPS	Catastrophic antiphospholipid syndrome
CLL	Chronic lymphocyte leukemia
CVID	Common variable immunodeficiency syndrome
EGPA	Eosinophilic granulomatosis with polyangiitis
GCA	Giant cell arteritis
GPA	Granulomatosis with polyangiitis
IFNγ	Interferon-γ
ITP	Immune thrombocytopenia
IVIg	Intravenous immunoglobulin
MG	Myasthenia gravis
MS	Multiple sclerosis
MuSK	Muscle-specific tyrosine kinase
PR3	Proteinase 3
PRCA	Pure-red cell aplasia

B. Godeau, MD
Internal Medicine Unit, Reference Center of Adults' Autoimmune Cytopenia, CHU Henri Mondor, APHP, UPEC, 94010 Créteil, France
e-mail: bertrand.godeau@aphp.fr

P. Imbach (ed.), *Antibody Therapy*, https://doi.org/10.1007/978-3-319-68038-5_21

pSS	Primary Sjögren's syndrome
RA	Rheumatoid arthritis
RBC	Red blood cell
SLE	Systemic lupus erythematosus
SSc	Systemic sclerosis
TNF-α	Tumor necrosis factor-α
TPO-Ras	Thrombopoietin receptor agonists
wAIHA	Warm autoimmune hemolytic anemia

21.1 Introduction

Autoimmune diseases (AIDs) are a heterogeneous group of conditions with diverse clinical manifestations and complex pathogenesis. Steroids and immunosuppressants are always the cornerstone of treatment of the severe form of most AIDs, but biologic therapies have become a new weapon in the treatment. Biologic therapies have deeply changed the natural history of diseases such as rheumatoid arthritis (RA) and other inflammatory arthritis diseases and antineutrophil cytoplasmic antibody (ANCA)-associated vasculitis. However, although life-changing in some AIDs, the adverse effects accompanying biologic therapy, such as infection and immunogenicity, and the often disappointing long-term effects with high risk of relapse remain important issues. We still need to identify new candidate targets.

Context	Autoimmune diseases
Immunohematology	Immune thrombocytopenia (ITP)
	Warm autoimmune hemolytic anemia (wAIHAI)
	Cold-agglutinin disease (CAD)
	Autoimmune neutropenia (AIN)
	Pure-red cell aplasia (PRCA)
	Acquired hemophilia
	Acquired thrombocytopenic purpura (TTP)
Common variable immunodeficiency (CVID) syndrome	Immune cytopenia (ITP, wAHAI, Evans syndrome)
Systemic autoimmune diseases and connective tissue diseases	Systemic lupus erythematosus (SLE)
	Antiphospholipid syndrome (APS)
	Sjögren's syndrome
	Systemic sclerosis (SSc)
	Inflammatory muscles diseases
	Rheumatoid arthritis
Systemic vasculitis	ANCA-associated vasculitis
	Cryoglobulinemia
	Giant cell arteritis and Takayasu arteritis
Nervous system	Multiple sclerosis (MS)
	Myasthenia gravis

B cells play an important role in the immune response (Godeau and Stasi 2014). Their major role is to produce antibodies. B cells are also efficient antigen-presenting cells for T cells and secrete various cytokines such as interleukin-1 (IL-1), IL-10, IL-6, interferon-γ (IFNγ), and tumor necrosis factor-α (TNF-α), which activate macrophages, dendritic cells, and immunoregulatory cells. B cells have an important role in the pathophysiology of AIDs, and a rational approach to AID treatment involves B-cell depletion.

Human CD20 is a non-glycosylated phosphoprotein exclusively expressed in the B-cell hematopoietic lineage but not in hematopoietic stem cells or plasma cells. Rituximab is a human-to-mouse chimeric anti-CD20 monoclonal antibody that induces rapid, profound, and prolonged B-cell depletion. It was initially developed 20 years ago to treat lymphoma but is now used to treat various AIDs.

Here, we discuss the use of rituximab in treatment of the most frequent AIDs.

21.2 Rituximab and AIDs

21.2.1 Immunohematology and Hemostasis

21.2.1.1 Immune Thrombocytopenia (ITP)

Clinical Manifestations

ITP is a heterogeneous disease with a complex pathophysiology, involving enhanced platelet clearance as well as impaired platelet production. ITP remains a diagnosis of exclusion, and primary (or isolated) ITP and secondary ITP are commonly differentiated. ITP manifests by bleeding, which usually occurs with platelet count <30 G/L.

Rules of Treatment

Steroids and intravenous immunoglobulin (IVIg) are the first-line treatments. They are highly effective, but relapse occurs in most adults, and second-line treatments are frequently required. Second-line treatments include thrombopoietin receptor agonists (TPO-RAs), dapsone, danazol, rituximab, and splenectomy. Each approach has benefits and risks that should be considered carefully. Unlike the availability of international guidelines, consensus remains lacking on the treatment of ITP and should be personalized.

Results of Rituximab

More than 15 years ago, in an open prospective study, Stasi et al. (2001) gave rituximab to adults with chronic ITP according to the infusion regimen used for lymphoma (i.e., 4 weekly infusions of 375 mg/m^2 rituximab). They reported an overall response rate of 52%. In view of these encouraging results, other groups conducted uncontrolled studies. In a prospective multicenter registry of 248 adult patients with ITP treated with rituximab, 61% showed an overall initial response and at a median follow-up of 24 months, and 39% showed a lasting response (Khellaf et al. 2014).

The pattern of response was similar with the two rituximab regimens (four infusions of 375 mg/m^2 and two fixed 1-g infusions 2 weeks apart), and reassuring data were obtained on the safety of the treatment. In a prospective double-blind randomized study, Ghanima et al. (2015) compared rituximab with placebo and standard care as a second-line treatment for ITP without splenectomy. The rate of complete response at 24 weeks was greater with rituximab than placebo, with a trend toward a lower rate of splenectomy in the rituximab arm. However, rituximab did not reduce the rate of treatment failure. The modest long-term effect of rituximab was confirmed in a retrospective study of 72 adults and 65 children finding 5-year estimates of 21% and 26% persistent response, respectively (Patel et al. 2012).

Comments and Perspectives

With its benefit/risk ratio, rituximab used off-label is a valid option for treating persistent or chronic ITP. However, relapses are frequent, and the long-term response appears modest. Therefore, strategies to ameliorate the long-term efficacy of the treatment must be developed. Several options that may be tested include giving rituximab first or early on after ITP diagnosis, maintenance treatment with repeated infusions, and combining rituximab with other treatments such as dexamethasone or anti-B-cell activating factor (BAFF, also called BLyS) monoclonal antibody for a synergistic effect.

21.2.1.2 Warm Autoimmune Hemolytic Anemia (wAIHA)

Clinical Manifestations

AIHA is a rare AID in which autoantibodies directed toward red blood cell (RBC) antigens lead to their accelerated destruction. The diagnosis of AIHA mainly relies on the direct antiglobulin test. The classification of AIHA is based on immunochemical properties and especially on the thermal amplitude of the autoantibody ("warm" or "cold" type), which in clinical practice mainly relies on the interpretation of the direct antiglobulin test pattern but also on the presence or not of an underlying condition or disease (i.e., secondary versus primary AIHA). The distinction between AIHA due to warm antibody (wAIHA) and cold antibody is crucial because it affects both the prognosis and treatment.

wAIHA can be isolated or associated with various diseases, including mainly systemic lupus erythematosus (SLE) and chronic lymphocyte leukemia (CLL).

The clinical presentation of AIHA is usually subacute and may be rather insidious anemia. An abrupt onset with the presence of dark reddish urine reflecting the presence of intravascular hemolysis and hemoglobinuria is rarely observed.

Rules of Treatment

RBC transfusion is indicated in patients with disabling symptoms of anemia and/or a serious underlying cardiovascular condition.

The first-line treatment of primary wAHAI remains corticosteroids given at an initial daily dose of 1–1.5 mg/kg. The total duration of treatment lacks consensus, but the likelihood of early relapse is very high if the treatment is prematurely stopped, so corticosteroids should be maintained at least 3 months after a complete response.

Management for stage A CLL and active hemolysis should be as for primary wAIHA. However, progressive CLL must be treated more aggressively, with combined regimens such as rituximab + cyclophosphamide and dexamethasone (R-CDex).

Results of Rituximab

Two open randomized controlled studies (Barcellini et al. 2012; Birgens et al. 2013) and one double-blind controlled study (Michel et al. 2017) using a different pattern of rituximab administration gave promising data and demonstrated the efficacy of rituximab in primary wAHAI. In a prospective study with a placebo, the overall response rate at 1 year was 75% with rituximab versus 31% with placebo.

Comments and Perspectives

The data from the literature support, whenever possible, the use of rituximab off-label for patients refractory to corticosteroids and those with a chronic active and/or relapsing primary wAIHA who need to be maintained on prednisone (or prednisolone) at a daily equivalent or >15 mg to maintain at least partial remission.

21.2.1.3 Cold Agglutinin Diseases (CADs)

Clinical Manifestations

Primary chronic CAD is a clonal lymphoproliferative B-cell bone-marrow disorder. The immune hemolysis is complement dependent, mediated by activation of the classical pathway and phagocytosis of erythrocytes opsonized with complement protein C3b. CAD can be an indolent disease, but typical clinical features include episodes of transient anemia that can be acute and severe and frequently associated with cold-induced ischemic symptoms ranging from mild to disabling.

Rules of Treatment

In the indolent disease form, no treatment is required, but patients should avoid exposure to cold. Pharmacologic treatment should be offered for symptom-producing anemia or disabling circulatory symptoms. Corticosteroids usually give disappointing results and the indication of steroids for CAD is still debatted. Splenectomy is not a good option because hemolysis in CAD is intravascular. Successful CAD therapy targets the pathogenic B-cell clone.

Results of Rituximab

Rituximab monotherapy can induce partial remission in about 50% of patients (Berentsen 2013; Berentsen et al. 2017). Those with relapse after previous treatment with rituximab may respond to a second or even a third series of monotherapy, and the treatment is well tolerated. Despite a somewhat disappointing median response duration of about 1 year, single-agent therapy with rituximab should still be considered first-line treatment in some patients.

Comments and Perspectives

Combination therapy with fludarabine and rituximab is more efficient, resulting in remission in approximately 75% of patients and complete response in 20% and a median response duration of more than 5 years. However, because of the toxicity profile, this treatment should be reserved for the more severe forms of CAD in patients showing failure of remission with rituximab monotherapy. Recent study suggests that Bendamustine could also be a good option.

In the near future, complement-modulating agents seem promising.

21.2.1.4 Autoimmune Neutropenia (AIN)

Clinical Manifestations

AIN is a rare and heterogeneous group of diseases with variable clinical manifestations from asymptomatic to severe forms associated with infectious complications (Autrel-Moignet and Lamy 2014). It is caused by antibodies directed against neutrophil-specific antigens. It includes primary and secondary autoimmune neutropenia. Acute autoimmune neutropenia can be related to drug-induced mechanisms or viral infections. Chronic autoimmune neutropenias occur in the context of AIDs such as SLE or Sjögren's syndrome, hematologic malignancies such as large granular lymphocyte leukemia, primary immune deficiency syndromes, or solid tumors.

Rules of Treatment

The therapeutic management depends on the etiology. Granulocyte growth factor is an option and can be transiently used in cases of symptomatic profound neutropenia. The question of their long-term safety is debated. Corticosteroids or immunosuppressive therapy (mainly cyclophosphamide, methotrexate, or cyclosporine) are indicated in infection-related autoimmune neutropenia or with symptomatic autoimmune disease or large granular lymphocytic leukemia.

Results of Rituximab

Rituximab has been only occasionally used, with disappointing results, and does not seem a valid option except when autoimmune neutropenia is associated in a setting of Evans syndrome (association of autoimmune neutropenia with ITP and/or wAHAI).

Of note, transient profound neutropenia, which is usually asymptomatic, is a complication of rituximab. This adverse event is mainly observed when rituximab is used for treating CLL or malignant lymphoma but is rarely observed in the setting of AIDs.

21.2.1.5 Pure-Red Cell Aplasia (PRCA)

Clinical Manifestations

PRCA is a rare syndrome caused by isolated erythropoietic hypoplasia with severe normocytic and reticulocytopenic anemia and a normally cellular bone marrow but devoid of erythroblasts. PRCA is often diagnosed in conjunction with a variety of diseases, such as lymphoproliferative disorders (mainly CLL), viral infections (parvovirus B19, HIV), wAHAI, rheumatologic disorders, and allogeneic stem cell transplantation.

Rules of Treatment

Acquired PRCA is managed as an AID, by immunosuppressive therapy with corticosteroids and cyclosporine A as first-choice treatments.

Results of Rituximab

Only isolated case reports suggested that rituximab could be effective in PRCA. Good response has been reported in a setting of PRCA associated with various diseases such as SLE or CLL or after allogenic bone-marrow transplantation.

Comments and Perspectives

Rituximab should be reserved as rescue treatment for patients who are refractory to steroids and immunosuppressive therapy such as cyclosporine A, and it cannot be considered as first-line treatment (Tendas et al. 2016).

21.2.1.6 Acquired Hemophilia

Clinical Manifestations

Acquired hemophilia is an AID caused by the development of specific autoantibodies that inhibit factor VIII (FVIII). It is associated with a high mortality rate, usually between 10 and 30%. Hemorrhagic manifestations of acquired hemophilia occur as acute, spontaneous, or traumatic in patients with no prior history of bleeding. The most common clinical findings are profuse cutaneous bleeding. Acquired hemophilia can complicate pregnancy and can be associated with many diseases such as various AIDs (SLE, Sjögren's syndrome, etc.), hematological diseases including lymphoid hemopathy, myelodysplastic syndrome, solid tumors, chronic viral infection (hepatitis B and C virus [HBV, HCV]), and allergic reaction to drugs.

Rules of Treatment

It consists of two parts: treatment targeting abortion or preventing bleeding episodes and that aimed at eradicating the autoantibody. As bypassing agents, two drugs are used for this indication: recombinant activated factor VII (rFVIIa [NovoSeven®]) and activated prothrombin complex concentrates (APCC [FEIBA®]).

The first-line immunosuppressive treatment most commonly used and recommended is based on corticosteroids (1 mg/kg/day) alone or associated with cyclophosphamide given at low doses (1–2 mg/kg/day), for between 3 and 5 weeks. The combination of immunosuppression and comorbidities, due to patient age and comorbidities, leads to the occurrence of cytopenias and secondary infections in almost half of all patients.

Results of Rituximab

Most reviews and guidelines point to rituximab as the alternative of choice with failure of first-line treatment. The usual pattern involves the administration of weekly doses of 375 mg/m^2/week for 4 weeks. Rituximab requires several weeks or months to achieve eradication of the inhibitor. For the more severe forms of acquired hemophilia, particularly with high titers of inhibitors, some authors consider that rituximab should be combined with other immunosuppressive drugs (Collins et al. 2012).

Comments and Perspectives

A large controlled prospective study is in progress in France to better define the place of rituximab in primary acquired hemophilia.

21.2.1.7 Acquired Thrombotic Thrombocytopenic Purpura (TTP)

Clinical Manifestations

Acquired autoimmune TTP is a severe form of thrombotic microangiopathy characterized by the association of a microangiopathic hemolytic anemia with a peripheral thrombocytopenia, organ failure of variable severity due to thrombi in microvasculature, and antibody-mediated severe deficiency (<10% of normal activity) in the von Willebrand-factor-cleaving protease ADAMTS13.

TTP can complicate pregnancy and can be associated with many diseases such as various AIDs (SLE, Sjögren's syndrome, etc.), viral infection (HIV, etc.), reaction to drugs (cyclosporine A), and bone-marrow transplantation.

Rules of Treatment

Daily therapeutic plasma exchange, which addresses the ADAMTS13 deficiency and to a lesser extent removes serum anti-ADAMTS13 antibodies and possibly pro-aggregant substances, has transformed the prognosis of TTP, with current overall survival rates of 80–85%. Because acquired TTP is now considered an AID, immunosuppressive drugs are also involved in the therapeutic strategy. In addition to the development of plasma exchange, rituximab has been a major breakthrough in managing this disease.

Results of Rituximab

For the acute phase of TTP, most studies reported that remission was achieved in most cases, typically in <4 weeks (Froissart et al. 2015). Rituximab is now routinely recommended during the acute phase, typically in patients with a suboptimal response to plasma exchange, or even as a first-line therapy. However, whether rituximab should be reserved for patients with suboptimal response to standard treatment or used as a first-line therapy for all patients with autoimmune TTP is still debated.

Comments and Perspectives

At least 40% of patients experience a recurrence of TTP. Each relapse exposes the patient to risk of death and to complications related to plasma exchange. ADAMTS13 activity represents a reliable marker of disease activity because patients who remain with severe enzyme deficiency are at high risk of relapse. Preliminary reports suggested that infusions of rituximab could prevent TTP relapse in patients with severe persistent ADAMTS13 deficiency and otherwise in clinical and hematologic remission. These findings argue for regular systematic assessments of ADAMTS13 activity during follow-up, to identify at an early stage those patients at risk of relapse. Preemptive rituximab represents a promising strategy that could modify the long-term prognosis.

21.2.2 Autoimmune Manifestations of Common Variable Immunodeficiency (CVID) Syndrome

21.2.2.1 Clinical Manifestations

CVID is a primary immune deficiency characterized by reduced serum levels of IgG, IgA, and/or IgM with reduced or absent specific antibody production. The diagnosis is typically between the ages of 20 and 40 years, but about 20% of patients are younger than 20. Infectious complications are the disease hallmark, but in two thirds of patients, granulomatous disease or one or more inflammatory and autoimmune manifestations develop. Inflammatory manifestations involve mainly the lung with progressive chronic lung diseases. ITP and wAHAI are the most common AIDs and complicate the CVID outcome. Lymphoma or other malignancies can occur in about 10% of patients.

21.2.2.2 Rules of Treatment

Substitutive treatment based on repeated IVIg infusion is the cornerstone of CVID and prevents infectious complications. However, this treatment is ineffective in treating autoimmune manifestations and particularly ITP and wAHAI. In this case, prolonged treatment with steroids and splenectomy should be avoided because of the risk of infection.

21.2.2.3 Results of Rituximab

In a retrospective study of 33 patients with CVID and ITP and/or wAHAI treated with rituximab, the overall initial response rate to rituximab was 85% (Gobert et al. 2011). After a mean follow-up of more than 3 years, ten of the initial responders showed relapse, and retreatment with rituximab was successful in seven out of nine responders. Severe infections occurred after rituximab in eight adults (24%), four not on IVIg replacement therapy. In conclusion, rituximab appears to be highly effective and relatively safe for managing CVID-associated severe immune cytopenias. However, it should be systematically associated with IVIg replacement to limit the risk of infectious complications.

21.2.2.4 Comments and Perspectives

TPO-RAs are very effective in primary ITP. They could be a good option for treating ITP associated with CVID. The respective places of TPO-RAs and rituximab in this setting are still debated.

21.2.3 Systemic Autoimmune Diseases and Connective Tissue Diseases: "Lupus Group"

21.2.3.1 Systemic Lupus Erythematosus (SLE)

Clinical Manifestations

SLE is a chronic autoimmune condition with unpredictable course, intermingled with flares and periods of remission. It can affect the skin, muscles and articles, heart, lung, kidney, and peripheral and central nervous system. Blood manifestations are frequent, and autoimmune cytopenias, including ITP and wAIHA, can be severe.

Rules of Treatment

Treatments may include nonsteroidal anti-inflammatory drugs, corticosteroids, immunosuppressants, and hydroxychloroquine. Although the prognosis has improved in the past decades, current therapies are still associated with treatment-related complications. Recently, there has been major progress in understanding the pathogenesis of SLE, paving the way for the development of new biologic agents, potentially revolutionizing the treatment of SLE.

Results of Rituximab

The use of rituximab in patients with SLE has been investigated in two randomized controlled trials, EXPLORER (the Exploratory Phase II/III SLE Evaluation of Rituximab) (Merrill et al. 2010) and LUNAR (Lupus Nephritis Assessment with Rituximab) (Rovin et al. 2012), with negative results regarding superiority to conventional treatment. However, before concluding that rituximab is not effective in SLE, a critical evaluation of the design of the EXPLORER and LUNAR trials is required. The results of these two trials suggested that the use of rituximab in SLE may be controversial, but it is still extensively used "off-label," especially in cases refractory to standard treatment (Cobo-Ibanez et al. 2014; Duxbury et al. 2013; Sciascia et al. 2015). Rituximab is effective in autoimmune cytopenia associated with SLE, with severe kidney involvement in case of failure of "conventional treatment" such as cyclophosphamide, mycophenolate mofetil, and azathioprine. A prospective, observational, single-center cohort study evaluated the effectiveness of treating lupus nephritis with rituximab and mycophenolate mofetil but no oral steroids (Condon et al. 2013). After 1 year of follow-up, overall response rate was >80%, which demonstrates that oral steroids can be safely avoided in treating lupus nephritis.

Rituximab could be associated with risk of fatal multifocal progressive leukoencephalopathy due to JC virus infection in the setting of SLE treated with rituximab. However, this risk appears exceptional.

Today, unlike in the absence of a license, rituximab can be proposed for SLE patients with lupus nephritis resistant to conventional treatment or autoimmune cytopenia.

Comments and Perspectives

Other B-cell-targeted therapies that inhibit BAFF currently being assessed include belimumab, tabalumab, and blisibimod. Belimumab received a license for non-severe SLE (without central system or kidney involvements).

21.2.3.2 Antiphospholipid Syndrome (APS)

Clinical Manifestations

APS is characterized by recurrent thrombosis and/or obstetric complications with the presence of antiphospholipid antibodies (lupus anticoagulant, anti-cardiolipid antibodies, anti-beta2-GP1 antibodies). It can be isolated and considered "primary" or associated with SLE.

The most frequent clinical manifestation is deep venous thrombosis, whereas cerebrovascular accident is the most prevalent manifestation of arterial thrombosis. Fetal losses (early and late), prematurity, and preeclampsia are the most frequent obstetric manifestations. The catastrophic variant of the antiphospholipid (APL) syndrome (CAPS) is characterized by thrombosis in multiple organs developing over a short time. The prognosis of CAPS is severe, and mortality remains high.

Rules of Treatment

The treatment for thrombotic APS is based on control of vascular risk factors, acetylsalicylic acid as primary thromboprophylaxis, and long-term anticoagulant treatment as secondary thromboprophylaxis.

The combined treatment with anticoagulation therapy plus glucocorticoids plus plasma exchange and/or IVIg results in a high recovery rate in patients with CAPS.

Results of Rituximab

For APS, we have only few data focused on the interest of rituximab in this setting. Some case reports suggested that rituximab could be effective for treating some non-thrombotic manifestations associated with APS, such as thrombocytopenia of skin necrosis (Ponsa et al. 2015).

For CAPS, despite the reduced mortality with treatment, some patients are refractory, such as those who die despite first-line treatments or those with recurrent episodes of CAPS. A review of the literature reported 20 patients with CAPS treated with rituximab (Berman et al. 2013). The number of patients was too low to draw firm conclusions, but 75% of patients recovered from the acute CAPS episode and 20% died. These results suggest that rituximab could have a role in treating APL-positive patients, especially those with refractory CAPS.

21.2.3.3 Sjögren's Syndrome

Clinical Manifestations

Primary Sjögren's syndrome (pSS) is a systemic autoimmune disease that involves the exocrine glands and internal organs. pSS leads to the destruction and loss of secretory function due to intense lymphoplasmacytic infiltration. In most patients, the outcome is benign, and symptoms are limited to sicca syndrome. However, in some patients, pSS may have systemic involvement, including the pulmonary, renal, vascular, central, and/or peripheral nervous systems. Autoimmune cytopenia is a known complication. The risk of non-Hodgkin lymphoma is higher than in the general population.

Rules of Treatment

Therapeutic options include mainly symptomatic and supportive measures, and traditional immunosuppressant drugs have shown no effectiveness in randomized trials. The use of systemic therapies for dryness, chronic pain, or fatigue is not warranted. The management of pSS should be organ specific, with low-dose steroids in patients with moderate systemic activity, limiting the use of high-dose steroids and second-line therapies to refractory or potentially severe cases.

Results of Rituximab

The number of published articles on rituximab used to treat pSS has been growing. However, most identified studies are case reports or series of specific systemic manifestations, and only a few randomized studies of rituximab have compared the effectiveness of this drug to placebo or other drugs (Souza et al. 2016). Because of multiple biases due to the design of most of these studies, drawing firm conclusions is difficult. The effect on improving lacrimal gland function appears modest, and we have no proof of the potential of this drug for improving salivary flow. Also no level of evidence suggests improvement of oral dryness. In particular, a double-blind prospective controlled study conducted in France that compared rituximab and placebo and included 120 patients confirmed that rituximab did not alleviate symptoms or disease activity in patients with pSS at week 24, although it alleviated some symptoms at earlier time points (Devauchelle-Pensec et al. 2014).

Comments and Perspectives

Rituximab is not indicated in pSS but can be discussed for some extraglandular manifestations such as autoimmune cytopenia.

21.2.3.4 Systemic Sclerosis (SSc)

Clinical Manifestations

SSc is characterized by diffuse microangiopathy and accumulation of collagen and other matrix constituents in the skin and target internal organs. Typical SSc symptoms can be skin ulcers, pulmonary arterial hypertension, and/or renal scleroderma crisis with fibrotic cutaneous and visceral organ involvement affecting particularly the heart and lung. Autoimmunity may contribute to both vascular and fibrotic SSc manifestations.

Rules of Treatment

The effect of nonselective immunosuppressive treatments, usually used during the early phases of SSc to control skin and lung inflammation, is often unpredictable. High-dose steroids should be avoided because of the risk of severe renal scleroderma crisis. These treatments tend to lose their efficacy once the disease enters a chronic phase, and consequently long-term treatment is not recommendable, considering the potential severe side effects.

Results of Rituximab

Small open studies and case reports suggested that rituximab could act on skin and lung fibrosis (Giuggioli et al. 2015). However, multiple biases are present, so one cannot conclude on the interest of rituximab in SSc. A multicenter prospective case-control study conducted in Europe included 63 patients receiving rituximab (Jordan et al. 2015). The comparison of rituximab-treated versus untreated matched-control SSc patients demonstrated improved skin fibrosis and prevention of worsening lung fibrosis, which supports the therapeutic concept of B-cell inhibition in SSc.

Comments and Perspectives

The results of the European Scleroderma Trial and Research (EUSTAR) group remain preliminary and need to be viewed with caution, recognizing the spontaneous regression of skin thickening that may occur early during the disease, and other studies are required before proposing rituximab as first-line treatment for severe pSS.

21.2.3.5 Inflammatory Muscle Diseases

Clinical Manifestations

To date, four main groups of idiopathic inflammatory myopathies (IIMs) have been identified—polymyositis, dermatomyositis, immune-mediated necrotizing myopathy, and sporadic inclusion body myositis—on the basis of clinical presentation and muscle pathology. Important phenotypical differences (muscular and/or extramuscular manifestations) persist within a group. We now have routine access to assays for detecting different antibodies, and all groups of myositis may present one of those autoantibodies. Most allow for identifying homogenous patient groups more precisely than with the classical international classifications of myositis.

Rules of Treatment

High-dose steroids remain the first-line treatment for inflammatory muscle diseases except for sporadic diseases including body myositis, for which steroids are ineffective. IVIg is indicated, particularly in dermatomyositis associated with dysphagia. Immunosuppressive treatment such as methotrexate, mycophenolate mofetil, and cyclophosphamide could be associated with steroids as a first-line treatment in the more severe forms of diseases or in patients refractory to steroids.

Results of Rituximab

We have only few data on the effectiveness of rituximab in IIMs. Most of the reported studies are retrospective and included a small number of patients. Moreover, they grouped different types of IIMs. Drawing firm conclusions is difficult, and the exact role of rituximab in the therapeutic strategy of IIMS is still a matter of debate, but these data suggest that rituximab could be effective in all IIMs (Hervier and Benveniste 2015). The delay of action is sometimes long, and at least 4 months may be needed before a response is seen. Rituximab should not be proposed alone but should be associated with steroids and/or immunosuppressive drugs. Relapses are frequent. In case of relapse, a new course of rituximab could be proposed.

Comments and Perspectives

Despite these relatively modest results, rituximab may play a role in the treatment of IIMs. All other available biotherapies such as anti-IL-1, anti-IL-6, and anti-IFN-α therapies have been not studied, and anti-TNF-α agents are contraindicated with myositis, at least in patients with positive myositis-specific autoantibodies.

21.2.3.6 Rheumatoid Arthritis (RA)

Clinical Manifestations

RA is a systemic autoimmune disease characterized by joint inflammation that often evolves into erosive joint damage with significant disability.

Rules of Treatment

Methotrexate remains the first-line treatment. Prolonged steroid treatment should be avoided. The development of anti-TNF agents has completely revolutionized the natural history of the disease and should be rapidly associated with methotrexate in cases of lack of response.

Results of Rituximab

Some patients show an inadequate response to anti-TNF agents. Rituximab is indicated in such cases (Cohen and Keystone 2015; Rossi et al. 2015. Several randomized controlled prospective studies compared two infusions of rituximab 1000 mg to placebo. Methotrexate was used in both. Treatment with rituximab has been clearly demonstrated as more effective than placebo in treatment-naïve patients and those with anti-TNF treatment failure. Rituximab is more effective in "seropositive" patients. It has been studied in combination with anti-TNF agents, and the numerical risk of serious adverse events was only slightly increased but without a significant increase in efficacy. The optimal rituximab dose is controversial. The 2 × 1000- and 2 × 500-mg doses may be equivalent in terms of improvement in signs and symptoms, but the 2 × 1000-mg dose showed better outcomes and should be used. Relapses are frequent, and the duration of the effect is quite variable. So, the optimal timing for retreatment is difficult to predict. A review of retreated patients from the clinical trials suggested that the fixed-interval (24 week) treat-to-target strategy was superior to retreatment at the discretion of the physician. The latest European consensus statement suggests that retreatment in initial responders should be considered at 24 weeks for patients who do not achieve low disease activity or remission and that it should be delayed otherwise until disease activity flares.

The incidence of human anti-chimeric antibodies varied from 2.7 to 7.1%, but the clinical significance of the antibodies is still debated.

Comments and Perspectives

Rituximab has been a significant addition to the short list of biologic agents approved for treating RA. The safety is reassuring, but as with all biologics for RA, further information regarding the safety of rituximab over longer periods is critical.

21.2.4 Systemic Vasculitis

21.2.4.1 ANCA-Associated Vasculitis (AAV)

Clinical Manifestations

AAV includes granulomatosis with polyangiitis (GPA), eosinophilic granulomatosis with polyangiitis (EGPA), and microscopic polyangiitis (MPA), which are small-vessel vasculitides associated with the presence of ANCAs to proteinase 3 (PR3-ANCAs) or myeloperoxidase (MPO-ANCAs). The clinical manifestations of GPA range from limited upper respiratory tract inflammatory disease to severe lower respiratory tract, renal, and nervous system vasculitis. MPA involves necrotizing systemic vasculitis of the respiratory tract, kidneys, and nervous system. EGPA clinical manifestations include asthma, nasal polyps, peripheral blood eosinophilia, and systemic vasculitis of the respiratory tract, skin, heart, and nervous system.

Rules of Treatment

The management of AAV is in accordance with the disease severity and is based on extensive clinical trial and clinical practice data. High-dose steroids associated with immunosuppressive drugs (mainly cyclophosphamide as attack treatment and methotrexate or azathioprine as maintenance treatment) have been considered the cornerstone for treating the most severe forms for a long time. Plasma exchange is also indicated in life-threatening situations such as pulmonary hemorrhage or acute renal failure.

Results of Rituximab

In two multicenter, prospective, randomized controlled studies, at 6 months, rituximab was found to be not inferior to cyclophosphamide for inducing remission of GPA and MPA. From these two studies, the US Food and Drug Administration accorded marketing authorization for rituximab as remission-induction and maintenance treatment for these two AAVs. In Europe, rituximab has been authorized for only induction therapy. Now, rituximab is considered as a first-line treatment, even for life-threatening GPA and MPA (Lutalo and D'Cruz 2015), except in France, where the recommendation is to continue to use cyclophosphamide for severe acute renal failure or pulmonary hemorrhage (Charles et al. 2013). For maintenance treatment, rituximab has been found superior to azathioprine. A fixed-interval rituximab protocol, with a single 1-g infusion administered every 6 months for 2 years, has been shown to reduce the rate of clinical relapse as compared with rituximab retreatment at the time of relapse in patients with severe relapsing, refractory AAV.

Indications

For EGPA, studies comparing conventional treatment and rituximab are in progress. To date, rituximab is not recommended in this setting, but some case reports and retrospective data suggest that rituximab could be effective in severe cases refractory to conventional treatment, with systemic vasculitis as the predominant clinical manifestation.

Comments and Perspectives

Rituximab has clearly completely revolutionized the therapeutic strategy of GPA and MPA. However, relapses are not rare, and the best maintenance treatment with repeated infusions or combining rituximab with other treatments should be determined.

21.2.4.2 Cryoglobulinemia

Clinical Manifestations

Cryoglobulinemia is characterized by the presence of cryoglobulins in serum. It has two main subgroups: type I, in which the cryoglobulins are monoclonal, and types II and III, in which the cryoglobulins are composed of a mixture of monoclonal IgM and polyclonal IgG (type II) or only polyclonal IgG (type III). Type I is seen exclusively in clonal hematologic diseases, whereas type II/III, named "mixed" cryoglobulinemia, is seen in hepatitis C virus infection and systemic diseases such as B-cell hemopathy and connective tissue disorders.

Clinical manifestations are various and include arthralgia, skin purpura, skin ulcers, renal involvement, and peripheral neuropathy. Life-threatening manifestations with heart or central nervous system involvement are rarely seen. Occasionally, when the cryocrit is high, hyperviscosity syndrome may occur, with oronasal bleeding, blurred vision, deafness, headache, confusion, and heart failure.

Rules of Treatment and Place of Rituximab

Only symptomatic cryoglobulinemia should be treated (Muchtar et al. 2017).

For the rare severe forms with hyperviscosity syndrome, plasma exchange is indicated.

Treating the underlying cause is important. Thus, in type I, the major goal is to treat the clonal hematologic disease, and in this field, chemotherapy is the cornerstone of treatment. In this case, rituximab is rarely indicated and may cause IgM flare and development of hyperviscosity syndrome.

For mixed cryoglobulinemia, with HCV infection, antiviral treatment is indicated. Rituximab can be associated with antiviral therapy in the most severe forms.

In noninfectious mixed cryoglobulinemia, with severe manifestations, treatment is required (i.e., cutaneous ulcers, glomerulopathy, debilitating neuropathy). The respective indications of rituximab associated with steroids or cyclophosphamide plus steroids are debated.

21.2.4.3 Giant Cell Arteritis (GCA) and Takayasu Syndrome

Clinical Manifestations

GCA is a large-vessel vasculitis characterized by a granulomatous involvement of the aorta and/or its major branches that usually affects people older than 50 years. It is frequently associated with polymyalgia rheumatica and manifests by headache and proximal myalgia. There is a risk of arteritic ischemic optic neuropathy, which can result in blindness. In one quarter of patients, the aorta and its major branches are involved.

Takayasu arteritis is a rare large-vessel vasculitis affecting the aortas and its large branches including proximal portions of renal, coronary, and pulmonary arteritis. It affects young patients (younger than 40 years), and it manifests by claudication of the extremities, myalgia, decreased brachial artery pulse over the subclavian, or abdominal aorta. Stroke is a complication of the most severe forms.

Rules of Treatment

Steroids remain the first-line treatment of GCA and Takayasu arteritis. Immunosuppressive drugs are indicated with lack of response to steroids or with relapse when decreasing the steroids dose. Methotrexate is the immunosuppressive treatment most frequently used in this setting. Recently, biologic therapy based on tocilizumab, an anti-IL-6 monoclonal antibody, showed promising results.

Results of Rituximab

We have only a few data for a small number of patients with Takayasu arteritis treated with rituximab (Loricera et al. 2015). In view of the small number of cases, we cannot draw definite conclusions, and so far the role of rituximab in the therapeutic strategy of ANCA-negative systemic vasculitis is marginal.

21.2.5 Nervous System

21.2.5.1 Multiple Sclerosis (MS)

Clinical Manifestations

MS is a chronic inflammatory demyelinating disease caused by an autoimmune response against central nervous system structures. MS attacks the myelin of the brain and spinal cord, causing inflammation and often damaging the myelin in patches. The disease results in a wide variety of symptoms such as dizziness, bladder dysfunction, gait, optic neuritis, and sensory impairment, depending on what part or parts of the central nervous system are affected. The symptoms improve during periods of remission.

Rules of Treatment

Treatment is very complex and should be personalized. Many treatments now available include IFN-β, teriflunomide, fingolimod, mitoxantrone, and monoclonal antibodies such as natalizumab and alemtuzumab. The choice of drug used for initial therapy or escalation of therapy should be based on a benefit/risk evaluation and tailored to the individual patient's requirements. Patients should ideally receive treatment by a specialized multidisciplinary team.

Results of Anti-CD20 Antibody Therapy

There is evidence for B-cell involvement in the pathophysiology of MS, and at the present, three therapeutic monoclonal antibodies are in clinical phase II and III trials (rituximab, ocrelizumab, and ofatumumab) (Bittner et al. 2017). Recent controlled studies demonstrated that ocrelizumab which is a monoclonal antibody directed against B cells was more effective than IFN (Hauser et al. 2017; Montalban et al. 2017).

21.2.5.2 Myasthenia Gravis (MG)

Clinical Manifestations

MG is an autoimmune neuromuscular junction disorder. It manifests by fluctuating fatigable weakness involving specific muscle groups. Ocular weakness with asymmetric ptosis and diplopia is the most common presentation. Oropharyngeal and limb weakness are less common. Antibodies against acetylcholine receptor (AchR) or muscle-specific tyrosine kinase (MuSK) are always present and are useful for the diagnosis.

Rules of Treatment

Treatment must be individualized. Cholinesterase inhibitors are the first-line treatment. Immunosuppressive treatment including steroids, azathioprine, cyclosporine, or mycophenolate mofetil is indicated in the most severe disabling forms. Thymectomy can be occasionally indicated. Plasma exchange or IVIg is required in an emergency for myasthenic crisis and life-threatening situations.

Results of Rituximab

Tandan et al. (2017) recently reviewed the efficacy and safety of rituximab in 169 MG patients from case reports and series. A response was observed in 72% of patients with MuSK antibodies and in only 30% with AchR antibodies. More than 50% of patients could have a relapse within a mean of 1.5 years after rituximab infusions (Robeson et al. 2017). These results suggest that rituximab could be an attractive option in severe MG.

Comments and Perspectives

Unlike these promising results, experts who recently published international consensus guidance for MG management concluded that no formal consensus could be reached concerning the place of rituximab in the therapeutic strategy.

Conclusions

Rituximab is used frequently for treating most AIDs. It has deeply changed the treatment strategy in AAV, and a license was obtained for the treatment of RA. However, for most AIDs, the drug is used off-label, and randomized controlled studies are often lacking. It is well tolerated, even if infectious complications are possible, particularly if associated with steroids. One important caveat is the risk of relapse. For the future, how to obtain better long-term results remains a crucial issue. Maintenance treatment with repeated rituximab infusions, association of rituximab with other biologic therapies or dexamethasone, and recognition of predictors of long-term sustained response could be different options to better select patients with AIDs who could receive rituximab and to hope for better long-term results.

References

Autrel-Moignet A, Lamy T. Autoimmune neutropenia. Presse Med. 2014;43:e105–18.

Barcellini W, Zaja F, Zaninoni A, et al. Low-dose rituximab in adult patients with idiopathic autoimmune hemolytic anemia: clinical efficacy and biologic studies. Blood. 2012;119:3691–7.

Berentsen S. Therapy for chronic cold agglutinin disease: perspective for further improvements. Blood Transfus. 2013;11:167–8.

Berentsen S, Randen U, Oksman M et al. Bendamustine plus rituximab for chronic cold agglutinin disease: results of a Nordic prospective multicenter trial. Blood. 2017;130:537–41.

Berman H, Rodríguez-Pintó I, Cervera R, et al. Rituximab use in the catastrophic antiphospholipid syndrome: descriptive analysis of the CAPS registry patients receiving rituximab. Autoimmun Rev. 2013;12:1085–90.

Birgens H, Frederiksen H, Hasselbalch HC, et al. A phase III randomized trial comparing glucocorticoid monotherapy versus glucocorticoid and rituximab in patients with autoimmune haemolytic anaemia. Br J Haematol. 2013;163:393–9.

Bittner S, Ruck T, Wiendl H, Grauer OM, Meuth SG. Targeting B cells in relapsing–remitting multiple sclerosis: from pathophysiology to optimal clinical management. Ther Adv Neurol Disord. 2017;10:51–66.

Charles P, Bienvenu B, Bonnotte B, et al. Rituximab: recommendations of the French Vasculitis Study Group (FVSG) for induction and maintenance treatments of adult, antineutrophil cytoplasm antibody-associated necrotizing vasculitides. Presse Med. 2013;42:1317–30.

Cobo-Ibanez T, Loza-Santamaria E, Pego-Reigosa JM, et al. Efficacy and safety of rituximab in the treatment of non-renal systemic lupus erythematosus: a systematic review. Semin Arthritis Rheum. 2014;44:175–85.

Cohen MD, Keystone E. Rituximab for rheumatoid arthritis. Rheumatol Ther. 2015;2:99–111.

Collins P, Baudo F, Knoebl P, et al. Immunosuppression for acquired hemophilia A: results from the European Acquired Haemophilia Registry (EACH2). Blood. 2012;120:47–55.

Condon MB, Ashby D, Pepper RJ, et al. Prospective observational single-centre cohort study to evaluate the effectiveness of treating lupus nephritis with rituximab and mycophenolate mofetil but no oral steroids. Ann Rheum Dis. 2013;72:1280–6.

Devauchelle-Pensec V, Mariette X, Jousse-Joulin S, et al. Treatment of primary Sjögren syndrome with rituximab: a randomized trial. Ann Intern Med. 2014;160:233–42.

Duxbury B, Combescure C, Chizzolini C. Rituximab in systemic lupus erythematosus: an updated systematic review and meta-analysis. Lupus. 2013;22:1489–503.

Froissart A, Veyradier A, Hié M, Benhamou Y, Coppo P. Rituximab in autoimmune thrombotic thrombocytopenic purpura: a success story. Eur J Intern Med. 2015;26:659–65.

Ghanima W, Khelif A, Waage A, et al. Rituximab as second-line treatment for adult immune thrombocytopenia (the RITP trial): a multicentre, randomised, double-blind, placebo-controlled trial. Lancet. 2015;385(9978):1653–61.

Giuggioli D, Lumetti F, Colaci M, Fallahi P, Antonelli A, Ferri C. Rituximab in the treatment of patients with systemic sclerosis. Our experience and review of the literature. Autoimmun Rev. 2015;14:1072–8.

Gobert D, Bussel JB, Cunningham-Rundles C, et al. Efficacy and safety of rituximab in common variable immunodeficiency-associated immune cytopenias: a retrospective multicentre study on 33 patients. Br J Haematol. 2011;155:498–508.

Godeau B, Stasi R. Is B-cell depletion still a good strategy for treating immune thrombocytopenia? Presse Med. 2014;43:e79–85.

Hauser SL, Bar-Or A, Comi G, et al. Ocrelizumab versus interferon beta-1a in relapsing multiple sclerosis. N Engl J Med. 2017;376:221–34.

Hervier B, Benveniste O. Rituximab in inflammatory myopathies: "a neolithic revolution". Rev Med Interne. 2015;36:505–8.

Jordan S, Distler JH, Maurer B, et al. Effects and safety of rituximab in systemic sclerosis: an analysis from the European Scleroderma Trial and Research (EUSTAR) group. Ann Rheum Dis. 2015;74:1188–94.

Khellaf M, Charles-Nelson A, Fain O, et al. Safety and efficacy of rituximab in adult immune thrombocytopenia: results from a prospective registry including 248 patients. Blood. 2014;124:3228–36.

Loricera J, Blanco R, Hernández JL, Pina T, González-Vela MC, González-Gay MA. Biologic therapy in ANCA-negative vasculitis. Int Immunopharmacol. 2015;27:213–9.

Lutalo PMK, D'Cruz DP. Biological drugs in ANCA-associated vasculitis. Int Immunopharmacol. 2015;27:209–12.

Merrill JT, Neuwelt CM, Wallace DJ, et al. Efficacy and safety of rituximab in moderately-to-severely active systemic lupus erythematosus: the randomized, double-blind, phase II/III systemic lupus erythematosus evaluation of rituximab trial. Arthritis Rheum. 2010;62:222–33.

Michel M, Terriou L, Roudot-Thoraval F, et al. A randomized and double-blind controlled trial evaluating the safety and efficacy of rituximab for warm auto-immune hemolytic anemia in adults (the RAIHA study). Am J Hematol. 2017;92:23–7.

Montalban X, Hauser SL, Kappos L, et al. Ocrelizumab versus placebo in primary progressive multiple sclerosis. N Engl J Med. 2017;376:209–20.

Muchtar E, Magen H, Gertz MA. How I treat cryoglobulinemia. Blood. 2017;129:289–98.

Patel VL, Mahévas M, Lee SY, et al. Outcomes 5 years after response to rituximab therapy in children and adults with immune thrombocytopenia. Blood. 2012;119:5989–95.

Ponsa I, Espinosab G, Cervera R. Efficacy and safety of rituximab in the treatment of primary antiphospholipid syndrome: analysis of 24 cases from the bibliography review. Med Clin (Barc). 2015;144:97–104.

Robeson KR, Kumar A, Keung B, et al. Durability of the rituximab response in acetylcholine receptor autoantibody–positive myasthenia gravis. JAMA Neurol. 2017;74:60–6.

Rossi D, Modena V, Sciascia S, Roccatello D. Rheumatoid arthritis: biological therapy other than anti-TNF. Int Immunopharmacol. 2015;27:185–8.

Rovin BH, Furie R, Latinis K, et al. Efficacy and safety of rituximab in patients with active proliferative lupus nephritis: the lupus nephritis assessment with rituximab study. Arthritis Rheum. 2012;64:1215–26.

Sciascia S, Talavera-Garcia E, Roccatelloa D, Baldovino S, Mengatti E, Cuadrado MJ. Upcoming biological therapies in systemic lupus erythematosus. Int Immunopharmacol. 2015;27:189–93.

Souza FB, Porfírio GJ, Andriolo BN, Albuquerque JV, Trevisani VF. Rituximab effectiveness and safety for treating primary Sjögren's syndrome (pSS): systematic review and meta-analysis. PLoS One. 2016;11:e0150749.

Stasi R, Pagano A, Stipa E, Amadori S. Rituximab chimeric anti-CD20 monoclonal antibody treatment for adults with chronic idiopathic thrombocytopenic purpura. Blood. 2001;98:952–7.

Tandan R, Hehir MK 2nd, Waheed W, Howard DB. Rituximab treatment of myasthenia gravis: a systematic review. Muscle Nerve. 2017;56(2):185–96. https://doi.org/10.1002/mus.25597.

Tendas A, Niscola P, Scaramucci L, Cupelli L, Perrotti AP, de Fabritiis P. Primary acquired chronic pure red cell aplasia refractory to standard treatments: remission with rituximab. Blood Res. 2016;51:133–47.

MIX
Papier aus verantwortungsvollen Quellen
Paper from responsible sources
FSC® C105338

If you have any concerns about our products,
you can contact us on
ProductSafety@springernature.com

In case Publisher is established outside the EU,
the EU authorized representative is:
Springer Nature Customer Service Center GmbH
Europaplatz 3, 69115 Heidelberg, Germany

Printed by Libri Plureos GmbH
in Hamburg, Germany